Social Work in a Glocalised World

This engaging and timely volume contributes new knowledge to the rapidly emerging field of globalisation and social work. The volume brings together cutting-edge interdisciplinary scholarship from countries such as Australia, Finland, Japan, South Africa, the Philippines and Sweden. It proposes 'glocalisation' as a useful concept for re-framing conditions, methodologies and practices for social work in a world perspective.

Part I of the volume, 'The Glocalisation of Social Issues', deals with major environmental, social and cultural issues – migration and human rights, environmental problems and gendered violence. Part II, 'Methodological Re-Shaping and Spatial Transgressions of Glocal Social Work', develops an epistemology of situated knowledge and methodologies inspired by art, creative writing and cultural geography, focusing on physical, material and emotional spatial dimensions of relevance to social work. Part III, 'Responses from Social Work as a Glocalised Profession', examines how social work has responded to specific social problems, crises and vulnerabilities in a glocalised world.

Mona Livholts is an Associate Professor of Social Work at the Department of Social and Welfare Studies at Linköping University, Sweden, Adjunct Associate Professor at the Centre for Social Change, University of South Australia, and Founder and Coordinator of R.A.W., The Network for Reflexive Academic Writing Methodologies.

Lia Bryant is an Associate Professor at the School of Psychology, Social Work and Social Policy, University of South Australia and is Director of the Centre for Social Change. She is Associate Professor in Social Work and Sociology.

'Mona Livholts and Lia Bryant's *Social Work in a Glocalised World* is a wonderful and timely book. A glocalised perspective is a whole way of framing social work, which we can no longer ignore. This volume walks the reader through the many ways in which the global and the local come together in forms of knowledge, practice and research methodology, drawing from diverse geopolitical regions, and weaving legal, economic, policy and discursive arguments together. The volume has a strong feminist voice. It expands social work views to include chapters on writing, participatory arts, and on film-making. I learned a lot from it, and I highly recommend it for teachers, students, practitioners, policy-makers and post-disciplinary learners.'

Adrienne Chambon, Ph.D., Professor Emerita,
University of Toronto, Factor-Inwentash
Faculty of Social Work

'*Social Work in a Glocalised World* makes an important contribution to global discourse and the dialogues that flow from it. Too often social work's involvement in global issues winds up masking or reproducing the very concerns that motivated its involvement. In large part, this is due to the application of traditional analyses and understandings and the absence of innovative critical approaches. In contrast, this book challenges such ways of thinking and the knowledge it produces and proposes alternative approaches to knowledge generation such as through new forms of writing and the arts. In doing so, the authors of this book make an important contribution to our understanding of global issues and open a space where new and more relevant responses to these issues can be developed.'

Stanley L. Witkin, Professor, Department of Social Work,
University of Vermont, Burlington, Vermont,
USA and President, Global Partnership
for Transformative Social Work

Routledge Advances in Social Work

New Titles

Social Work in a Global Context
Issues and Challenges
Edited by George Palattiyil, Dina Sidhva and Mono Chakrabarti

Contemporary Feminisms in Social Work Practice
Edited by Nicole Moulding and Sarah Wendt

Domestic Violence Perpetrators
Evidence-Informed Responses
John Devaney and Anne Lazenbatt

Transnational Social Work and Social Welfare
Challenges for the Social Work Profession
Edited by Beatrix Schwarzer, Ursula Kämmerer-Rütten, Alexandra Schleyer-Lindemann and Yafang Wang

The Ecosocial Transition of Societies
The Contribution of Social Work and Social Policy
Edited by Aila-Leena Matthies and Kati Närhi

Responsibilization at the Margins of Welfare Services
Edited by Kirsi Juhila, Suvi Raitakari and Christopher Hall

Forthcoming Titles

Homelessness and Social Work
An Intersectional Approach
Carole Zufferey

Supporting Care Leavers' Educational Transitions
Jennifer Driscoll

Social Work in
a Glocalised World

Edited by Mona Livholts and Lia Bryant

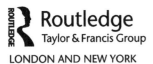
Routledge
Taylor & Francis Group

LONDON AND NEW YORK

First published 2017
by Routledge

2 Park Square, Milton Park, Abingdon, Oxfordshire OX14 4RN
52 Vanderbilt Avenue, New York, NY 10017

*Routledge is an imprint of the Taylor & Francis Group,
an informa business*

First issued in paperback 2020

British Library Cataloguing in Publication Data
A catalogue record for this book is available from the British Library

Library of Congress Cataloging in Publication Data
A catalog record for this book is available from the Library of Congress

ISBN: 978-1-138-64499-1 (hbk)
ISBN: 978-0-367-11211-0 (pbk)

Typeset in Times New Roman
by Deanta Global Publishing Services, Chennai, India

For students and teachers in the course Global and Transnational Social Work at Linköping University, Sweden, with great affection.

For Zeffie Summerton, for tirelessly working for social justice.

Contents

Figures

List of Contributors

Editors

Mona Livholts is an Associate Professor of Social Work at the Department of Social and Welfare Studies at Linköping University, Sweden, Coordinator of R.A.W., The Network for Reflexive Academic Writing Methodologies, and Adjunct Associate Professor at the Centre for Social Change, University of South Australia. She has published monographs and co-edited and edited volumes in Swedish and English, including: *'Women', Welfare, Textual Politics and Critique: An Invitation to a ThinkingWriting Methodology in the Study of Welfare* (2011, Lambert Academic Publishing); *Emergent Writing Methodologies in Feminist Studies* (2012 (ed), Routledge); and *Discourse and Narrative Methods: Theoretical Departures, Analytical Strategies and Situated Writing* (2015, co-authored with M. Tamboukou, Sage); and a trilogy of untimely academic novellas: *The Professor's Chair, The Snow Angel and Other Imprints* and *Writing Water*.

Lia Bryant is an Associate Professor at the School of Psychology, Social Work and Social Policy, University of South Australia and is Director of the Centre for Social Change. She is Associate Professor in Social Work and Sociology. She has published extensively in academic journals and her books include *Gender and Rurality* (2011, co-authored with Barbara Pini, Routledge); *Sexuality, Rurality and Geography* (2013 (eds) Gorman Murray, A., Pini, B. and Bryant, L., Lexington Books); *Women Supervising and Writing Doctoral Theses: Walking on the Grass* (2015, Bryant, L. and Jaworski, K. Lexington Books; Bryant, L. (ed) *Critical and Creative Research Methodologies in Social Work* and Bryant, L. with George, J. *Water and Rural Communities, Local Meanings, Politics and Place* (2016, Routledge).

Chapter Authors

Charlotte Åberg is a visual artist with a master's degree in Fine Arts from the Faculty of Art, Umeå University, Sweden. Her works pivots around issues of representation, and several of her works deal with personal stories, dreams, clothes and gender issues. Åberg is a co-founder of the artist organisation

ArtAgent, Stockholm. Together with Lott Alfreds, she has implemented inter-disciplinary art projects based on dialogue and participation. She has been co-leader for the EU-funded project 'Visualize the Invisible', 2013–2014. Publications include *Sossial Sculptur: A Collection of Dreams from Ali Demi Prison* (with Alfreds, 2010, Harakulla Press), and *Visualize the Invisible* (edited with Alfreds 2014, Art Agent Press).

Mary Lou Alcid is Professor of Social Work at the University of the Philippines. She has extensive experience in social development as a community organ-iser, trainer, founder, administrator and trustee of non-government organisa-tions engaged in promoting the rights and well-being of Indigenous Filipinos, fisherfolk, farmers, women and overseas Filipino workers. She was part of the pioneering initiatives for orienting social work academic programs towards practice in rural communities. She served as president of the Philippine National Association for Social Work Education from 2008–2012.

Lott Alfreds, MFA Visual Art, Royal Art Academy, Stockholm, is a co-founder of ArtAgent, an artist organisation in Stockholm. Alfreds has worked together with artist Charlotte Åberg on several projects exploring participatory art prac-tices with vulnerable groups in multicultural urban settings as well as mak-ing her own exhibitions. In 2013–2014 she was co-leader of the EU-funded artistic research project 'Visualize the Invisible'. Publications include *Sossial Sculptur: A Collection of Dreams from Ali Demi Prison* (with Åberg, 2010, Harakulla Press); and *Visualize the Invisible* (edited with Åberg 2014, Art Agent Press, Stockholm).

Els-Marie Anbäcken is an Associate Professor of Social Work, School of Health, Care and Social Welfare, Mälardalen University, Sweden. With a PhD in Japanology, Els-Marie has been involved in cross-cultural comparative studies in Japan and Sweden on themes of ageing and care, social policy and the role of formal and informal actors. Existential issues have come to occupy several of her studies. In 2008–2012, Els-Marie held a professorship at Kwansei Gakuin University in Japan where she encountered both research and volunteer activi-ties related to earthquake disaster.

Bridget Garnham, PhD, is a research fellow at the Centre for Social Change, School of Psychology, Social Work and Social Policy at the University of South Australia. Her recent research writing takes up the problem of rural sui-cides through understandings of distress that help to materialise the sociopo-litical, cultural and moral conditions of possibility that shape subjectivity and emotions. More broadly, her research foci are connected to themes of ageing, 'older' subjectivities, cosmetic surgery and social justice and inclusion in rela-tion to wellbeing.

Lucas Gottzén is an Associate Professor in Social Work and Senior Lecturer at the Department of Child and Youth Studies, Stockholm University, Sweden. His research primarily focuses on gendered and generational aspects of family life, masculinity and violence against women and embodied action and identity-making of children, youth and violent men.

Sabine Gruber is a lecturer in social work at the Department of Social and Welfare Studies, Linköping University, Sweden. Her research is primarily on migration and ethnic relations in welfare institutional practices, and the restructured welfare state. She has done ethnographic research on ethnicity and gender in primary health care and special residential homes for young people, and schools' responses to honour-related violence. Her current research is on ethnicity in foster care.

Jeff Hearn is Guest Research Professor at the Faculty of Humanities and Social Sciences, based in Gender Studies, Örebro University, Sweden; Professor of Sociology, University of Huddersfield, United Kingdom; and Professor Emeritus, Hanken School of Economics, Finland. He has published extensively on sociology, social policy, gender, men and masculinities, sexuality, violence, organisations, management, ICTs and cultural studies. His current research focuses on men, gender relations, organising and transnationalizations, along with violation and autoethnography.

Sindi F. Gordon, PhD, is an award-winning filmmaker, writer and tutor of creative writing and life narrative courses. She has worked with a range of international organisations including the 2nd Johannesburg Biennale and South African Broadcast Corporation (SABC, South Africa), UNESCO (Zimbabwe), Radio WBAI and Public Broadcast Service (PBS, USA). She is currently a research fellow at the University of Sussex (United Kingdom); research interests include memory, inclusivity, embodiment, equity and education.

Shepard Masocha is a Lecturer in Social Work at the School of Psychology, Social Work and Social Policy at the University of South Australia, Australia. His research explores the ways in which social workers enact their discourses in everyday practice through language use, taking into cognisance that these local meanings are situated in wider discourses. His current research focuses on the critical study of social work with ethnic minorities, immigrants and asylum seekers, and the intersecting discourses of race, racism, culture and social citizenship.

Bob Pease is Professor of Social Work at the University of Tasmania, Australia. His main research interests are in the fields of men's violence against women, cross-cultural and global perspectives on men and masculinities, the interrogation of privilege, critical social work practice and the links between masculinity and global warming. His most recent books are *The Politics of Recognition and Social Justice: Transforming Subjectivities and New Forms of Resistance* (co-editor, Routledge, 2014); *Men, Masculinities and Disaster* (co-editor, Routledge, 2016); and *Doing Critical Social Work Practice* (co-editor, Allen and Unwin, 2016).

Kopano Ratele is a Professor at the Institute for Social and Health Sciences at the University of South Africa (Unisa) and a Researcher at the South African Medical Research Council-Unisa's Violence, Injury & Peace Research Unit. He is past president of the Psychological Society of South Africa and former chairperson of the board of Sonke Gender Justice. He writes mostly about boys, men and masculinity.

Tamara Shefer is Professor of Women's and Gender studies at the Faculty of Arts at the University of the Western Cape. Her research is primarily on youth, gender and sexualities, and includes work in the areas of HIV/AIDS, gender-based violence, masculinities, memory and post-apartheid, gender and care, and social justice in higher education.

Sonia Tascón is lecturer in the School of Social Work at Western Sydney University and her specialist interest in this discipline focuses on the critical engagement with the visual arts for social change. Sonia's research has traversed numerous glocal topics including migration and refugee studies, race and white privilege, human rights cinema, and film activism. Her most recent publications have included a sole-authored book, *Human Rights Film Festivals: Activism in Context*, followed by the 2017 title, *Activist Film Festivals: Towards a Political Subject*, in which she is author and co-editor. She is now preparing a new title for Routledge titled *Visual Power and Social Work Practice* in which she will explore the power of visual images and their growing potential for social work practice.

Päivi Turunen, PhD, is Assistant Professor of Social Work, Department of Social and Welfare Studies, Linköping University. Her research has been practice-orientated and carried out from social political perspectives on global, national and local societal changes concerning community work, societal entrepreneurship, deliberative methods and socio-spatial aspects of social work. Päivi Turunen's thesis, *Community Work in Scandinavia: Discourses and Practices in Transformation*, from 2004 is a comparative study of community work in four Nordic countries, also recounted in Hutchinson (2009) *Community Work in the Nordic Countries – New Trends*.

Nilan Yu, PhD, is Lecturer in Social Work and Program Director on the Master course on Social Work at the University of South Australia. Nilan has been teaching social work for more than 15 years. His teaching and research interests include community development and human rights, labour migration, disability and critical social work practice. He co-edited the volume *Subversive Action: Extralegal Practices for Social Justice* (2015, Wilfrid Laurier University Press). He is a member of the editorial committee of the *Asia Pacific Journal of Social Work and Development* and the Asia Advisory Board of the journal *Social Work Education*.

1   Introduction

Social Work in a Glocalised World

Mona Livholts and Lia Bryant

Across the world, people are on the move – international students, highly skilled workers, economic migrants, retirees, refugees, nomads, those within global care chains and those whose unauthorised status leaving them vulnerable to all sorts of human rights violations, including slavery.

(Williams & Graham 2014, p. il)

The relevance of outside boundaries and borrowings is one entry point into a discussion on the nature of a discipline and the identity of a field. The activities at the borders of a field are concrete manifestations of movements in knowledge in the academic sense [...]. The thesis put forward is that social work has had a phased history of alternating expansion and contraction of its knowledge base. [...]. Shifts occur with changes in knowledge from within the discipline, and very much from broader scholarly influences. But importantly, in an applied discipline, these knowledge changes are very much shaped by economic, social, and political conditions of societies [...].

(Chambon 2012, p. 1)

Social issues emerge in the intersection of local, national and global contexts and as the citations above from social work scholars illustrate, social work as a discipline and profession 'works' across, within and between these spheres. At the time of writing this book, social inequalities are increasing and the dignity and worth of people as well as human rights issues are of central concern for societies in 'a world on the move' (Williams & Graham 2014, p. il; see also Hughman 2008; Dominelli 2010a, 2012; Kamali 2015; Pease 2010). The complexity of contemporary social issues raises profound questions like how to work with communities of people whose citizenship rights are stripped in their country of origin and whose human rights require assertion in their place or journey towards settlement.

Further, the propensity for western dominance equally raises difficult questions about how to constitute collective social work values and standards and promote collective activism. In these ways, social work becomes increasingly interspatial but also finds itself caught within multiple understandings of social justice and cracks in state systems, their policies and their ideologies that can remain inflexible to social concerns that move across borders, like climate change or asylum seeking (Dominelli 2012; Welbourne 2009). Therefore, social work is confronted by how, as an academic discipline and profession, it can respond to contemporary globalised challenges theoretically, methodologically and in practice. In the context of environmental changes and the role of 'green social work', interaction between people and their environments becomes increasingly vital. In relation to green social work, for example, Dominelli (2012, p. 8) argues that there are diverse capacities for social workers to act as 'advocates; mobilizers and organizers of people, communities and resources; lobbyists who can influence policy makers; and therapeutic workers who can respond to individual distress'. It is at the juncture of praxis that this volume examines how contemporary movements and border crossings in society and academia are linked with the re-shaping of social work as a globalised field for research, education and professional practice (Bryant 2015; Dominelli 2010a, 2012; Hugman 2010; Jönsson 2014a; Lyons *et al.* 2006). Our aim is to explicate the 'glocal', that is, the interstices between globalising conditions and forces and local contexts and conditions, in two ways. The first is by examining economic, political and social interconnections and power asymmetries that shape interspatial social issues. The second is to extend the 'social reach' of social work to promote theoretical and methodological renewal to understand that lives and the creating of knowledge are increasingly subject to glocal influences (Bryant 2015; Chambon, 2013; Livholts 2010b, 2012).

However, the role of social work in a changing world perspective is socio-historically contained, bringing into focus both 'old' and 'new' questions, tensions and debates that reach back to the history of social work. Writing the history of social work in a western context, Hugman (2010) and Righard (2013) describe how colonialism, social rights movements, wars and conflicts influenced social work in different socio-historic periods and contexts, showing the continuing pertinence of debates about the global positioning of social work. Indeed, social work has been shaped by western colonialisation from the late eighteenth century and onwards, creating a colonial past and (post)colonial present (Ranta-Tyrkkö 2011; Chambon 2013). Dominating relations of power have been evident in 'professional imperialism' (Midgely 1981), through which social work has contributed to oppressive structures in regard to marginalised and Indigenous populations. Further, models for social development were transported from countries in the North and imposed on countries in the South. Despite these hegemonic impositions of western dominance, movements also occur from the periphery to the centre; however, such movements are often obscured in the way knowledges are produced (Abu-Lughod 1991; Appadurai 2013). Equally, social work has worked, albeit slowly, towards critiquing and dismantling hegemonic western views by turning to contributions from Indigenous knowledges on sustainability, ecology and spirituality and models for family support (Dominelli 2010a; Hugman 2010). For example, as Dominelli (2010a, p. 609) argues, Indigenous practices around 'Maori family group conferencing and redistributive justice systems' have been used in family therapy in the United Kingdom and Canada. Similarly, Hugman (2010, p. 143) has challenged social work to think about 'reversing the process' of knowledge construction, that is, 'if we are concerned with insuring that the influences from social work in the global North to the global South are appropriate, what of the transfer of ideas and practices in the other directions'.

As conceptualising the glocal is critical to methodology and development of social work and social issues in the context of dialectic spatial relations, we now turn to reviewing conceptualisations and applications of the terms 'international', 'global' and 'transnational' in social work. Following the examination of current states of knowledge, we move towards developing 'glocalisation' as an emergent theoretical and methodological framework for social work.

Contextualising Concepts: International, Global and Transnational Social Work

Social work as an international or global phenomenon in the west has been given currency from as early as 1928, with inspiration from the settlement movement (1860–1935) and Hull House 1889 in Chicago. The following international organisations in social work: IASSW (International Association of Schools of Social Work), IFSW (International Federation of Social Workers) and ICSW (International Council of Social Work) have established common internationally agreed goals for the discipline and profession. In a historical overview of the development of different conceptualisations, Righard (2013) shows how new conceptualisations emerge as a result of critique and discussion of existing ones at the same time as they co-exist with established understandings as opposed to replacing them.

The 'international' foci of social work begun in the late 1800s and developed organisationally as a result of the first international social work conference in Paris, France in 1928 (Righard 2013). At this time, the three international organisations of social work (IASSW, IFSW and ICSW) were founded. They were strengthened by the establishment of the United Nations Relief and Rehabilitation Administration (UNRRA) in 1943 and the welfare division in 1946. In a western context, international social work emerged during the 1940s after the Second World War as a response to social workers working across state boundaries with refugees in addition to sending resources for refugees across borders. During the 1960s and 1970s, a growing critique towards western hegemony and westernised models of social work grew. International development during the next two decades (from the 1980s to the 1990s) raised questions about otherisation of migrants or 'us' and 'them' divisions within and across nations.

Contrastingly, in globalisation studies, Steger has argued that (2010, p. 1): '[…] the term "international" need[s] to be replaced by "global" since the nation-state … [can] no longer serve as the basic unit of analysis'. Steger has shown how the emergence of the interdisciplinary field of global studies has raised different issues, definitions and methodologies in critiquing, examining and understanding the 'global'. However, like many globalisation scholars, he excludes the social within his fields of analyses conflating the social with the economic, political, cultural and ecological spheres of social life. Social work as a discipline extends globalisation theories by centralizing the social. Social work as a globalised field of knowledge draws attention to how power asymmetries such as class, gender, race, sexuality, able-bodiedness and age shape conditions of life and actualise marginalisation, threat and violence. These actualisations occur in different local contexts, shaped by national regulations of law and normative praxis (see Chapters 2, 3, 4, 12 and 13), and are central to the geopolitics of social work scholarship, methodological re-shaping and spatial transgression (see Chapters 6–10). Thus, there is a need to continue to develop theoretical frameworks for the globalised field of the discipline and the profession.

In social work, this shift in conceptualisation from international to global is especially manifested in 2001 in the international organisations of social work agreement on an *international* definition of social work, which was revised in 2014 to a *global* definition of social work. Further, in 2012 'The Global Agenda for Social Work and Social Development' was agreed upon with long term goals within four prioritised areas: social and economic inequalities within countries and between regions; dignity and worth of the person; environmental stability; and the importance of human relationships (The Global Agenda 2012). The first report of the global agenda for social work and social development (Jones & Truell 2012), shows diversity and complexity in the way social work is practised across regions and locally within countries in Africa, Asia-Pacific, Europe, Latin America and the Caribbean and North America. Increasing inequalities between the 'haves' and 'have nots' caused by unequal distribution of resources, social inequality and social problems have caused consequences for both individuals and societies. There is evidence both from research and social work practitioners 'that people are happier and their well-being greater in more equitable societies. And when economic growth is not linked to improving social conditions, suffering and wellbeing can worsen' (Jones & Truell 2012, p. 7). In this world perspective, challenges for social work scholarship, research, education and professional practice are located in unequal distributions of resources, effects of colonial legacy, migration, conflict and war and environmental changes and disasters. In this way, contemporary social work knowledge emphasises that international agencies cannot 'develop' other communities, acknowledging the necessity for locally driven solutions to social problems.

There is some debate about what distinguishes social work as *global*. Hugman (2010) suggests that the international organisations in social work are 'global' as they bring together social work organisations and knowledge from different parts of the world and emphasise international differences as well as international linkages. Healy, however, suggests a divergent understanding of international and global arguing:

> [...] *global* means pertaining to or involving the whole world, whereas *international* can mean any of the following: between or among two or more nations, of or pertaining two or more nations or their citizens, pertaining to the relations between nations, having members or activities in several nations, or transcending national boundaries or viewpoints.
>
> (Healy 2008, p. 7)

Thus, for Healy, 'international' draws on relations between nation states whilst Hugman reflects on the nature of organisations as international enterprises. The global definition of the social work profession approved by the IFSW General Meeting and the IASSW General Assembly in July 2014 formulates the following common basis:

> Social work is a practice-based profession and an academic discipline that promotes social change and development, social cohesion, and the empowerment and liberation of people. Principles of social justice, human rights, collective responsibility and respect for diversities are central to social work. Underpinned by theories of social work, social sciences, humanities and indigenous knowledge, social work engages people and structures to address life challenges and enhance wellbeing.
> The above definition may be amplified at national and/or regional levels.
>
> (IFSW 2012)

Both the global agenda and the definition have been debated in terms of the possibilities and limitations of creating a common foundation from which social work in different contexts across the world can both incorporate and depart. In terms of values and perspectives, some scholars argue these remains western-centric (Jones & Truell 2012). In this volume, authors critically analyse and discuss how the postcolonial legacy of imperialism exercised by 'First World' western nation states continues to be a challenge for social justice and social change (see Chapters 4, 5, 6, 9, 12, 13 and 14).

Within the academy, Dominelli (2010b) has been influential in bringing attention to 'globalizing' influences in social work in three critical ways. Firstly, she documented the *inter*national diffusion of neoliberal management regimes occurring in the global North which has altered service delivery models and social work practice by 'increasing the techno-bureaucratic nature of practice through performance measures aimed at maximizing the use of limited resources for the greatest number of people' (Dominelli 2010b, p. 602). This model of welfare which centralises the market as welfare funding is sourced outward to non-government agencies or to private corporations with service users constituted as consumers who take on individual responsibility to navigate and acquire services. Secondly, Dominelli (2010b) has interrogated broad globalising changes that impact on regions, localities, communities and individuals, like, for example, the global financial crisis, war, environmental changes and disasters, migrations of peoples (including those seeking asylum), human trafficking and international adoption. Thirdly, she has raised attention to knowledge hierarchies and western knowledge claims which are articulated as 'truths', delimit or ignore Indigenous ways of knowing and continue to colonise through the hegemony of western social work models (Dominelli 2010b).

Since the mid-2000s, central to the work of scholars like Dominelli (2010a), Healy (2008) Hugman *et al.* (2010) and Lyons *et al.* (2006), globalisation has been critiqued in relation to how it has been applied in social work as a governing monolithic force that produces effects at the local level and '[produces] a one way movement of social work knowledge and practice from the North to the South' (Hugman *et al*. 2010, p. 108). Increasing attention has been directed to the intersections between globalising processes and agency. Glocalising care work in Nordic countries, for example, illustrates globalising market-driven models of care that are reliant on flexible low-paid migrant female labour but also shows local differences among Nordic states and at the institutional level within states (Wrede & Nare 2013). As Wrede and Nare (2013, p. 57) argue, 'the glocalisation argument calls attention to the fact that the characteristics of the social embeddedness of care work regimes are not fixed'. They remind us that 'the impact of globalisation ... may be best understood as convergence and divergence' (Wrede & Nare 2013, p. 57).

Like the term international, *transnational* social work is somewhat limiting. Righard (2013) emphasises that transnationalism is more limited as a conceptual practice than the concept 'global' and focuses on how people live their lives in and orient towards a place in two or more countries. Thus, globalisation affects social relations translocally and in a hierarchical way. Furman *et al*. (2008) suggest that transnational social work includes a number of practices, which he describes in the following way:

> Transnational social work is an emerging field of practice that (a) is designed to serve transnational populations; (b) operates across nation-state boundaries, whether physically or through new technologies; and (c) is informed by and addresses complex transnational problems and dilemmas.
>
> (Furman *et al*. 2008, p. 8)

The way Furman describes the transnational practices of social work brings into focus ways in which social workers become engaged in the life situations of people whose everyday lives are shaped by connectivity across national boundaries. For Furman, there are three elements to transnational social work. The first refers to transnational populations like asylum seekers, migrant workers, human trafficking and international adoptions. The second element indicates how social work practice may transgress national borders and the associated complexities that emerge for international collaboration, especially given the operation of different legal frameworks. The third aspect raises questions about how to understand and respond to social problems and dilemmas which cannot be identified solely within a single national context.

Glocalisation: An Emergent Theoretical Framework for Social Work

In this book we suggest that glocalisation is an emergent theoretical framework for social work which, alongside established concepts such as international, global and transnational, enrich complex understandings of interconnections, power asymmetries and interspatial social issues. To operationally define and introduce glocalisation, we draw on the influential work of sociologist Roland Robertson (1992, 1995, 2012) and, in addition, build on literature in the creative arts, geography and social work. As Robertson (2013) suggests in one of his recent publications, the term glocal is today widely discussed and used in a range of disciplinary fields such as anthropology, economy, geography and sociology. There are disputes about the origin and disciplinary basis of the term glocalisation. Robertson argues (1995, 2013) that the term originates from Japanese media and business in the late 1980s, illustrating how products were marketed to adapt into new local contexts. In an alternative explanation, Roudometof (2015, p. 775) claims that the term was originally coined in the Global Change Exhibition (opened 30 May 1990) at the German Chancellery in Bonn through Benking's 'Rubik's Cube of Ecology' which 'aimed towards better understanding and communication about multi-disciplines like ecology'. Roudometof refers to Dr Manfred Lange, director of the touring exhibit, who named the cube 'glocal' to capture the range of micro-, meso- and macro-scales that characterised its construction. Despite disputes over origin, we contend that increasing interest in the complex relationship between economic, political, social and cultural systems, multi-scalar spatialities, science and the creative arts, has led us to an interest in the term glocalisation that is fruitful for understanding theories, methodologies and responses in social work in a globalised context.

One of Robertson's key arguments was that globalisation neglects the ways in which the local is, to a large degree, constructed on a global basis (1992, 2012) and he regards the dialectal asymmetrical power relation of the global-local nexus as one that places locality in opposition to the global. In one of his early texts, Robertson (1995) rejects counterpoising the global as the larger entity which incorporates the local. He writes:

> […] the global is not in and of itself counterpoised to the local. Rather, what is often referred to as the local is essentially *included* within the global. In this respect globalization, defined in its most general sense as the compression of the world as a whole, involves the linking of localities. But it also involves the 'invention of locality', in the same general sense of the idea of the invention of tradition.
>
> (Robertson 1995, p. 35)

Our understanding of this 'invention of locality' is that it represents glocalisation as a process, intimately intertwined with the postmodern rejection of grand narratives, and simultaneously includes fragmentation, interdependency and transgression. Distinctions between the local and the global have also had theoretical and practice implications for understanding the social. Such distinctions have created limitations to understanding heterogeneity, particularity and universalism, and time and space dimensions both for academic scholarship and activist movements (Robertson 2012). As we have shown in the previous section, social work scholarship mainly employs the terms international, global and transnational to conceptualise local-global relations, while the term glocalisation is less common.

However, some recent social work studies discuss and develop glocalisation. Kamali (2015, p. 148) argues in his book on war, violence and social justice that 'global social problems' should be replaced with the more accurate term '*glocal social problems*', [italics in original] 'in order to address the complexity and multi-edged nature of social problems [...]'. Thus, a framework for the glocalisation of social work calls for acknowledging the variety of such interconnections and their consequences. Jönsson (2014b) makes use of the concept of 'localised globalities' to investigate globalised social problems in the context of west-centric modernity and neo-liberal globalisation showing how complex patterns of colonial legacy create global social problems such as undocumented migrants in Sweden, micro-credits in India and EU fishing in West-African waters. This creates challenges for local communities and social work within and beyond national borders. Departing from the expression 'think globally act locally' inspired by Lyons (2006), Hong and Song (2010, p. 53) link the challenges of social justice to the diminishing responsibilities of welfare to all citizens in many countries, and state that 'social work has become fragmented, disrupted and dislocated in a postmodernist world of globalization where established assumptions and consensus about social welfare has been shattered'. They call for new social actors and structures as a response to globalising forces of inequality and propose a model for global social policy. Romanov and Kononenko (2014) account for processes of glocalisation in Russian social work which created a departure after the socialist regime. In Russia, professional social work was institutional from the 1990s and onward.

In critiquing the concept of globalisation, Robertson (2005, no page reference) has also argued that the term has often been employed in ways that neglect spatial dimensions. He writes:

> Thus to speak of glocalisation is meant to ensure that the general discussion of globalisation encompasses the cross-cutting dimensions of locality along spatial lines. In other words, the relative inattention to spatiality is, when we look back, a conspicuous feature of sociology [...].

Indeed, inattention to spatiality and therefore the problematisation of social space has also been given limited attention in social work. Spatial analyses have an important contribution in analysing the physical, material and emotional dimensions of social work. Chambon, in particular, has made contributions to spatiality and social work by arguing for the creation of new spaces in the production of social work knowledge. She emphasises the force of telling to create movements and asks her readers to re-think how places for encounters in social work are not neutral. She asks (Chambon 2005, pp. 4–5): 'Is the middle a neutral place? Or a wish for a neutral place? [...] Moving from behind the desk, moving outward. Moving towards knowledge, "what do I want to know?" What do I not want to know? What am I moving away from?' Following Chambon (2005), this edited collection seeks to reflexively examine metaphoric 'movements', and the chapters in this volume show how spaces are vital for the current re-shaping of social work in a glocalised world. The spatiality of glocal social work is one where all spheres of the discipline and profession are intimately intertwined in micro-, mezzo- and macro levels (see Chapters 7, 11 and 13). In this volume we view what Chambon (2012, p. 10) refers to as dialogues at the borders between social work and other disciplines, as crucial to theoretical and methodological renewal. She shows, for example, how the political economy was influential on social work development in Toronto and England, while sociology influenced social work in the United States. Chambon (2012, p. 10) describes how these areas 'did not dilute the specificity of social work. They were used instead as catalysts [...] and promoted social work to a central knowledge position [...]'. In this volume, we wish to contribute to the creation of spaces for what we propose is an emergent theoretical and methodological field of glocal studies in social work by inviting contributions from emergent theoretical lenses of glocalisation and less common areas such as art, creative writing and cultural geography.

Glocalising Methodologies: Situated Body Politics and Story Telling

While becoming a social worker is influenced by past histories and western-centric values, as Cree (2013) puts it, increasingly it is shaped by cross-national experiences of social work and personal experiences of living transnational lives. Reflecting on her work as editor of a book on the theme of global narratives, she writes:

> Perhaps the strongest impression I am left with in reading the chapters again is the degree to which people writing in this book demonstrate the impact of globalisation. Travel, journeys, cross-cultural understandings features in a significant number of chapters. This highlights the reality that many of those who are living and working in the UK today were born in another country; many UK authors have worked (or are working) overseas; many authors from the Global 'South' travelled to the Global 'North' for their education; some have returned to their country of origin, while others have not. A small number have made multiple journeys over the years. Of course, this in part, reflects some of the choices I made in inviting people to tell their stories; I wanted to interrogate the global nature of social work today. However, I believe it also demonstrates a wider truth: that we are living in a global world, and social work is affected by globalisation (for good and bad) as we all are, in all areas of life.
>
> (Cree 2013, p. 215)

The merging forms of interconnectivity between place, experiences and realities that Cree illustrates create the body politic of social work as a profession. It is this change in professional constitution that this volume contributes to in developing a knowledge base for social work in a world, which is international, local and global and, as we suggest, 'glocal'. We acknowledge that 'world' is a word that is as problematic as 'global', taking into account the risk of homogenisation and generalisation. Our intention is to develop a knowledge base for social work that actualises the possibility to provide multiple stories and sites of writing to re-shape this knowledge base (see Chapters 6, 8 and 9). We will show that 'there is not one unitary story about social work, but many' (Dominelli 2010a, p. 10). Dominelli also argues that the partial and limited narratives of social work remind us of both its emancipatory and oppressive role in a western world perspective. Thus, we can make explicit use of our limited and situated knowledge claims and show awareness about how we make ideas of the world 'worldly' and critically examine the theoretical lenses for 'what we learn how to see' (Haraway 1988, p. 581; Chapter 6, this volume).

Interwoven with this situated departure is the emergence of critical, creative and reflexive methodologies in glocalised social work as tools to promote social justice and anti-discriminatory practices in research, education and professional practice. We have noted that, while there is a growing field of scholarship in social work that uses such methodologies (see for example Bryant 2015; Chambon 2005; Gunaratnam 2007; Livholts 2015), literature in the field of globalisation and social work (e.g. Bettman *et al.* 2013; Dominelli 2010a, 2012; Healy & Link 2012) rarely places its emphasis on the relationship between methodological challenges and emergent global problems linked with local, national and global contexts. In this volume, we argue that the creative arts and creative writing provide social work with a lens through which to critique and analyse social spaces across local and global contexts (see also Bryant & Livholts 2013, 2015; Livholts 2010b, 2012). Contributing authors interrogate the glocalised nature of emergent issues, methodologies and responses in social work through established forms of writing and representation as well as by introducing creative forms of writing and visual representation.

As Gunaratnam (2007, p. 271) puts it, 'art can touch people and convey complex and incoherent notions of difference and otherness'. By making use of a personal narrative style, poetic writing and photography in the area of care and social welfare, Gunaratnam challenges the dominant paradigm of representation and actualises important issues for the social work professions and service users in a glocalised world. Gunaratmam questions expertise in relation to the unspoken, the blurring between structure and improvisation, the predictable and unexpected, and suggests that researchers and teachers challenging dominant paradigms and using creative forms will enable a movement between academia and other sectors. These movements will also allow the participation of new audiences. The poem below is an example of such movements, and this poem invites readers to consider various and entangled representations of the body, emotions, race and masculinity through the experience of illness:

> Intent concern accompanied the glinting blade
> that sliced from hip to hip.
> A tributary
> meandering down into dry recesses of manliness.
> A cut so deep, so low

folds of distinction reopen.
Hard layers. Moist untouched spaces.
Shiny black skin. Striated muscle.
Prowess
flow into tired, needy sinews of a pure new
softness.

(Gunaratnam 2007, p. 280)

Leavy (2009, p. 3), exploring the relationship between the social sciences and art, emphasises the interconnectivity between the subject positions and/or the practice locations of the artist, researcher and teacher to create a position for a/r/tography where 'these three roles are integrated creating a *third space* [italics in original] [...]' in which 'practitioners occupy "in-between" space'. We suggest a third space has multiple meanings: it can be a position between formal and informal structures or a newly carved space for imagining, creating and thinking (see Chapters 6, 9, 10 and 11; see also Livholts 2010a, 2010b). Our interpretation of the global standards in social work education (Sewpaul & Jones 2004a, 2004b) is that personal and professional development and reflective practice need to work with what Patel and Lynch (2013, p. 223), in glocalised pedagogy, refer to as 'framing of local and global community connectedness in relation to social responsibility, justice and sustainability'.

The Glocal and The Micro: Bringing into Focus Agency and the Body

The intersecting connectivity that gives life to the concept of 'glocal' enables examination of interstices between the macro-meso and micro and, therefore, social agency, that is, engagement, activism and change by individuals and communities to state and globalising processes. Agency has been employed by social work scholars to show possibilities for engagement and contestation through social movements or challenges to the state at the local level. As Dominelli (2010a) argues:

The contestation of space and place includes those who 'migrate' virtually by exploring the internet; those doing so in reality through migration, those who remain to defend their sense of the local – as in the case of Indigenous people living in colonized territories; those segments of majority populations that feel threatened by newcomers to their lands.

(Dominelli 2010a, p. 120)

Inherent in Dominelli's statement is that agency is also enacted through fears, desires, cultural identification and ways of being. In these ways, globalising forces are glocalising in ways that are deeply entrenched in bodily politics (Ahmed 2004). Questions of the body and affect in relation to the glocal have gained increasing attention in disciplines like gender studies, cultural studies and cultural and social geography but have yet to receive significant attention in social work.

It is surprising, given social work's focus on locating individuals within systems, that few social work accounts begin their analyses with the most local of local spheres: the body. An exception is Alphonse *et al.*'s (2008) theoretical examination of identity in India using Gidden's conceptualization of individualisation to identify how globalising forces created movements of people from rural to urban areas and the need for the construction of new identities. There are, however, few empirical in-depth examples that begin with the self and analyse multidirectional processes shaping the contexts and conditions in which people live.

Moosa-Mitha and Ross-Sheriff (2010) have drawn interesting parallels between 'transnational' or 'international' social work and the early waves of feminist theorising, focusing in particular on the universalising of social categories evident in each. However, there are further lessons that can be gained from feminism. Most notably, feminist theorising on temporality and spatiality which takes into account the spatial body, that is, dialectically linking everyday lived experiences with glocal processes in time and space (e.g. Massey 2005; Simonsen 2007). The spatial body and, as such, bodily politics locate affect into analyses of the glocal. As Ahmed (2004, p. 1) argues using the example of discourses of threat in relation to asylum seekers, emotions are politically produced and worked to 'shape the surfaces of individual and collective bodies'. Inscribed fleshy bodies in turn shape and transgress the production of social space. Using the asylum example again, we have seen glocal responses where subjects and professional associations have mobilised and talked back discursively, emotionally and performatively to the nation state. We suggest that, by approaching the glocal from body politics, social work as a discipline can contribute a nuanced account to globalising issues and process which 'takes the practices of "ordinary" people and organizations ... as a starting point' as opposed to beginning analyses from 'above' (Listerborn 2013, p. 294). This book uniquely contributes to developing theorisations from the body to understand the dialectics of the glocal (see Chapter 2, 4, 7, 9, 12, 13). Further, it examines how unequal power relations are created in the glocal through the circulation and consumption of images in human rights films (see Chapter 5) and the discursive otherisation of asylum seekers as a risk and a threat in the context of nations (see Chapter 4).

Glocal Social Challenges and Responses from Social Work

One of the most multifarious and complex contemporary human rights issues for social work is that the epitome of glocal forces, contexts and conditions is associated with the re-settlement of asylum seekers. The majority of refugees and asylum seekers suffer from displacement and unauthorised status, threatening human rights: threatening health, safety, dignity and worth. These contraventions to human rights are evident in the increasing number of unaccompanied minors displaced (and some orphaned) from country and family (Dominelli 2010a), and women being the target of human trafficking for sexual exploitation (Hodge 2008;

Hodge & Lietz 2007). Today, social workers experience dilemmas, possibilities and challenges in working with people, families and communities with origins in another country and societal hostilities which are discursively embedded in institutional practices towards refugees and migrant workers which actualise the continuous need for critical and anti-discriminatory perspectives in social work (Dominelli 2012; Jönsson 2014a; Williams & Graham 2014). Thus, dilemmas for social work occur in the context of social work values and welfare systems of particular countries that may deny migrant workers, asylum seekers and refugees their status and citizen rights (Williams & Graham 2014). As Hugman writes:

> [...] the form of social work that is possible in any particular location is struc-
> tured by the type of welfare regime in that country. Thus it can be argued that
> the possibilities for social work are circumscribed by national borders and
> that this is the case, even if we are talking about 'international' social work.
>
> (Hugman 2010, p. 8)

However, exclusionary practices are linked with the discrimination of people with different ethnic backgrounds, disabilities, gender and sexuality (Pease 2010). These structural dimensions of power actualise questions about homeland and belonging in the everyday and this is most apparent in relation to people seeking asylum. Mediatised otherisation is increasingly common, whereby 'refugees' are portrayed in party politics and through the mass media as a social problem and a burden (Ahmed 2004). In this way, questions of 'otherisation' are intimately intertwined within language and representation and give rise to public threat and emotion (Ahmed 2004). They are inherent at the discursive level of speech and sto-ries, creating practices and emotions of location and dislocation. These discursive practices, which simultaneously dislocate and locate, are rarely nuanced, rarely allow for differences within communities of people seeking asylum and submerge lived experiences of war and colonisation. In this volume, authors seek to examine how mediatised otherisation discursively comes into being (see Chapter 4), how it can be challenged by making use of human rights film (Chapter 5) and how colonialism and imperialism shape contemporary situations of and social work responses to migration (see Chapters 4, 12 and 13).

Overview of the Book

This international collection has three sections: the first provides exemplars of social issues that are glocal, the second considers methodological re-shaping and spatial transgressions of glocal social work and the third examines how social work as a glocalised profession responds to glocal concerns and agendas.

Part I: The Glocalisation of Social Issues

In section one, the focus is on major structural political, economic, social and cul-tural issues for social work such as migration, human rights and humanitarianism and gendered violence to self and others. This section examines the multiscalar dimensions of social issues, the globalising trends and practices that set in train multiscalar concerns, the responses to and development of social issues by nation states and how bodies affectively experience the issues in question. Part I begins with Bryant and Garnham's exploration of farmer suicide: an area of enquiry where social work has remained absent. Chapter 2 brings attention to the distressed body and the affect, practices and experiences that work to undo subjectivities. The authors examine how globalising political, economic and environmental conditions are re-articulated, responded to and navigated at the local level in space and time. In this way, this chapter takes the concept of the glocal as fundamental to understanding the conditions and contexts to distress and suicide. The ways farmers' bodies are enmeshed within political and moral economies and communities are interspatial dimensions that occur across geopolitical borders, shaping the possibility for farmer suicide. The authors propose a number of potential reasons why social work remains absent in understandings of farmer suicide – one of which is that the agri-political economy has not been a traditional sphere for social work engagement.

While Chapter 2 focuses on men's self-harm through suicide, Chapter 3 examines the problem of men's violence and violent masculinities. Specifically, Hearn, Ratele and Schefer examine the diverse locations and intersectional gendering of men, as the major doers of violence. In addition, the authors explore why men are disproportionately represented as victims of homicidal violence. They situate their analyses within global/local intersections, as part of transversal, postcolonial feminist/profeminist politics. The authors work across, in and between Africa and Europe and focus on three transnational examples, all framed in relation to violence and violation. These three examples include global, international and transnational violences; interpersonal violence in intimacy; and engaging men and boys in global and local anti-violence initiatives. This chapter illustrates a complexity about diverse forms of gendered violence and provides a lens through the examples portrayed in the text to examine how violence can come into being in the context of globalising forces, institutional, local and interpersonal contexts. The authors connect theoretical and social work practice complexities which require consideration in working in the field of gendered violence.

Glocalisation is taken up in Chapter 4 to examine how nation state policies and, in particular, those in the United Kingdom and Australia have responded to the global forced migration of people seeking asylum. As Masocha argues, 'Asylum seekers' presence in western countries represents an intrusion of global issues into everyday lives at the local level'. Like Bryant and Garnham in Chapter 2, Masocha extends social work thinking into this domain by explicating how political economy shapes lived experience and, in particular in the case of asylum seekers, how North-South disparities in relation to income and wealth contribute to conflicts and forced migration. He shows that common approaches to asylum seekers in the United Kingdom and Australia underscore surveillance and control to reduce, if not stop, entry of those seeking asylum. Drawing on the governmentality risk thesis, Chapter 4 shows how asylum seekers are discursively constructed as risky and threatening, with threat being constituted in the context of ideologies of nationhood. In these ways, the bodies of asylum seekers are othered. Masocha illustrates glocality through the global nature of forced migration and the glocal responses to asylum seekers framed in discourses of nationhood. Social work practice, the author suggests, has focused on local responses to asylum seekers. However, by doing so, it remains situated in practices that respond and reinforce 'othering' discourses. Instead, it is timely for social workers to move beyond the local to work collectively across borders to advocate for the human rights of people seeking asylum.

The question of human rights and othering and how we respond to these issues as social workers is also given attention in Chapter 5. Tascón examines the 'humanitarian gaze' as constituted through moving images. She critiques current representations in film of people deemed as 'suffering' or 'struggling' and critiques how these images become tools to draw attention to human rights issues and make them palatable to the public. She suggests that social workers in social work education and elsewhere often deploy these images. She encourages social workers to analyse our practice and that of our students of 'looking' and the discursive power of meanings associated with 'humanitarianism'. Tascón suggests that these discursive meanings emerge from global discourses which can be undone at the local level, that is, subverted by social workers. Chapter 5 provides an interesting lens through which to examine the economic and political dimensions that create the glocal, likening it to modern forms of colonialism or neo-colonialism. Her focus is on how unequal power relations in the glocal are created, circulated and consumed as images. She provides examples of discursively produced understandings of humanitarianism represented through images in documentaries shown as part of the Human Rights Watch International Film Festival in 2011. Chapter 5, like other chapters in this section, brings attention to political and moral economies and social and cultural systems. The chapters in this section examine lived experiences and policies to consider how glocality is shaped; Chapter 5 contributes an additional dimension, the relationships between viewers and subjects and how social workers can work to subvert these.

Part II: Methodological Re-Shaping and Spatial Transgression in Glocalised Social Work

Within the second section, chapters elaborate on topics related to spatial dimensions of relevance to social work including physical, material and emotional spaces. This sparsely elaborated field enables a re-shaping of social work knowledge to further develop spatial dimensions that take into consideration inter/transdisciplinary contributions from cultural geography. The creative arts and creative writing provide social work with a new lens through which to critique and analyse social spaces across local and global contexts.

Chapter 6 methodologically situates social work and the glocal in relation to a politics of location, that is, from geographically and historically located relations of power. Livholts uses situated writing to bridge and intersect interdisciplinary positions and epistemological spaces, opening up a new space for social work. This new methodological space is given shape by the disciplines of social work, art, geography and creative writing. Social work in this space is one where questions of self/other, relationships of power, privilege and subordination are central to critical analytical reflexivity. In this chapter, Livholts provides examples of situated writing that show the reader critical analytical reflexivity in action. She uses situated intersectionality to examine diverse orders of stratification from neighbourhood to household, city, state, region, global, national, regional and local.

The theme of spatiality and glocality as a methodological lens for social work is also taken up in Chapter 7 where Gottzén, following Deleuze and Guattari, explores gendered violence and bodies in material spaces. He uses case studies with children and young people, who have been exposed to domestic violence, to examine affective atmospheres: how spaces are infused with emotions across different locales. Hence, the globally identified issue of gendered domestic violence is experienced and felt in multiscalar ways (in and through the body, in rooms and buildings) and responded to differently across borders in relation to the possibility of refuge, shelter and laws on the safety and protection of women and children. Gottzén's theorisation brings to the fore a new methodological approach to glocal and social work in relation to gender through the concept of 'atmosphere', that is, multiple spaces filled with power relations and affect but also safe spaces. Safety, he argues, is an atmosphere which is produced differently in different spaces. For social workers, analysing safe spaces as an affective atmosphere enables practice that takes into account what might be made possible by the inclusion of sensorial and affective safe spaces for women and children who have experienced domestic violence.

Anbäcken uses autoethnography to explore loss and grief in the context of a climatic disaster, which is now becoming increasingly a part of the natural and social landscapes in a number of countries. Chapter 8 takes as its focus the tsunami which hit northeastern Japan on 11 March 2011 and which Anbäcken witnessed. Autoethnography, as a method, enables the reader to enter into the text affectively, to visualise the loss of buildings, homes and people – to feel the sense of panic as discrepancies between stories from the media and local people unfold about the impact of radiation. This chapter argues that social work has remained largely absent from examining loss and grief, especially in relation to disasters, and that the discipline has a practice-based role to play in understanding how to respond to disasters especially as, with disaster, chaos and fear require trained responses.

Autoethnography as well as written storytelling is also given methodological priority in the next chapter (Chapter 9). Gordon uses creative writing as a community-based participatory approach to explore how memory and imagination are used in writing to change personal narratives. Using bell hooks' experience of reflecting on her past through fictionalising her memories, Gordon used this method to work collaboratively with clients of a salon/barbershop in the United Kingdom. The glocal in this context is finding a 'third' space for an ethnically diverse group of women and men in Britain. This third space was an affectively safe space, as Gottzén in Chapter 7 suggests, but was also a space that encouraged and enabled people to connect with their feelings, imagination and memories in a convivial atmosphere. A material and affective space emerged where, through autobiographical fiction writing, participants drew on experiences about their settlement in the United Kingdom and experiences of belonging in addition to feeling 'othered'. This chapter, like the section which follows, enables social workers to not only facilitate the opening up of spaces for growth but also opens innovative methodological spaces for community engagement.

Responsiveness to social issues is a core theme of Chapter 10. Alfreds and Åberg, artists involved in community development, discuss participatory art projects they have worked on in Kosovo, Macedonia and Albania. They use art and, in particular, social sculpture, film and installations to collaboratively form dialogue and facilitate personal and social change. They worked with prison workers in Albania using social sculpture to depict their dreams to open up ways of talking about and working through gendered workplace stress. This chapter provides case studies of several examples of working with communities to establish understandings and knowledge production which moves beyond 'cultural barriers'. In Alfreds and Åberg's words: 'in a global context, the "immaterial materials" such as thoughts, feelings and imagination can be part of a social force and form new collective patterns against the state or market-driven interests'. Chapter 10 is an exemplar of transgressing boundaries and finding new spaces and interdisciplinary ways of working for what is increasingly glocal social work.

Part III: Responses from Social Work as a Glocalised Profession

The third section of the book focuses on responses from social work as a glocalised profession related to emergent social problems, crises and social vulnerability. Collectively, these chapters reconceptualise community work.

Chapter 11, like Chapter 10, builds on the conceptualisation of the 'third space' in relation to social work activity in the community development sphere where community development becomes a deliberate response to socio-spatial segregation and economic and social vulnerability. In this chapter, Turunen's third space is contextualised as a space emerging between governmental and non-governmental sectors in Sweden with reference to housing development. Specifically, the third space is but one which in neoliberal economies are embedded in entrepreneurial social innovation. Turunen takes the reader through the history of community development in Swedish social work. She shows knowledge production as globally produced and, in part, locally reconstituted. She notes that the globalising presence of entrepreneurial individualistic notions of community moves analyses away from glocal poverty and reduces collective action.

Yu and Alcid, in Chapter 12, take the issue of migration raised in Chapter 4 and focus especially on the human rights of foreign workers, in particular Filipino workers. While there are 10 million Filipino workers working as overseas contract workers, their plight remains at the vagaries of employers and they remain excluded from protective national industrial laws. Yu and Alcid show how this global issue is lived in glocal contexts, pointing to economic, sexual, physical and emotional exploitation and abuse including trafficking, forced labour and non-payment of wages. Chapter 12 shows the complexity of social work practice across geopolitical borders and, as Yu and Alcid argue, 'with the globalisation of labour and employment comes the need for a global social work response'. This chapter, like many of the chapters of this book, argues that social work practice and education need to develop knowledge, as well as drive activism around global imbalances of power and resources that deem some lives as less worthy.

Chapter 13, like Chapters 4 and 12, focuses on international migration. Gruber brings attention to new occupations in Sweden that have emerged through international migration, and these are bridge-builder (brobyggare), health communicator (hälsokommunikatör), cultural interpreter (kulturtolk) and doula (doula). She explains that these professionals are tasked with bridging linguistic and cultural differences by facilitating meetings between the Swedish welfare institutions (such as schools, healthcare and social services) and clients with a migrant background. Gruber focuses especially on the role of doulas in maternity and obstetric care and explores how doulas are expected to handle 'the gap' between the global and local. Specifically, doulas are expected to bridge the border between a nationally oriented welfare institution and patients with another national, cultural and/ or linguistic background. She shows how this bridging is a problematic space for doulas caught between the institution and patients.

Chapter 14 focuses on the practice of social work as discipline and profession across geopolitical spaces. Pease employs the concept of transnationalism to examine how social work transcends national borders. He encourages us to think about western-centric philosophies, knowledge production and ways of working that shape social work, reproducing social work practice and education as white western masculine forms of knowing and doing. Whilst this chapter sets the challenge for social workers (particularly those in the global north) to rethink their privilege, it also challenges that this frame is homogenous. Pease argues for the validation of local and Indigenous ways of knowing and contributing to social work knowledge, calling for a critique of 'global' social work agendas that reinforce western neoliberal ideologies.

Collectively, this edition aims to encourage further dialogue about what constitutes social work within and across geopolitical spaces. It explores how to foster social work that is critical of political and moral economies and societies and how to encourages debate about ways of producing knowledge and practice that speak to the 'third spaces', encouraging diverse forms of social community engagement and activism.

References

Abu Lughod, J (1991), 'Going beyond global babble', in King, D (ed) *Culture, Globalisation and the World-System*, Palgrave, New York, pp. 131–138.

Ahmed, S (2004), *The Cultural Politics of Emotion*, Edinburgh University Press, Edinburgh.

Alphonse, M, Purnima, G & Moffatt, K (2008), 'Redefining social work standards in the context of globalisation', *International Social Work*, vol. 5, no. 2, pp. 145–158.

Appadurai, A (2013), *The Future as Cultural Fact. Essays on the Global Condition*, Verso, London and New York.

Bettman, JE, Jacques, G & Frost, CJ (eds) (2013), *International Social Work Practice. Case Studies from a Global Context*, Routledge, London and New York.

Bryant, L (ed) (2015), *Critical and Creative Research Methodologies in Social Work Research*, Ashgate, Farnham.

Bryant, L & Livholts, M (2013), 'Location and unlocation. Examining gender and telephony through autoethnographic textual and visual methods', *International Journal of Qualitative Methods*, vol. 12, pp. 403–419.

Bryant, L & Livholts, M (2015), 'Opening the lens to see', in Bryant, L (ed) *Critical and Creative Research Methodologies in Social Work*, Ashgate, Farnham, pp. 109–130.

Chambon, A (2005), 'Social work practices of art', *Critical Social Work*, vol. 6, no. 1, pp. 1–11.

Chambon, A (2012), 'Disciplinary borders and borrowings: Social work knowledge and its social reach, a historical perspective', *Social Work and Society*, vol. 10, no. 2, pp. 1–12. Available online at www.socwork.net/sws/article/view/348/700 (accessed 4 September 2016).

Chambon, A (2013), 'Recognising the Other, understanding the Other: A brief history of social work and Otherness', *Nordic Social Work Research*, vol. 3, no. 2, pp. 120–129.

Cree, V (2013), *Becoming a Social Worker. Global Narratives*, 2nd edition, Routledge, London.

Dominelli, L (2010a), *Social Work in a Globalizing World*, Polity Press, Cambridge.

Dominelli, L (2010b), 'Globalization, contemporary challenges and social work practice', *International Social Work*, vol. 53, no. 5, pp. 599–612.

Dominelli, L (2012), *Green Social Work: From Environmental Crises to Environmental Justice*, Polity Press, Cambridge.

Furman, R, Nalini N, Schatz, M & Jones, S (2008), 'Transnational social work. Using a wraparound model', *Global Networks*, vol. 8, no. 4, pp. 496–503.

Gunaratnam, Y (2007), 'Where is the love', *Journal of Social Work Practice*, vol. 21, no. 3, pp. 271–287.

Haraway, D (1988), 'Situated knowledges: The science question in feminism and the privilege of partial perspective', *Feminist Studies*, vol. 14, no. 3, pp. 575–599.

Healy, LM (2008), *International Social Work: Professional Action in an Interdependent World*, Oxford University Press, New York.

Healy, L & Link, R (eds) (2012), *Handbook of International Social Work. Human Rights, Development, and the Social Profession*, Oxford University Press, New York.

Hodge, DR & Lietz, CA (2007), 'The international sexual trafficking of women and children, Affilia', *Journal of Women and Social Work*, vol. 22, no. 2, pp. 63–74.

Hodge, DR (2008), 'Sexual trafficking in the United States: A domestic problem with transnational dimensions', *Social Work*, vol. 53, no. 2, pp. 143–52.

Hong, PYP & Song, H (2010), 'Glocalisation of social work practice: Global and local responses to globalization', *International Social Work*, vol. 53, no. 5, pp. 656–670.

Hugman, R (2008), 'Ethics in a world of difference', *Ethics and Social Welfare*, vol. 2, no. 2, pp. 118–132

Hugman, R (2010), *Understanding International Social Work. A Critical Analysis*, Palgrave MacMillan, London.

Hugman, R, Moosa-Mitha, M & Moyo, O (2010), 'Towards a borderless social work: Reconsidering notions of international social work', *International Social Work*, vol. 53, no. 5, pp. 629–643

Jones, DN & Truell, R (2012), 'The global agenda for social work and social development: A place to link together and be effective in a globalized world', *International Social Work*, vol. 55, no. 4, pp. 454–472.

Jönsson, JH (2014a), 'Local reactions to global problems: Undocumented immigrants and social work', *British Journal of Social Work*, vol. 44, pp. 35–52.

Jönsson, JH (2014b), *Globalised Localities and Social Work: Contemporary Challenges*. Mid Sweden University Doctoral Thesis 177, Sweden.

Kamali, M (2015), *War, Violence and Social Justice. Theories for Social Work*, Ashgate, London.

Leavy, P (2009), *Method Meets Art. Art-Based Research and Practice*, The Guilford Press, New York.

Listerborn, C (2013), 'Suburban women and the "glocalisaiton" of everyday lives: Gender and glocalities in underprivileged areas in Sweden', *Gender, Place and Culture*, vol. 20, no. 3, pp. 290–312.

Livholts, M (ed.) (2012), *Emergent Writing Methodologies in Feminist Studies*, Routledge, New York and London.

Livholts, M (2015), 'Imagine transfiguration: The chapter exhibition as a critical and creative space for knowledge in social work and media studies', in Bryant, L (ed) *Critical and Creative Qualitative Research Methodologies for Social Work*, Ashgate, Farnham, pp. 131–158.

Livholts, M (2010a), 'The professor's chair. An untimely academic novella', *Life Writing*, vol. 7, no. 2, pp. 155–168.

Livholts, M (2010b), 'The snow angel and other imprints. An untimely academic novella', *International Review of Qualitative Research*, vol. 3, no. 1, pp. 103–124.

Lyons, K (2006), 'Globalization and social work: International and local implications', *British Journal of Social Work*, vol. 36, pp. 365–380.

Lyons, K, Manion, C & Carlsen, M (eds) (2006), *International Perspectives on Social Work*, MacMillan, Hampshire.

Massey, D (1991), A Global Sense of Space, *Marxism Today*, vol. 38, pp. 365–380.

Massey, D (2005), *For Space*, Sage, London.

Midgley, J (1981), *Professional Imperialism: Social Work in the Third World*, Heinemann, London.

Moosa-Mitha, M & Ross-Sheriff, F (2010), 'Transnational social work and lessons learned from transnational feminism', *Affilia*, vol. 25, no. 2, pp. 105–109.

Patel, F & Lynch, H (2013), 'Glocalization as an alternative to internationalization in higher education: Embedding positive glocal learning perspectives', *International Journal of Teaching and Learning in Higher Education*, vol. 25, no. 2, pp. 223–230.

Pease, B (2010), *Undoing Privilege: Unearned Advantage in a Divided World*, Zed Books, London.

Ranta-Tyrkkö, S (2011), 'High time for postcolonial analysis in social work', *Nordic Social Work Research*, vol. 1, no. 1, pp. 25–41.

Righard, E (2013), 'Internationellt social arbete. Definitioner och perspektivval i historisk belysning', *Socialvetenskaplig Tidskrift*, no. 2, pp. 127–146.

Robertson, R (1992), *Globalization: Social Theory and Global Culture*, Sage, London.

Robertson, R (1995), 'Glocalization: Time-space and homogeneity-heterogeneity', *Global Modernities*, vol. 2, pp. 25–45.

Robertson, R (2005), 'The conceptual promise of glocalization: Commonality and diversity', *ART-e-FACT: Strategies of Resistance*, vol. 4. Available online at http://artefact.mi2.hr/_a04/lang_en/theory_robertson_en.htm (accessed 4 September 2016).

Robertson, R (2012), 'Globalisation or glocalisation?', *The Journal of International Communication*, vol. 18, no. 2, pp. 191–208.

Robertson, R (2013), 'Situating glocalisation: A relatively autobiographical intervention', in Drori, GS, Höllerer, MA & Walchenbach, P (eds) *Global Themes and Local Variations in Organization and Management*, Routledge, New York, pp. 25–36.

Romanov, P & Kononenko, R (2014), 'Glocalization processes in Russian social work', *International Social Work*, vol. 57, no. 5, pp. 435–446.

Roudometof, V (2015), 'The glocal and global studies', *Globalizations*, vol. 12, no. 5, pp. 774–787.

Sewpaul, V & Jones, D (2004a), 'Global standards for social work education and training', *Social Work Education*, vol. 23, no. 5, pp. 493–513.

Sewpaul, V & Jones, D (2004b), 'Global standards for the education and training of the social work profession', The General Assemblies of IASSW and IFSW, Adelaide, Australia, pp. 1–24.

Simonsen, K (2007), 'Practice, spatiality and embodied emotions: An outline of a geography of practice', *Human Affairs*, vol. 17, pp. 168–181.

Steger, MB (2010), 'Globalization', *The Encyclopedia of Political Thought*, 1st edition, John Wiley & Sons Ltd, New York.

The Global Agenda for Social Work and Social Development: Commitment to Action, (2012), IFSW. Available online at http://cdn.ifsw.org/assets/globalagenda2012.pdf (accessed 4 September 2016).

Wrede, S & Näre, L (2013), 'Glocalising care in the Nordic countries', *Nordic Journal of Migration Research*, vol. 3, no. 2, pp. 57–62.

Welbourne, M (2009), 'Social work: The idea of a profession and the professional project', *Locus SOCI@L*, vol. 3, pp. 19–35.

Williams, C & Graham, M (2014), '"A world on the move": Migration, mobilities and social work', *British Journal of Social Work*, vol. 44, pp. 1–17. Available online at http://bjsw.oxfordjournals.org/content/early/2014/05/28/bjsw.bcu058.short (accessed 4 September 2016).

Part I

The Glocalisation of Social Issues

2 Glocal Terrains of Farmer Distress and Suicide

Lia Bryant and Bridget Garnham

Introduction

The landscape of farmer suicide has, on the whole, remained absent from social work examination. Academic focus on farmer suicide has been situated within the 'psy' and medical disciplines and the social science disciplines of geography, sociology and suicidology (Bryant and Garnham 2013). These foci have tended to produce knowledge which constitutes farmer suicide as causally associated with diminished individual resilience that arises due to downward spirals in economic circumstances and climatic conditions. As a consequence, farm viability and hence subjectivity, heritage and wellbeing become threatened due to externalising, uncertain and uncontrollable forces.

Disciplines like social work and critical geography enable a more nuanced examination of farmer distress and suicide, tracing the multiple interwoven threads which enmesh the subject in broader globalising and local contexts and conditions. Bryant and Garnham, in a series of papers (2013; 2015; and Garnham and Bryant 2014), have argued that the terrain of farmer distress and the possibility of suicide is contoured by the interstices between subjectivity and the political, cultural, social, economic and climatic conditions in which farming occurs (Bryant and Garnham 2013). We argue that subjectivity is informed by masculinities, as in Australia, men predominantly claim the occupational identity of farmer and inherit farming properties. Farmers, through the business of farming, are enmeshed in globalising practices of transnational corporations, international markets, national policies of the state and local community politics. Hence, conditions which lead to farmer distress and suicide are related to multi-scalar phenomena that are affectively and viscerally lived at the scale of the body, compounded by 'glocal' contexts and conditions that create distress. Specifically, we contend that bodily encounters are mediated by glocal contexts and conditions, and that these are 'negotiated in the moment' (Wilson 2016: 5) with actions, reactions and emotions brought forth enabling the moment (e.g. Ahmed 2000; 2004a; Askins and Pain 2011).

The problematisation and production of farmer suicide as a glocal phenomenon can be traced to how suicide is defined and distress treated. Categorisation and treatment are informed by global medicalised knowledge that pathologises distress in medical texts and diagnostic manuals. Suicide statistics, however, come into being as a result of the enumerative practices of states which result in the publishing of national suicide mortality data. This data is often collected from coroner's reports, which become privileged sites for examining suicide (Münster 2015). In turn, suicide statistics become internationalised as international data sets are used to compare occupations and demographics at risk of suicide. Farmers, in particular, have been identified as a 'high risk' occupation or as 'suicide prone' (e.g. Tiesman *et al.* 2015). Statistics are then reproduced in the media, often removed from the context in which they were collected and the definitions that spurned their production. They become the basis for sensationalist media accounts and headlines which then politicise and incite calls for action. One such account by an Australian televised news site reported that 'Sixty per cent of Queensland is in drought, and farmers are facing the prospect of losing their livelihood in order to pay back crippling debts ... [the reporter] spent a week in far north Queensland where farmers are now taking their own lives at a staggering rate' (SBS Two 2014). This same news report quoted what has become a frequently reported statistic, that is, that one in four farmers commit suicide every day. Over the last few years, this statistic has been scrutinised, showing that it had been taken from research produced over a decade ago (e.g. Page and Fragar 2002) without recourse to variations associated with time, agricultural industry or region in Australia.

In this chapter, to contextualise the extent of the phenomenon of farmer suicide, we review international literature on farmer distress showing that suicide is a substantial issue for farmers across the global south and north. To explicate the multiple glocal encounters with the body, we draw on an Australian case study of farming men from a region in South Australia. As analyses of suicide face a 'lacunae of primary evidence' (Feldman 2010: 305), we are limited in terms of 'what we can know' about the contexts and conditions within which farmers decide to suicide. As Munster suggests, 'All that is available to the ethnographer are representations – second-hand rationalizations of an act that ultimately remains a black box for the researcher' (Münster 2015: 1600). Like Feldman (2010), however, we argue that

> we need to appreciate, as a complement to evidentiary materials available directly from [those] who have committed suicide, the normative assessments and regulatory practices that historicize and contextualize their everyday lives.
>
> (Feldman 2010: 306)

Thus, the approach we have taken does not directly focus on suicide and so does not seek to illuminate the subjective experiences of those who are suicidal. Rather, it aims to contribute to understanding how political, economic, social, ethical and emotional conditions underpin and generate distress and thus render suicide a possibility for farmers. It also aims to examine why social work as a discipline has largely remained absent in understanding farmer distress and suicide.

Farmer Suicide: A Global or Interspatial Problem?

Disproportionately high rates of suicide have been reported in the literature for the United States, Canada, United Kingdom, France, India, Japan, Brazil and Australia (Arnautovska *et al*. 2014; Behere and Bhise 2009; Bossard *et al*. 2013; Hounsome *et al*. 2012; Stark *et al*. 2006; Sturgeon and Morrissette 2010; Tiesman *et al*. 2015). Whilst the argument that farmers are disproportionately at risk of suicide is clearly stated across the literature, there is very little data that clearly outlines the extent of the phenomenon in each of the countries identified. Claims are often based on ageing data (e.g. Miller and Burns 2008; Page and Fragar 2002) or the rates for this population are embedded in overall rates for rural areas. A recent study of suicide mortality for farmers in France revealed that the rate of suicide amongst farmers is between 20 per cent and 30 per cent higher than the population rate for men (Bossard *et al*. 2013). In Australia, using data from the Australian Institute of Health and Welfare, Hogan *et al*. (2012: 119) state that 'the suicide rate for non-indigenous males in non-metropolitan areas in Australia is 25 per cent to 40 per cent higher than that of males living in major cities and proportionately 48 per cent higher for male farmers'. The highest rate of farmer suicide appears to occur in India, where the phenomenon constitutes an ongoing epidemic with more than 100,000 farmer deaths over the past 10 years (Münster 2015).

Explanations for farmer suicide are situated within two opposing approaches, which privilege the macro or micro factors and contexts associated with distress and suicide. Micro approaches focus on individualistic accounts of suicide and aim to produce aggregate risk factors. The dominant discourses in the literature shape understandings of suicide in terms of *individual mental states*, particularly stress and depression, and correlate this with intentional self-harm and suicide (e.g. Faria *et al*. 2014; C. E. Fraser *et al*. 2005; Freire and Koifman 2013; Hounsome *et al*. 2012; Judd *et al*. 2006b; Stark *et al*. 2006). This *particular rendering of risk for suicide* provides the basis for the state to respond through pastoral apparatus intended to intervene in mental health and suicide prevention. Whilst making an important contribution to the knowledge on suicide, this dominant positivist and 'psy' framework also operates to limit and exclude other possible renderings of farmer suicide and thus narrows the frame of possible prevention strategies.

Identifying the risk factors for farmer suicide constitutes a 'surface' to understanding suicide, but one that is fragmented, reductive and circumscribed. As Price and Evans (2005: 45) argue, the 'psy' disciplines 'tend to focus on the dramatic outcomes of processes of stress in the form of suicide rather than the dynamics of social processes themselves which form the underlying causes of stress'. Since 'suicidal behaviour does not begin with the 'precipitating factor' and end with the 'suicidal act', but extends deep into individual and collective pasts and futures' (Staples and Widger 2012: 199), we need to examine the contexts and conditions in which suicide is embedded.

Macro foci are informed by the discipline of sociology, in particular, and the seminal work of Emile Durkheim. This literature also remains largely positivist and considers social rates of suicide, making comparisons between farmer suicide and other occupations (e.g. Stark *et al.* 2006; Nishimura *et al.* 2004; Tiesman *et al.* 2015) and rural to urban populations (Handley *et al.* 2011; Hirsch 2006; Judd *et al.* 2006a; Kapusta *et al.* 2008; McPhedran and Leo 2013; Middleton *et al.* 2003; Sankaranarayanan *et al.* 2010; Singh and Siahpush 2002) and, most recently, by occupation and location (Arnautovska *et al.* 2014). In addition, there are studies that examine suicide mortality by method and demographic factors and through psychological autopsy (Malmberg *et al.* 1997). There is also a suite of studies focused on variables correlated with risk and gendered methods of self-harm and varying lethality (Guiney 2012; Page and Fragar 2002). Given the positivist methodologies informing much of this research, the knowledge produced on farmer suicide is largely descriptive. As a result, as Hogan *et al.* argue, 'Conceptually this literature is fragmented. It lacks a theoretically-informed framework through which one can both better understand this phenomena and work toward preventing its occurrence' (Hogan *et al.* 2012: 120).

Over the last decade, the international literature spanning these poles situates farmer suicide in the context of economic conditions and, in particular, indebtedness, which delimits possibilities for futures. For example, in Australia, a dominant narrative in research and policy on farmer suicide is the centralisation of drought as a causative factor for economic hardship with economic distress causing suicide. The problem with this dominant narrative is that governments then have to respond to suicide prevention for farmers in a linear way, focusing on financial packages for drought relief precluding or reducing the possibilities of other preventive strategies. This raises a number of problems, the first being that drought is not a 'natural' condition but is determined by official definitions of the state (Bryant and George 2016), and so if drought is not declared, financial relief is unlikely to follow. Secondly, other market conditions lead to financial stress, like fluctuating commodity prices, disease to crops and other climatic conditions like floods. Similarly, in India, a monolithic narrative circulates which constitutes farmer suicides as a form of political protest in response to 'the structural violence of globalization and neoliberal reform' (Münster 2015: 1582). Here, social discourses inscribe farmer's enumerated bodies with multiple discourses of agrarian distress in ways that erase individuality and specificities of distress (Kaushal 2015; Münster 2015). In the examples above and across geographical borders, 'economic reductionism' has become the nucleus for understandings of farmer suicide with multiple and intersecting factors decentred from analyses (Münster 2015: 1589).

Farmer Suicide: Bodies Enmeshed in Political and Moral Economies/Communities

We have extensively argued that, to understand farmer suicide, micro and macro approaches need to be bridged (see Bryant and Garnham 2013; 2014; 2015). To do so, we suggest that analyses begin with an understanding of the interstices between farmer subjectivities and the political and moral economies and communities in which farmers live. This position affirms an understanding of space which is produced, inter-related and scaled (Lefebvre 1991). Hence, the glocal in this context refers to a 'global-local dialectic' and an excavating of the '*processes* that are operating' (Listerborn 2013: 294 – original emphasis). Commonly, however, glocal research has tended to exclude daily experiences or the view from the body focusing on globalising trends and forces and their interaction with local economies, policies and practices. The local then takes on a particular meaning which can exclude the everyday practices, emotions and imaginaries of people. As such, feminist geographers have called for a scaling that begins with the body (Simonsen 2007; Nielson and Simonsen 2003, Listerborn 2013; Pain 2009). Simonsen (2007: 174 – original emphasis), drawing on Lefebvre (1991) and Merleau-Ponty (1962), contends that 'An important precondition of the production of space is ... that each living body *is* and *has* its space; it produces itself in space at the same time as it produces space'. Australian farmer's bodies, which are mostly male bodies, are inscribed with particular hegemonic masculinities that render their bodies as physically strong, stoic, resilient and enshrined in the concept of 'battler' (Bryant and Garnham 2015). The farmer's body is pitted against the elements attempting to control nature and animals, battling for food production and the reproduction of farm and family (Bryant and Garnham 2015).

Using the body in the context of the 'glocal' as a methodological approach is not simply a matter of 'scaling down' analyses but enables 'new ways to refocus on different interconnected sites simultaneously' (Pain 2009: 2). The body, as lived in the glocal, provides a way in which to envision these simultaneous interconnections worked through subjectivities that are enmeshed in political and moral economies and communities. Beginning with the body enables spatial understandings to emerge from the perspective of farmers; it is their discursive, experiential and imagined glocal in which we begin to build our understanding of political and moral economies/communities. Distress, however, is not a passive response to glocal contexts and conditions. Rather, farmers and communities accept or partially accept discourses by making moral judgements about themselves and others; that is, they react to glocal conditions through bodily distress but also create conditions of blame and shame that may produce the possibility for distress in others. At the same time, they act on their own distress and their distress at seeing their community members become mentally unwell or suicide. Action is taken in the form of lobbying government to change drought policies to offer financial assistance to farmers (see Bryant and George 2016 for further discussion) and by establishing community support networks (Bryant *et al.* 2006). Hence, at times, distress is used to mobilise bodies and create change in social and cultural contexts.

Wine Grape Growers in The Riverland, South Australia: A Case Study

The Riverland is used as a case study, that is, as a 'framing device' (Schostak 2002: 22) to allow in-depth analysis of the glocal contexts and conditions that shape farmer distress. A case study enables the examination of broad phenomena in relation to bounded terrain (Schostak 2002). Our study focused on farming men, locally known as 'blockies', from The Riverland, a 330 km long region of South Australia that surrounds the Murray River. The Riverland wine region has approximately 1,100 wine grape growers who in 2012 produced over 411,000 tonnes of grapes (Riverland Wine Industry Development Council 2009). The wine industry is characterised by family-owned properties (94 per cent of wine grape growing businesses are family owned and operated) where grapes are grown for sale to wine companies. We have drawn on data from two studies. The first involved 30 in-depth qualitative semi-structured face-to-face interviews held in 2006 and the second consisted of 24 in-depth qualitative semi-structured face-to-face interviews repeated annually over three years from 2010–2012 (see Bryant and Garnham 2013 and 2015 for a detailed discussion of research design). Participants were asked a series of questions focused on demographic details about their families and farms and were encouraged to discuss personal wellbeing, industry changes and economic, social and political conditions occurring in farming. Transcripts were analysed using thematic analysis to identify key recurring themes, relationships between themes and non-patterns occurring in the data (Minichiello *et al.* 2008).

Distressed Bodies

The work of Price and Evans (2009) has been pivotal in conceptualising distress, noting the overuse of the medicalised conceptualisation of stress and clarifying the difference between stress and distress. The concept of 'distress' allows for analyses that take into account the lived actualities within the social, cultural and political contexts in which farming takes place. Price and Evans (2009) and Bryant and Garnham (2013; 2014; 2015) have demonstrated that distress in farming is a gendered, emotional, physical and psychological experience. However, distress comes into being through multiple and interwoven dimensions occurring from the socio-historic conditions of family farming. In countries like Australia and the United Kingdom, the subject position of farmer is constituted and reconstituted within the macro politics of farming. This approach recognises that whilst emotional, mental and physical distress is a subjective experience, there are social, cultural and ethical dimensions that provide the conditions of possibility for individual emotional experience and impact on wellbeing (e.g. Ahmed 2004b; Probyn 2004; 2005). Thus, in this way, distress is lived as:

> visceral
>   *I thought I was dying of cancer …*
> and emotional
>   *I couldn't stop crying, I was bluing [arguing] with the wife*
> as well as mental
>   *I'm a loser*
> and gendered
>   *… didn't want to be the one who loses the farm*

When farm viability is threatened, subjectivity is threatened: bodies are threatened. As Coldwell (2009: 988) suggests, 'the struggle to survive in farming is, for many men, a struggle to maintain their masculine identity'. The subject position of farmer is not an occupational identity alone but historically woven into the continuance of farm and family through patrilineal succession (Brandth and Haugen 2005; Bryant 1999). As has been discussed in detail elsewhere, to farm means to enact masculinity through being the embodied conduit of family heritage and succession. In Australia, 'the idealized notion of the farming man as hero emerges from the romantic agrarian mythology of the "Aussie battler"' (Bryant and Garnham 2015: 75). Hence, to battle means to be strong and resilient against environmental, economic and political conditions. For Australian farmers, masculine pride is connected to battling and self-sacrifice, which have become cultural virtues. For example, a farmer explained, 'there's a real element of pride and people on the land don't want to admit defeat, it's just not what you do, you try to battle on' (Bryant and Garnham 2015: 35).

To fail in business is to fail as a farmer – and as a man. As Ramirez-Ferrero (2005) suggests:

> Men who have based their subjectivity and pride upon these agrarian discourses experience their own cultural and emotional devaluation and sub-jugation. As a result, some farmers withdraw. Some may turn to violence.
>
> (Ramirez-Ferrero 2005: 121)

Farmer's moral value of self-worth becomes threatened through embodied feelings of shame which, while felt at the scale of the body, are culturally and socially constructed. Sayer aptly (2005) draws attention to the social conditions and norms which constitute feelings of shame, arguing:

> Shame is a complex emotion evoked by failure of an individual or a group to live according to their values or commitments, especially ones concerning their relation to others and goods which others value, so they believe them-selves to be defective.
>
> (Sayer 2005: 152–153)

For farmers, shame is constituted through the neoliberal discourse of economic 'success' and 'failure' as encapsulated in the concept of the entrepreneur – the rational, free agent driven by skills that, if used appropriately, deliver success. In this economic positioning, farmers are then individually responsible for managing risk. The sections below critique the notion of success and individual respon-siveness to the market and demonstrate that community norms, responses of the nation state and global markets create a political and moral economy that impli-cates the subject in feelings of shame.

Bodily Encounters with Political and Moral Economies

Political economy refers to the intersection between the government and the economy through policies and legislation that are designed to support and promote economic activity. Australian agriculture is broadly regulated according to neoliberal rationalities of government. These neoliberal rationalities provide the framework for a 'free market'. Therefore, with the introduction of neo-liberal government, a range of state policies that were supportive of family farming was abolished (Pritchard *et al.* 2007). The rationale underpinning the withdrawal of state support is that, in order to avoid economic distortion, 'farm units should persist only to the extent that they are sustained by the market' (Pritchard *et al.* 2007: 79).

Within the structures of the political economy of agri-business, a moral economy operates. Essentially, moral economy refers to a framework of norms and ethical principles governing social relations within economic systems (Sayer 2000; 2001; 2005; 2007). The notion of a moral economy is useful for drawing attention to the ways in which economic processes are embedded within normative social and cultural aspects of the 'lifeworld' (Sayer 2001). As Sayer (2000: 49) observes, 'Notions of reciprocity and regard, trust and obligation, among other ethical and moral concerns, permeate business transactions'. Such an approach enables the examination of social and economic (in)justice at the level of interactions between corporations and households (Sayer 2000; 2001).

Farmers' bodies located within the political and moral economy bring into focus bodily reactions and actions in the moment of encounter. Wilson (2016) demonstrates how the concept of bodily encounters has been used in multiple ways, particularly in social and critical geography. In short, she suggests that the concept of encounters is often employed to critique power relations bringing things, bodies and places together (e.g. Gibson 2010). Scholars examining cities have also suggested that places are made from a series of encounters, whether they be chance encounters with other bodies or mediated encounters, as in enduring gendered or class relations. This particular passage in Wilson's article, drawing on Gibson (2010), is of relevance to farming bodies in political and moral economies. She argues:

> … encounters can enable a better grasp of the contradictions, entanglements and momentary extensions of power that undermine such essentialist thinking and can thus 'sharpen ethical concepts'.
>
> (Gibson 2010: 521)

For farmers who participated in our research, contradictions and entanglements emerged from changing market conditions as a result of a worldwide oversupply of grapes. This grape glut occurred in the first decade of the new millennium, bringing new embodied encounters for farmers with transnational corporations. According to participants, the oversupply of wine grapes was a result of increased planting funded by corporate investment that in turn was stimulated by government tax incentives to drive growth in the wine industry. State intervention in the market was therefore perceived as producing economic distortion through an oversupply of produce. The tax incentives were revoked in 2004 amidst concerns of oversupply (Nipe *et al.* 2010) but the economic effects were a rapid and significant downturn in prices which, in the short term, meant operational losses, and in the long term threatened business viability. At the time of interview, many of the growers were in the midst of experiencing large financial losses (hundreds of thousands of dollars) and were cutting back on farming practices to reduce expenditure, taking up paid employment off the land to cover day-to-day living expenses, working long hours and considering options for exiting the industry.

The neoliberal political economy shapes a micro-politics of agri-business at the level of relations between farmers, corporations and the state. One of the ways in which agri-business has been transformed through neo-liberal discourses is through a reduction of state intervention in the commercial interaction between growers and processing companies (Pritchard *et al.* 2007). In response, the wine industry has adopted the use of contracts between primary producers and wineries to coordinate supply and manage risk (Fraser 2005). During times of success and economic growth, growers and wineries had enjoyed long-term contracts of approximately 15 years and an expectation that these would be unproblematically rolled over into new, lengthy contracts. At the time of the interviews (2006), however, the oversupply of grapes had severely impacted on the contracted business relationships between growers and wineries.

In this space of encountering 'ethics' in business, relationships were brought into focus in a new way for farmers. A number of the farmers we interviewed revealed that the wineries with which they had agreements had included a clause that had enabled them to suspend their contracts, which meant that the wineries would not accept and pay for the grapes produced under the contract but neither could the growers sell the produce on the open market because they had been contracted. This meant that growers had to accept the operational and production losses from producing the grapes which, for many, meant substantial annual economic deficits. It was also evident from the interviews that in some cases wineries were delaying or withdrawing payment for grapes that had already been accepted and processed.

The impact of delayed payment or non-payment on small family-owned businesses, already economically vulnerable, was in many cases threatening viability. Issues of contract suspension and delayed payment impacted on farmers' perceptions of ethical conduct within the social relations in the supply chain and many described breaches of trust and loyalty. Indeed, their personal treatment by wineries, with whom they had a longstanding relationship, was particularly distressing for farmers. Farmers expressed sentiments of moral outrage, anger, disappointment and hurt.

According to neoliberal policy, which requires market-sustainable agri-business, the state's directive is for farmers facing unviability to 'walk off the land'. However, there are social, economic and practical constraints that limit farmer's autonomy in this respect by restricting choice – for instance, banks refusing to take over landholdings or farmers being unable to sell their properties. For farmers experiencing these conditions, narratives of feeling trapped and doing whatever it takes to survive day by day were the norm. Farmers reported that feeling 'trapped' economically and emotionally produced extreme distress. As Ahmed

(2004b: 31) has argued, emotions are embodied experiences which are 'shaped by ... contact with objects, rather than being caused by objects', that is, how encounters are evaluated as hurtful or not involves 'reading the encounters in a certain way'. These encounters 'reopen past encounters' (Ahmed 2000: 8) and, for farmers, what is wrenched open is being at risk in the political and moral economy and its relational threat to the self.

Bodies in Situ: Rural Communities

As Liepins (2000) states, rural communities are 'both a discursive and material phenomenon of social connection and diversity'. Physically situated in a geographical place, the social fabric of rural communities is woven through intersections between heterogeneous subjectivities and social, economic, cultural, political and moral discourses and practices that shape social relations in rural places. Hence, the body in the rural is relational – shaping and being shaped by glocal spaces. However, the body provides 'a specific form of relationality' (Abrahamsson and Simpson 2011: 336, quoted in Wilson 2016: 6). In rural communities, intensely ingrained ideologies and normative judgments circulate and are reproduced through everyday social interaction that shapes ethical subjectivity and practice. In the following sections, we show the body in situ and the doing of encounter. We examine how the body recognises itself intersubjectively through norms and ideologies but also through practices that sustain and exclude. We show bodily encounters working through moral discourses that circulate through everyday social interaction and comprise an 'ordinary ethics' in rural communities. These discourses provide the normative values that underpin judgements about ethical selfhood and the moral worth of farmers. However, this discursive and lived space is a contradictory one which lends itself to belonging and exclusion, through binaries of self-assertion in space and self-loathing, collectivity of farming almost as a 'brotherhood' and individual action/reaction to social, political and climatic conditions.

We examined the operation of moral discourses in the Riverland farming community at a time when the community was experiencing water shortages and changes to water trading policy. Social policy was introduced with the provision for exit grant packages for eligible farmers to assist them to leave farming through advice, infrastructure removal and re-training. In neoliberal economic terms, the decision of whether to remain in farming during a period when the viability of the farm is threatened is one shaped by figures of profit and loss and predicted and anticipated economic recovery. However, for farmers, this decision constitutes a moral dilemma. What emerged during the interviews when farmers were discussing exit packages and the decisions of others in the community to either stay or leave were judgements of blame connected to moral discourses about farming.

Small landholders and those judged as not being 'real' or 'respectable' farmers were charged with a moral responsibility to exit from farming to allow neighbouring farmers to grow and thrive (Bryant 2016). Moral discourses also operated to differentially position farmers facing financial hardship as either morally responsible, and hence blameworthy, or as moral agents with mitigating circumstances. These judgements hinged upon conservative financial values and whether the economic management of farm profits was perceived as appropriate and necessary to the business.

Farmers who accepted an exit grant and chose to move away from the rural community were subject to blame for the perceived economic and social decline of the community. This judgement of blame emerges from rural values of 'active citizenship', that is, an ongoing participation in local community social and economic affairs. Active citizenship is located within a moral framework that positions farmers' rural community participation as contributing to a 'greater good' and, specifically, the sustainability of rural communities.

Farmers who accepted an exit grant to leave their farms were blamed for the environmental consequences and perceived degradation of land fertility of their properties and neighbouring properties. This withdrawal was framed as a moral transgression of farming values that renders farmers who leave as 'unethical'.

Farmers spoke of 'cracks' in the community, driven by emotions of resentment connected to the ascription of blame and perceived injury. This illustrates the importance of moral discourses and normative evaluation in shaping the social dynamics of rural communities in the context of economic and socio-political issues connected to agri-business. These moral discourses and judgements surface in the social fabric of everyday life during 'fleeting encounters and mundane conversations' for those living in rural communities and provide a vital dimension to understanding threats to wellbeing (Sayer 2011: 1). This is because complex intersections between moral discourses, ethical subjecthood, moral worth and possibilities for agency may generate distress for farmers who must navigate these positions in everyday life. At the level of community, perceived transgression of rural values designates farmers as blameworthy and may enact processes of social exclusion and reduce social standing. If these discourses become internalised through processes of subjectivation, there is a potential for farmers to experience loss of self-worth, shame and distress that provides the conditions of possibility for suicide.

Farmer Distress and the Absence of Social Work

The essence of social work is to bridge micro and macro contexts to enable a more complex understanding of social problems and create social change. Why has social work, as an academic discipline, remained largely absent in producing knowledge about farmer distress and suicide? We propose a series of contentions to explain social work's absence in this field. The first is that social work remains, in countries like Australia and the United Kingdom, predominantly an urban-centric discipline. As Pugh (2003: 67) argues, 'most British social work literature is written with the implicit assumption of an urban context, but large numbers of people still live in comparatively rural settings'. The urban-centric focus of social work in some nation states can be traced back to settlement patterns in countries like Australia and Canada with population density concentrated in urban areas.

In countries like Britain, the rise of city slums and poor health emerging from the growth of industrialised cities also focused social attention on the urban poor.

Our second contention is that, given that the profession of social work has a limited presence in rural areas in Australia, Canada and the United Kingdom, knowledge production about rurality and social work is likely to receive less interest than urban practice. The formula for social service provision is often calculated on the basis of population size, hence the centralisation of services in cities. In the United Kingdom, with greater population density across space, 'the most cited reason for these inequalities are the higher costs associated with the provision of rural services' (Pugh 2003: 74). In the early 1990s, Cheers (1992) drew attention to the proportionally increased economic and health disadvantage experienced in rural Australia. Alongside increased social need there remains extensive disparities between urban and rural access to social services in Australia.

Thirdly, rural disadvantage may have remained on the margins of social work as rural places have been idyllised in the global north (Pugh 2003). The conceptualisation of 'rural community' as places based on communitarian values and practices and quiet havens can obscure disadvantage, isolation and lack of health and social services (Bryant and Pini 2011).

Fourthly, knowledge production in social work education has privileged the urban. In more recent times, some social work textbooks are providing rural-based case studies for skill building in direct practice (e.g. Morgaine and Capous-Desyllas 2015; Walsh 2013). However, the majority of teaching texts for practice and research in social work rarely differentiate between urban and rural contexts, assuming practice occurs in cities. Cheers' (1992) argument from the early 1990s remains pertinent:

> ... Australian policy formulators, service planners and practitioners are socialised, trained, and work in an urban context, and are informed by urban-based research and literature from Australia and overseas. This is no less true of the social work profession.
>
> (Cheers 1992: 13)

Finally, farmers are not a traditional clientele for social workers. There is evidence to suggest that farmers are unlikely to access social services in rural places where such services exist (Alston 2012) and contrary evidence to suggest that when farmers experience emotional and psychological distress they seek out social services (Bryant *et al*. 2006). Further, many family farmers are business owners and belong in Marxist terms to the 'petty bourgeoisie' as they are owners of land and may hire farm workers. Social workers often work with the most 'marginalised' and 'vulnerable' and this translates to the most economically marginalised or vulnerable. However, farmers are often asset-rich but income poor, and therefore stand somewhat outside traditional social work understandings of clients and vulnerability.

We contend that social work as a discipline and as a profession has a skill set that enables the bridging of macro and micro contexts to enhance knowledge but also farmer suicide prevention strategies.

Conclusion

Farmer distress and the possibility of suicide are social concerns that explicate the concept of glocality. The context and conditions of distress intertwine across global and local economies, cultures and politics and are reacted and acted upon at the scale of the body. The glocal enables analyses of multidirectional global/ local conditions and encounters. As Roudometof (2015: 11) suggests, 'it is possible to map power relations and therefore to analyse local-global relationship[s] in terms of power differentials ... [but] ... with power [emanating and residing] in all actors participating in global-local interactions'. Our analyses of farmer distress and suicide show bodily encounters with political and moral economies whereby state policies shape access to funding and the entrepreneurial rules of the game, alongside transnational corporations who, for farmers, set the conditions for contracts. In these ways, farmers live with being at risk in the political and moral economy. Their bodily encounters with the state and corporations 'reopen past encounters' (Ahmed 2000: 8) and relational threats to subjectivity. How these threats are understood, imagined and experienced also shapes local encounters within rural communities and, in particular, how community members respond to farmers judged as 'progressive' and 'successful' or as 'failures'. Bodily and affective responses to community judgements for some farmers induce feelings of shame, social exclusion and loss of self-worth.

The conditions that create the possibilities for distress and suicide simultaneously provide the context and conditions for farmer activism. In South Australia, where the study was conducted, we have seen farmers attend government consultation forums to discuss drought policies. Famers have driven trucks and tractors to meetings and parked these across main streets in their local town, and filled town halls to such capacity that people remain standing in aisles with working bodies spilling onto the streets. These actions are a very embodied manner of registering protest.

Farmer's bodies, especially those marked by distress, have remained outside of social work encounters and, specifically, academic social work. Social work education remains urban-centric; however, rural social issues are beginning to receive some attention in academic textbooks. As we have argued, social work has specific macro and micro skills to offer in the development of knowledge about farmer distress and suicide prevention. As farmer distress and suicide are an increasing phenomenon located across geopolitical boundaries, social work has the potential to respond to this issue at the scale of the local and global and, as always, at the scale of the body.

References

Abrahamsson, S. and Simpson, P. (2011) 'The limits of the body: Boundaries, capacities, thresholds'. *Social and Cultural Geography* 12: 331–338.

Ahmed, S. (2000) *Strange Encounters: Embodied Others in Post-Coloniality*, London and New York: Routledge.

Ahmed, S. (2004a) *The Cultural Politics of Emotion*, New York: Routledge.

Ahmed, S. (2004b) 'Collective feelings – Or the impressions left by others'. *Theory Culture and Society* 21 (2): 25–42

Alston, M. (2012) 'Rural male suicide in Australia'. *Social Science & Medicine* 74 (4): 515–522. doi:10.1016/j.socscimed.2010.04.036

Arnautovska, U., McPhedran, S., and De Leo, D. (2014) 'A regional approach to understanding farmer suicide rates in Queensland'. *Social Psychiatry and Psychiatric Epidemiology* 49 (4): 593–599. doi:10.1007/s00127-013-0777-9.

Askins, K. and Pain R. (2011) 'Contact zone: Participation, materiality, and the messiness of interaction'. *Environment and Planning D: Society and Space* 29: 803–821.

Behere, P. B. and Bhise, M. C. (2009) 'Farmers' suicide: Across culture'. *Indian Journal of Psychiatry* 51 (4): 242–243.

Brandth, B. and Haugen, M. (2005) 'The gendered embodiment of agricultural work: Nature, machinery and patriarchy'. In *Gendered Bodies and Work*, edited by D. Morgan, B. Brandth and E. Kvande. Aldershot: Ashgate.

Bossard, C., Santin, G., and Guseva Canu, I. (2013) 'Surveillance of mortality by suicide among farmers: First results'. France: Institut de veille sanitaire.

Bryant, L. (1999) 'The detraditionalization of occupational identities in farming in South Australia'. *Sociologia Ruralis* 39 (2): 236–261.

Bryant, L. and Garnham, B. (2013) 'Beyond discourses of drought: The micro-politics of the wine industry and the mental health of farmers'. *Journal of Rural Studies* 32: 1–9.

Bryant, L. and Garnham, B. (2014) 'Economies, ethics and emotions: Farmer distress within the moral economy of agribusiness'. *Journal of Rural Studies* 34: 304–312.

Bryant, L. and Garnham, B. (2015) 'The fallen hero: Masculinity, shame and farmer suicide in Australia'. *Gender, Place & Culture* 22 (1): 67–82. doi:10.1080/0966369X.2013.855628.

Bryant, L. and George, J. (2016) *Water and Rural Communities: Local Politics, Meaning and Place*, London: Routledge.

Bryant, L, Hoon, E. and Silvestri, G. (2006) *Socio-Economic Impacts of Drought*, Adelaide: University of South Australia.

Bryant, L. and Pini, B. (2009) 'Gender, class and rurality: Australian case studies'. *Journal of Rural Studies* 25 (1): 48–56.

Bryant, L. and Pini, B. (2011) *Gender and Rurality*, New York: Routledge.

Butler, J. (1997) *The Psychic Life of Power: Theories in Subjection*, Stanford: Stanford University Press.

Cheers, B. (1992) 'Rural social work and social welfare in the Australian context'. *Australian Social Work* 45 (2): 10–21.

Coldwell, I. (2009) 'New farming masculinities "More than just shit-kickers", we're "switched on" farmers wanting to "balance lifestyle, sustainability and coin"', *Journal of Sociology* 43 (1): 87–103.

Faria, N. M. X., Fassa, A. G., and Meucci, R. D. (2014) 'Association between pesticide exposure and suicide rates in Brazil'. *NeuroToxicology* 45: 355–362. doi:http://dx.doi.org/10.1016/j.neuro.2014.05.003

Feldman, S. (2010) 'Shame and honour: The violence of gendered norms under conditions of global crisis'. *Women's Studies International Forum* 33 (4): 305–315. doi:http://dx.doi.org/10.1016/j.wsif.2010.02.004.

Fraser, C. E., Smith, K. B., Judd, F., Humphreys, J. S., Fragar, L. J., and Henderson, A. (2005) 'Farming and mental health problems and mental illness'. *Int J Soc Psychiatr* 51 (4): 340–349.

Fraser, I. (2005) 'Microeconometric analysis of wine grape supply contracts in Australia'. *The Australian Journal of Agricultural and Resource Economics* 49: 23–46.

Freire, C. and Koifman, S. (2013) 'Pesticides, depression and suicide: A systematic review of the epidemiological evidence'. *International Journal of Hygiene and Environmental Health* 216 (4): 445–460. doi:http://dx.doi.org/10.1016/j.ijheh.2012.12.003.

Garnham, B. and Bryant, L. (2014) 'Problematising the suicides of older male farmers: Subjective, social and cultural considerations'. *Sociologia Ruralis* 54 (2): 227–240.

Gibson, C. (2010) 'Geographies of tourism: (Un)ethical encounters'. *Progress in Human Geography* 34 (4): 521–527.

Guiney, R. (2012) 'Farming Suicides During The Victorian Drought: 2001-2007'. *Australian Journal of Rural Health* 20 (1): 11–15.

Handley, T. E., Inder, K. J., Kelly, B. J., Attia, J. R., and Kay-Lambkin, F. J. (2011) 'Urban-rural influences on suicidality: Gaps in the existing literature and recommendations for future research'. *Australian Journal of Rural Health* 19 (6): 279–283. doi:10.1111/j.1440-1584.2011.01235.x.

Hirsch, J. K. (2006) 'A review of the literature on rural suicide: Risk and protective factors, incidence, and prevention'. *Crisis: The Journal of Crisis Intervention and Suicide Prevention* 27 (4): 189–199. doi:10.1027/0227-5910.27.4.189.

Hogan, A., Scarr, E., Lockie, S., Chant, B., and Alston, S. (2012) 'Ruptured identity of male farmers: Subjective crisis and the risk of suicide'. *Journal of Rural Social Sciences* 27 (3): 118–140.

Hounsome, B., Edwards, R., Hounsome, N., and Edwards-Jones, G. (2012) 'Psychological morbidity of farmers and non-farming population: Results from a UK survey'. *Community Mental Health Journal* 48 (4): 503–510. doi:10.1007/s10597-011-9415-8.

Judd, F., Cooper, A., Fraser, C., and Davis, J. (2006a) 'Rural suicide – People or place effects?' *Australian and New Zealand Journal of Psychiatry* 40 (3): 208–216. doi:10.1080/j.1440-1614.2006.01776.x.

Judd, F., Jackson, H., Fraser, C., Murray, G., Robins, G., and Komiti, A. (2006b) 'Understanding suicide in Australian farmers'. *Social Psychiatry & Psychiatric Epidemiology* 41 (1): 1–10. doi:10.1007/s00127-005-0007-1.

Kapusta, N. D., Zorman, A., Etzersdorfer, E., Ponocny-Seliger, E., Jandl-Jager, E., and Sonneck, G. (2008) 'Rural-urban differences in Austrian suicides'. *Social Psychiatry & Psychiatric Epidemiology* 43 (4): 311–318. doi:10.1007/s00127-008-0317-1.

Kaushal, A. (2015) 'Confronting farmer suicides in India'. *Alternatives: Global, Local, Political* 40 (1): 46–62. doi:10.1177/0304375415581258.

Lefebvre, H. (1991) *The Production of Space*, Oxford: Blackwell Publishing.

Liepins, R. (2000) 'Exploring rurality through "community": Discourses, practices and spaces shaping Australian and New Zealand rural "communities"'. *Journal of Rural Studies* 16 (3): 325–341. doi:http://dx.doi.org/10.1016/S0743-0167(99)00067-4.

Listerborn, C. (2013) 'Suburban women and the "glocalisation" of everyday lives: Gender and glocalities in underprivileged areas in Sweden'. *Gender, Place and Culture* 20 (3): 290–312.

Malmberg, A., Hawton, K., and Simkin, S. (1997) 'A study of suicide in farmers in England and Wales'. *Journal of Psychosomatic Research* 43 (1): 107–111. doi:http://dx.doi.org/10.1016/S0022-3999(97)00114-1.

McPhedran, S., and Leo, D. D. (2013) 'Risk factors for suicide among rural men: Are farmers more socially isolated?' *International Journal of Sociology and Social Policy* 33 (11/12): 762–772.

Merleau-Ponty, M. (1962) *Phénoménologie de la Perception*, Routledge & Kegan Paul, London.

Middleton, N., Gunnell, D., Frankel, S., Whitley, E., and Dorling, D. (2003) 'Urban-rural differences in suicide trends in young adults: England and Wales, 1981–1998'. *Social Science & Medicine* 57 (7): 1183–1194.

Miller, K., and Burns, C. (2008) 'Suicides on farms in South Australia, 1997–2001'. *Australian Journal of Rural Health* 16 (6): 327–331. doi:10.1111/j.1440-1584.2008.01011.x.

Minichiello, V. R., Aroni, T. and Hays, T. (2008) *In-Depth Interviewing*, Third Edition, Sydney: Pearson Education.

Morgaine, K. and Capous-Desyllas, M. (2015) *Anti-Oppressive Social Work Practice: Putting Theory into Action*, Thousand Oaks, CA: Sage.

Münster, D. (2015) 'Farmers' suicides as public death: Politics, agency and statistics in a suicide-prone district (South India)'. *Modern Asian Studies* 49 (5): 1580–1605. doi:10.1017/S0026749X14000225.

Nielson, E. H. and Simonsen, K. (2003) 'Scaling from "below": Practices, strategies and urban spaces'. *European Planning Studies* 11 (8): 911–927.

Nipe, A., York, A., Hogan, D., Faull, J., and Baki, Y. (2010) *The South Australian Wine Cluster: Microeconomics of Competitiveness*, Cambridge: Harvard University.

Nishimura, M., Terao, T., Soeda, S., Nakamura, J., Iwata, N., and Sakamoto, K. (2004) 'Suicide and occupation: Further supportive evidence for their relevance'. *Progress in Neuro-Psychopharmacology and Biological Psychiatry* 28 (1): 83–87. doi:http://dx.doi.org/10.1016/j.pnpbp.2003.09.023.

Pain, R. (2009) 'Globalized fear? Towards an emotional geopolitics'. *Progress in Human Geography* 33 (4): 1–21.

Page, A. and Fragar, L. (2002) 'Suicide in Australian farming, 1988–1997'. *Australian and New Zealand Journal of Psychiatry* 36 (1): 81–85. doi:10.1046/j.1440-1614.2002.00975.x.

Price, L. and Evans, N. (2009) 'From stress to distress: Conceptualizing the British patriarchal family way of life'. *Journal of Rural Studies* 25 (1): 1–11.

Pritchard, B., Burch, D., and Lawrence, G. (2007) 'Neither "family" nor "corporate" farming: Australian tomato growers as farm family entrepreneurs'. *Journal of Rural Studies* 23: 75–87.

Probyn, E. (2004) 'Shame in the habitus 1'. *Sociological Review* 52 (S2): 224–248.

Probyn, E. (2005) *Blush Faces of Shame*, Minneapolis: University of Minnesota Press.

Pugh, R. (2003) 'Considering the countryside: Is there a case for rural social work?' *British Journal of Social Work* 33: 67–85.

Ramirez-Ferrero, E. (2005) *Troubled Fields: Men, Emotions and the Crisis in American Farming*, New York: Columbia University Press.

Riverland Industry Wine Development Council. (2009) *Submission to the October Tax Summit in Reference to Social and Environmental Taxes*, Unpublished report.

Roudometof, V. (2015) 'Theorizing glocalization: Three interpretations'. *European Journal of Social Theory*, 1–15. doi: 10.11771368431015605443.

Sankaranarayanan, A., Carter, G., and Lewin, T. (2010) 'Rural-urban differences in suicide rates for current patients of a public mental health service in Australia'. *Suicide & Life-Threatening Behavior* 40 (4): 376–382. doi:10.1521/suli.2010.40.4.376.

Sayer, A. (2000) 'Moral economy and political economy'. *Studies in Political Economy* 61: 79–103.

Sayer, A. (2001) 'For a critical cultural political economy'. *Antipode* 33 (4): 687–708. doi:10.1111/1467-8330.00206.

Sayer, A. (2005) 'Class, moral worth and recognition'. *Sociology* 39 (5): 947–963.

Sayer, A. (2007) 'Moral economy as critique'. *New Political Economy* 12 (2): 261–270. doi:10.1080/13563460701303008.

Sayer, A. (2011) *Why Things Matter to People: Social Science, Values and Ethical Life*, Cambridge: Cambridge University Press.

SBS Two (2014) *Farmer Suicide in Queensland*. 10th November, 2014. Available from: http://www.sbs.com.au/news/thefeed/story/farmer-suicide-queensland [Accessed 11th May, 2016].

Schostak J. F. (2002) *Understanding, Designing and Conducting Qualitative Research in Education*, Philadelphia: Open University Press.

Simonsen, K. (2007) 'Practice, spatiality and embodied emotions: An outline of a geography of practice'. *Human Affairs* 17: 168–181.

Singh, G. K. and Siahpush, M. (2002) 'The increasing rural-urban gradients in U.S. suicide mortality, 1970–1997'. *American Journal of Public Health* 92 (7): 1161–1167.

Staples, J. and Widger, T. (2012) 'Situating suicide as an anthropological problem: Ethnographic approaches to understanding self-harm and self-induced death'. *Culture, Medicine and Psychiatry* 36 (2): 183–203.

Stark, C., Gibbs, D., Hopkins, P., Belbin, A., Hay, A., and Selvaraj, S. (2006) 'Suicide in farmers in Scotland'. *Rural and Remote Health* 6 (1): 509.

Sturgeon, R., and Morrissette, P. J. (2010) 'A qualitative analysis of suicide ideation among Manitoban farmers'. *Canadian Journal of Counselling and Psychotherapy* 44 (2): 191–207.

Tiesman, H. M., Konda, S., Hartley, D., Menéndez, C. C., Ridenour, M., and Hendricks, S. (2015) 'Suicide in U.S. workplaces, 2003–2010: A comparison with non-workplace suicides'. *American Journal of Preventive Medicine* 48 (6): 674–682.

Walsh, J. (2013) *Theories for Direct Social Work Practice*, Stamford: Cengage Learning.

Wilson, H. F. (2016) 'On geography and encounter: Bodies, borders, and difference'. *Progress in Human Geography*: 1–21. doi:10.1177/039132516645958.

3 Gendered Globalization and Violence

Jeff Hearn, Kopano Ratele and Tamara Shefer

Introduction

Globalization has become an extremely well-used, perhaps over-used, concept in recent years, as a gloss on what is happening in the world. It is also frequently employed within a normative framing, either positively as a key to liberation, whether through political struggle or capitalist expansionism, or negatively as the source of current evils, as with some factions in anti-globalization movements. There is a wide range of influences that bear on these transnationalizing developments that have to be borne in mind in global/local social work. They include postcolonialism, neoliberalism, social movements, the spread of information and communication technologies (ICTs) and other technologies, the transformation of knowledge construction (albeit dominated by the global North), and the growing impact of transnational processes beyond, between and within nations (Hearn et al. 2013). Taking a broad, global view does, however, bring some risks. In short, such a translocal, transnational perspective cannot mean a perspective-less "god's eye" view.

In this chapter, we examine some of these key processes of gendered globalization, with special reference to the urgent problem of men's violence and violent masculinities and its significance for global and transnational social work. It arises from a medley of extensive empirical, political, and theoretical comparative, transnational, and collaborative work, especially in and between Africa and Europe. It also reflects the growing interest in macro-studies on gender equality and relations to violence, as well as the overlaps between the global and local, with numerous crossovers between research, policy development, and activism.

Meanings of Globalization

Although one of "the most important phenomena of our times" (Ritzer 2007, p. 1), globalization is highly debated, is polarizing, and means many different things. A concise definition is that provided by the Australian sociologist Malcolm Waters (1995), who defines globalization as a "social process in which the constraints of *geography* on social and cultural arrangements recede and in which people become increasingly *aware* that they are receding" (p. 3) (our emphases).

Bryan Turner (2007, p. 675) maintains that "'globalization' refers ... to the process by which the world becomes a single place, and hence the volume and depth of social interconnectedness are greatly increased."

In contrast to this emphasis on place, social processes, and consciousness, many commentators prioritize the development of transnational economic units. Waters himself notes that globalization also affects the movements of people, goods, services, and information, through material, political, and symbolic exchanges. However, importantly, in each case there are contradictions with tendencies toward both the local and non-local, national and transnational, and territorialized and non-territorialized social processes and entities. Indeed, the huge literature on globalization has failed to produce a consensus on what it is, and frequently involves contradictory accounts. For example:

> Roland Robertson (1995) asserted greater material interdependence and unity, but not greater integration, of the world; greater world consciousness; (while it is a single system) the promotion or 'invention' of difference and variety in globalization; and indeed 'clashes, conflicts, tensions and so on constitute a pivotal feature of globalization' (Robertson and Khondker, 1998: 29). Antony Giddens (1990) highlighted the nation-state, modernity (capitalism, surveillance, military order, industrialism), time-space distanciation[1] and reflexivity. Scott Lash and John Urry (1994) emphasized transcendence of the nation-state, and the increasing importance of signs, symbols, and transnational cultures. With anti-globalization, alternative economics and returns to the local have grown.
>
> (Hearn 2015a, pp. 63–64)

What is noticeable in what might be called this critical mainstream is the lack of attention to gender relations. The fact is that most, especially mainstream, texts on globalization fail to discuss gender relations or do so in a cursory way. Gendering globalization problematizes some of the more ambitious claims of globalization theses and adds greater gendered complexity to debates on global convergence or divergence in social work and beyond.

Gendering Globalization

So, how is globalization now gendered? Joan Acker (2004) summarizes the key processes as "gender as embedded in globalizing capitalism," "gendered construction of a division between capitalist production and human reproduction," "masculinities in globalizing capital," "gender as a resource for globalizing capital," and "the gendered effects of globalization." Even though the main focus in the chapter is on the gendering of globalization, it is also critical to note the globalization of gender conceptualizations and social relations. Characterized by both progressive and deleterious consequences, globalization condenses time-space for the exportation of understandings of gender and gender relations (usually, though not always) from the global North to the global South. Research indicates that intensified international trade liberalization may benefit women, but globalization can produce other disempowering gender understandings and effects as well as reinscribing other kinds of inequalities between and within countries (Black & Brainerd 2004; Kabeer & Mahmud 2004; Safa 2002).

Globalization is not new and indeed has long been incredibly gendered in its forms, demographics, and effects, whether it is the pioneering men and masculinities of imperialism, colonial settlement by families and communities, or gendered structurings of contemporary migrations – some mainly women, some mainly men, some gender-mixed. Globalizations make possible changing possibilities for gendered actors, individually and collectively. This may both facilitate and restrict certain gendered powers, for example, in the extension of some men's transnational intersectional power through ICTs, the loss of expected security and privilege for other men in moves to transnational decision-making and relocations, and further various forms of recouping of destabilized power. Important research areas across and beyond nation-states include feminist and gendered work on development, economics, international relations (IR), war and militarism, and the flexibilization of gendered labor. Yet, many of those that do attend to gender still translate gender as meaning women, with little if any explicit and developed analysis of men and global gender relations. Interestingly, gendered work on globalization, along with non-gendered notions of globalization, are criticized for freighting a globalizing coloniality of knowledge and power, seen to be constitutive of globalized modernity (Escobar 2004; Lugones 2007).

In some cases, critical gendered analyses of men and masculinities in globalization, sometimes informed by a world-centered perspective, have been developed (Connell 2014). Such analyses of men and masculinities within globalization processes and the "big picture" (Connell 1993) have opened up a whole range of possibilities for exploration and contestation, including conceptualizations of "global business masculinity" (Connell 1998) and "men of the world" (Hearn 1996, 2015a). Indeed, in recent years, there has been a surge of research studies, books, and other contributions with an explicitly gendered focus on men that looks beyond national borders in regional, international, global, or postcolonial terms or contexts. Many of these derive from the global South (for example, Cornwall & Lindisfarne 1994; Ouzgane & Coleman 1998; Jones 2006; Donaldson et al. 2009; Ruspini et al. 2011; Hearn et al. 2013; van der Gaag 2014).

On the other hand, there are some difficulties with the concept of globalization as few things are truly global; an alternative is to speak instead of transnationalization(s).[2] Transnational processes of change involve flows of people, money, or information across borders and the crossing and spanning of borders by social networks, organizations, and institutions. Multi-strandedness operates in economic, political, cultural, symbolic. and emotional realms. Transnationalism and transnationalizations emphasize multiple, often hybrid processes and institutions across geographical, cultural, and political borders. Such transnational moves have opened alternative, complex references and relations to nation-states and movements and formation of transnational social and cultural spaces.

These can be seen as arenas of transnational patriarchies, or transpatriarchies for short. Key contemporary arenas of global and transnational gender relations are

- transnational business corporations and governmental organizations, with the dominance of men at top levels along with their gender-segregated workforces;
- global finance, with their masculinization of capital market trading;
- militarism and the arms trade;
- international sports industries and their gender segregation;
- consumption and consumerism;
- transnational work-family/household/life relations;
- bio-, medical, and reproductive movements, for example, cosmetic surgery, surrogacy;
- migrations, refugees, flows, movements, care chains, circuits;
- ICTs, virtualization, information flows, image transfer and circulation;
- the sex trade, and sexualization in global mass media;
- cultural, political, religious, aesthetic social movements;
- transportation, water, environment, energy, climate;
- knowledge production, theory, and theorizing.

(Hearn 2015a, pp. 20–21)

All of these arenas bear on the question of violences and indeed anti-violence, if only indirectly. This means addressing the diverse locations and intersectional gendering of men, as the major doers of violence, as well as men being disproportionately represented as victims of homicidal violence. It also means addressing the question of epistemology and ontology: the nature and status of the concepts of globalization and gender. While research, policy, and activist work on gendered globalization and violence has ranged widely in relation to many sociopolitical arenas, here we focus on three transnational examples, all framed in relation to violence and violation and all of direct relevance to social work: global, international, and transnational violences; interpersonal violence in intimacy; and engaging men and boys in global and local antiviolence initiatives through broadly progressive (loosely "profeminist") activism.

Global, International, and Transnational Violences

There is a very wide range of violences that can be understood as global, international, or transnational in character, and as occurring across time and space. They have a very long history, as with the violences of genocide, colonialism, and imperialism. What might be called global violences include most obviously the ecological violences of environmental degradation that affect people, other species, and the planet. These violences care not for national boundaries and also tend to most affect those who are already the most deprived. As the IPCC (Inter-Governmental Panel on Climate Change, Chapter 19) wrote in an early report:

> ... poor people in wealthy countries may be more vulnerable to health impacts than those with average incomes in the same countries. ... The ability to adapt to and cope with climate change impacts is a function of wealth, technology, information, skills, infrastructure, institutions, equity, empowerment, and ability to spread risk. The poorest segments of societies are most vulnerable to climate change. Poverty determines vulnerability via several mechanisms, principally in access to resources to allow coping with extreme weather events and through marginalization from decision-making and social security ... . Vulnerability is likely to be differentiated by gender – for example, through the "feminization of poverty" brought about by differential gender roles in natural resource management ... . If climate change increases water scarcity, women are likely to bear the labor and nutritional impacts.
>
> (IPCC 2001)

Ecological violences intersect with, are paralleled by, and to a large extent are caused by the expansionism and polarizations of global capitalism and finance, patterns of consumption and waste, whether capitalist or not, and the structural economic and social inequalities, poverty, and dispossession that accompany these ways of organizing societies. These are, in short, structural violences on a wide, international scale. Societal trends toward greater inequality are increasing in many parts of the world. Moreover, the extent of the concentration of power and resources is staggering:

> Almost half of world's wealth is now owned by just 1% of population. The wealth of the one percent richest people in the world amounts to $110 trillion. That's 65 times the total wealth of the bottom half of the world's population. The bottom half of the world's population owns the same as the richest 85 people in the world.
>
> (Fuentes-Nieva & Galasso 2014, pp. 2–3)

According to Oxfam (2016), the situation is increasingly bleak as in 2015, 62 individuals had the same wealth as more than 3.6 billion people. However, these tendencies are not automatic or determined. Indeed there have, for example, been significant moves toward reductions in inequalities in Latin America in particular in recent years (Cornia 2012). Economic and social inequalities are both contexts of violence and qualified probabilistic determinants of violence. These international connections of inequality and violence can be examined at both societal and individual levels. There is now a well-established stream of research on the relations between societal inequality and the enactment of violence.

Both Sylvia Walby (2009) and Øystein Gullvåg Holter (2014) have recently examined the macro-relations between socioeconomic inequalities and violence. Holter has analyzed aggregate macro-level data at the national European or US state level, noting how in some respects greater societal gender equality, or less gender inequality, may be accompanied by less interpersonal violence, including violence against men. Walby has also developed an analysis relating inequalities to societal levels of violence, including militarism and the construction of state institutions, especially prisons, in a spiraling response to increased interpersonal violence and prosecuted crime. Framed thus, violence seen on an international scale is embedded in diverse economic, political, and social relations rather than being reducible to specific and immediate interpersonal, "domestic" and intimate partner violences.

A different kind of approach has been developed by the IMAGES (International Men and Gender Equality) survey on the preconditions of men's violence. Ruth Levtov and colleagues (2014) have based their investigations on individual-level data from eight low- and middle-income countries, aggregated by country and then compared across the countries. At an aggregate level, men's more gender-equal attitudes tend to be predictable from such factors as men's own educational attainment, the mother's education, men's reports of the father's domestic participation, family background of the mother alone or joint decision parents, and not witnessing violence against the mother. Men's self-reported attitudes are, in turn, predictors of men's gender-equal practices and less interpersonal violence.

Such conditions of equality and inequality present such a taken-for-granted backcloth to social work in different parts of the world that they may seem hardly worth mentioning. Societal contexts of inequality speak to all manner of global, transnational, ethnicized, and racialized hierarchies and differential statuses and valuations of marked regions, nations, groups of people, and individuals, live, violated injured, threatened, or dead. Indeed, violence is a form of inequality in itself.

Patterns of intergovernmental and para-state IR represent a further major way of broadening understandings of the relations of gendered globalization and violence. IR operates on a global and transnational scale and involves both extensions of and resistances to (post)imperialisms and (post)colonialisms, themselves enacted and structured through religion, education, media, governance, and ideology. These may be enacted through (post)imperial and (post)colonial "commonsense" and colonizations of the mind, sometimes with benevolent intent, at other times certainly not, and on different occasions conspiratorially. The contemporary period has seen major shifts in IR, for example in the Middle East, in East–West relations, and in the rise of BRICS nations (Brazil, Russia, India, China, South Africa), along with associated shifts in actual and potential violences and violations.

These matters become more clearly concretized when we turn to militarism, as one of the clearest arenas of transnational violence and violation. The size, power, scale, and impacts of the military worldwide are beyond belief. Estimates of deaths in the twentieth century *caused by humans* (mainly by men) range between about 188 million and over 262 million (circa 5 percent of total deaths). The world total for military spending was estimated as $1,738 billion in 2011, about 2.5 percent of global gross domestic product or $249 for each person (SIPRI 2012). In 2008, Stiglitz and Bilmes estimated the costs of the Iraq and Afghanistan wars at over $3 trillion. Estimates of the depleted uranium used in US bombing during the Iraq War stand as equivalent to about 28,000 Hiroshimas. Through globalization and technological innovation, militarism is being extended into new areas, oceans, the Arctic regions, and inner space.

While IR focuses on intergovernmental relations, including militarism, it is also vital to attend to the intersections of capital and government. A recent example is the massive subsidies of private corporations by the United States and other states in Iraq and elsewhere in supporting the military and the arms trade generally. There is extensive evidence of huge waste and overpayment to companies such as Halliburton, KBR, and Parsons and Bectel, and payments by the US government that were simply lost, stolen, or "unaccounted for" during the Iraqi War – according to some estimates as at least $23 billion. The use of "cost +" (CPA, all costs plus a percentage) in contract accounting partly explains the massive overspends (Boorstin & Nolan 2004; Bowen 2009).

IR, militarism, and such state-business relations provide the grounds of and for military violence that leads to the terrible violations and other effects of war. Both military veterans and civilian victims of war suffer physical and psychological damage, including trauma, violence, and sexual violence. Younger military recruits are at especially higher risk of alcohol problems, depression, and suicide (Forces Watch 2013). The casualties and victims of war may or may not be responded to by social work and related welfare and aid agencies. These are basic issues in considering the place of global and transnational social work, both in current, former, and potential war zones and neighboring regions, including with displaced persons, forced migration, ethnic cleansings, and refugees more generally, but also more generally in terms of the impact of militarism on what may appear "at home" as peaceful societies. Bringing together an analysis of different violences, such as military violence, rape, and violence against women in intimacy, is a major challenge for social work.

Finally, in this section, we highlight the transnational violences that can occur through the use of ICTs. These are being increasingly recognized, as in online harassments, threats, stalking, and indeed the more general sexism, racism, and homophobia that characterize many virtual environments. It is important to consider that we happen to have been living through a huge expansion of the sex trade. For example, the annual number of hardcore porn videos rentals in the United States rose from 79 million to 759 million between 1985 and 2001 (Hughes 2002). More recently, the 2014 EU Fundamental Rights Agency (FRA) found that 11 percent of women surveyed had experienced inappropriate advances on social websites or had been subjected to sexually explicit emails or texts/SMS, and 20 percent of women aged between 18 and 29 years had been victims of cyberharassment.

Violence Against Women in Intimacy

A global lens on violence against women that is located within a feminist critique of patriarchy interwoven with global forms of inequality, including contexts of postcoloniality and global capitalism steeped in neoliberal and consumerist imperatives, has been important for global and local struggles for gender justice. However, such a lens has not come without its disadvantages and challenges. In this section, we attempt to delineate some important contributions that transnational research and collaboration have played in understanding gender-based violences across the globe, but focus primarily on unpacking the "dangers" and "problems" that have come with these initiatives. While the imperatives of the largely global northern and western focus on the global South have mostly been steeped in well-meaning efforts, we argue that these unintentionally may reproduce some of the very discourses they seek to challenge and speak to the imperative of cautious, reflexive scholarship and programmatic work. Such arguments may resonate in both national (within countries on the basis of existing social divides and inequalities) and transnational contexts (across the globe on the basis of global divides and inequalities that relate to histories of colonization and their continuities in contemporary global politics). Such reflections are arguably especially important for a discipline like social work with both scholarly and pragmatic community-oriented goals.

In reflecting on the benefits of global collaborative efforts around sexual violence, obvious areas include international policy developments such as the United Nations (UN) agencies' work on developing policies, legal frameworks, and guidelines that become the international norm. Policy and international legal frameworks such as the Convention on the Elimination of all Forms of Discrimination Against women (CEDAW), adopted in 1979, have clearly been of some benefit in pressurizing different nation-states to conform to certain minimum standards and take seriously human rights abuses against women and children. Yet, such international frameworks are clearly limited, as Etienne (1995), representing one of the many critiques of such international interventions, elaborates:

> The Convention on the Elimination of all Forms of Discrimination Against Women, the United Nations' most comprehensive attempt to address gender bias, offers little more than a declaration of policy to advance the goals of greater equality and respect for women.
>
> (Etienne 1995, p. 170)

Within the research framework, increasing imperatives of "internationalization," arguably interwoven into increased consumerist and neoliberal pressures for global higher education and research agencies, have allowed for a proliferation of collaborations across continents and countries to become normative in contemporary research practices. Thus, within larger practices of international collaboration located in current global capitalist engagements, there have been increasing funds made available for researchers to collaborate across national boundaries on research projects. A small body of scholars has begun reflecting on such collaborations, their advantages, and their benefits (see, for example, Airhihenbuwa et al. 2011; Hearn 2014, 2015a, 2015b; Reddy et al. 2014; Shefer et al. 2015), but this remains a relatively marginal area where arguably far more work is required. Such resources have clear benefits for knowledge production through providing comparative data on gender-based violence across different contexts as well as, and possibly more importantly, facilitating a more complex understanding of male violence against women through a reading of a particular context through the lens of diverse contexts. The appreciation of intersectionality in the dynamics of violence is made more possible through the engagement with multiple contexts. As Shefer et al. (2015) report in their reflection on a recent transnational collaboration that brought together scholars in two different national contexts to reflect on young people's engagement in social justice goals:

> A key gain ... relates to the development of their [participants] own scholarship through deepened critical reflection. Respondents shared how the project has allowed for a *different vantage point* for reflecting on one's own research, in particular through seeing how those located outside of one's national context respond to our research, which allows for a clarification of one's own project in one's own context.
>
> (Shefer et al. 2015, p. 168)

However, the availability of funds for such transnational collaboration may also have reflected and served to rationalize and reproduce certain global power relations located within postcolonial frameworks of continued privilege of certain nations and subordination and the marginality of others. A kind of "academic tourism" is made possible, which is exploited in some cases, allowing for the global South to be the research laboratory for the North. Further, since material resources are still primarily located in the North (even when South–South collaborations are possible, they are usually with a Northern funder), patronizing and unequal relations may be endemic to these projects (for example, Ratele 2015; Shefer et al. 2015).

Some of the disadvantages of the scrutiny of the global South as well as the peripheries of highly industrialized Western European countries (for example, Eastern European countries), in global efforts related to sexual violence, are evident in the effects of scholarship that interrogates southern sexual and gender-based violence. Researchers in the global South have, for example, increasingly questioned the way in which African masculinities have been problematized both in global and national contexts (Ratele et al. 2011; Ratele 2014, 2015). The negative construction of men, boys, and masculinity, particularly migrant, black, and poor young men as the 'problem' and 'dangerous' in both scholarly and public responses to violence and other social issues, has been pointed out by a number of gender scholars (for example, Bhana & Pattman 2009; Pattman 2007; Ratele 2014; Shefer et al. 2010). Arguably reflecting an "outsourcing of patriarchy" (Grewal 2013), the emphasis on researching poor, migrant, and black communities within and across national boundaries may serve to fuel an othering of some sexualities. A similar effect has also been foregrounded by critiques of global discourses on HIV/AIDS (for example, Patton 1997; Jungar & Oinas 2004) and global practices of "racist sexualization" (for example, Lewis 2011; Ratele & Shefer 2013).

Perhaps a good example of such outsourcing is the proliferation of transactional sex in South African contexts, which has also focused almost exclusively on poor, black communities. Studies of globalized contexts of the materiality of intimacy and sex are of course very helpful since the transnational economies of care and selling of sex are key terrains that particularly speak to globalized gender inequalities (see, for example, Ehrenreich & Hochschild 2002). However, as critical scholars in the South have argued, the focus on transactional sex as facilitating unsafe and violent sexual practices in African contexts may bolster a northern "othering" and racist discourse on African sexualities (see, for example, Brouard & Crewe 2013; Shefer & Strebel 2013). Similarly, the global focus on women as victims of sexual violence has tended to hinge on and reinforce the stereotypic image of poor, subaltern women, which has arguably resulted in a stereotypic construction of poor, non-western women in a victim identity (for example, Shefer 2016). Yet, the attempt to reinstate such women as "agents" is equally problematic, serving to legitimize the huge inequalities that may shape their lives. Postcolonial feminist researchers Katarina Jungar and Elina Oinas (2004, 2010, 2011), for example, have consistently "troubled" dominant readings of HIV, sexuality, and gender, particularly those transferred from global Northern to global Southern contexts. They suggest that those in the privileged position of researchers who attempt to subvert the admittedly damaging picture of Southern women as passive, submissive victims, by an idealistic notion of powerful women, may then be denying the multiple inequalities and violences that constrain women's lives.

Thus, in our attempts to address gender inequality and the normative gender practices that shape inequitable sexual and other forms of male violence against women, our research may have functioned to reproduce the very discourses that underpin and rationalize such inequalities (see, for example, Shefer 2016, reflecting on heterosexualities research). In that way, rather than achieve more freedom, agency, and well-being for girls and women or challenge hegemonic masculinities, dominant notions of feminine vulnerability and passivity together with male dominance and inevitable violence may be reinstated. This further may legitimize a continued controlling and oppressive response to women and girls and female sexuality and desire and a demonization of boys and men, particularly specific groups of boys and men in global and local contexts. An overlapping concern is the way in which South African and other global South-based research on such violence may have served to reproduce an "othering" gaze on Southern sexualities, which in South Africa and in global contexts may serve to bolster racist representations of black and other non-western men.

Engaging Men and Boys in Global and Local Anti-Violence Initiatives

There are different histories, points of entry, approaches, and initiatives concerning men's involvement in anti-violence efforts. What distinguishes the projects and programs noted here is the connection they make between violence, on the one hand, and gender equality, on the other. Hence, much of this work tends to focus on sexual violence and gender-based violence against women and girls, in contradistinction to men's violence against other men and boys. War and legitimate and extrajudicial violence by states against their citizens and structural forms of violence are often occluded in these initiatives.

Some countries have a longer history of men's gender-critical anti-violence work while work in other countries has become visible only in the last two decades or so, possibly due to the apparent increased attention by multilateral organizations and big funding agencies on sexual and gendered violence against women. Some of the efforts have been transnational in character, but much of them remain highly localized and oriented toward in-country problems.

There is currently a growing number of such initiatives. However, many are locally focused and their work is not necessarily intended for wider dissemination or publication; as such, the initiatives referred to here are far from exhaustive or representative. On a global level, multilateral organizations like the World Health Organization (WHO) have taken on a growing interest in working with and on men and boys against violence. Among other things, the work of the WHO has been to call for policy approaches to build men's support for gender equality and promote health in women and men. The WHO has also supported work to assess the effectiveness of programs around the world aimed at engaging men and boys in achieving gender equality in health, among which are programs working on or with men to challenge sexual and gender-based violence (WHO 2007, 2010).

Another multilateral organization that has shown interest in engaging and supporting gendered work with men and boys against violence is UN Women.[3] While there have been criticisms on the initiative, the HeforShe campaign has garnered global support. Launched on 20 September 2014, HeForShe is meant to be a global movement focused on activating men and boys toward supporting gender equality. The initiative aims to accelerate the effectiveness of UN Women's strategic goals that include eliminating gender-based violence. HeForShe provides a platform through which, first and foremost, men and boys can prevent violence by observing and evolving their own attitudes, values, and behaviors toward women and girls, ensuring that they do not personally engage in discrimination or violence. In cases where violence has already been perpetrated, men can, through HeForShe, seek support to change their behaviors, breaking the cycle of violence.

The Swedish International Development Cooperation Agency (SIDA) has been active in funding and supporting global work related to engaging men and boys around gender equality and against sexual and gender-based violence. The agency's work around gender equality "is guided by Sweden's international policy for gender equality" (SIDA 2013), highlighting the global export of national conceptualizations of gender relations. Some of the work of the MenEngage Alliance (see below) has benefited from SIDA funding. The agency's focus and support for interventional work with men and boys, which began in the 1990s, has increased (SIDA 2014). However, while this global North-led work is readily viewed as important by some feminist and gender-critical social workers and others, both in the global North and South, the need for critical reflexivity about transnational and global North–South knowledge/economic power relations is a constant. Other key actors are Promundo, a Brazilian-originated non-governmental organization (NGO), now based also in the United States and working transnationally to engage men and boys in efforts toward gender equality and against sexual and gender-based violence[4]; and the South African-born NGO Sonke Gender Justice that works with men and boys across countries.[5] The White Ribbon Campaign,[6] Men's Action to Stop Violence Against Women,[7] and MenEngage[8] are relatively loose networks that have the elimination of sexual and gender-based violence as one of their goals. The White Ribbon Campaign was established in Canada with the aim of activating men and boys to work toward ending violence against women and girls. It originated in Canada in 1991 in response to what is known as the Montréal Massacre, in which fourteen women were killed. The campaign uses the symbol of a white ribbon to signal "a man's pledge to never commit, condone, or remain silent about violence against women".[9] Men's Action to Stop Violence Against Women is an alliance that could be mentioned – an Indian alliance of men and organizations founded in 2001. It uses cultural and advocacy campaigns to raise awareness and toward institutional changes in gender relations, focusing on working with men to react to and help reduce incidents of violence against women.

With a global secretariat in the United States, MenEngage is a global alliance of organizations and networks in several countries and across several world regions. MenEngage organized its first global symposium on engaging men and boys, which took place in Rio de Janeiro in March 2009, and its second in New Delhi in November 2014. Ending violence against women and girls is one of several topical areas in which members of the alliance work with or on men and boys. More broadly, MenEngage aims

> to provide a collective voice on the need to engage men and boys in gender equality, to build and improve the field of practice around engaging men in achieving gender justice, and advocating before policymakers at the local, national, regional and international levels.[10]

A criticism of many of these initiatives and networks is that they focus on one type of violence. Although men's violence against women and girls is a very serious issue spread across the globe, neglecting other forms of violence, as well as how sexual and gender-based violence intersects with other socioeconomic problems such as economic inequality and racism, can be regarded as problematic. There is also a need to retain some suspicions about the apparently positive support given to initiatives focused on changing men and boys by global organizations like the World Bank and UN as well as most states and global businesses. These doubts arise in light of the support that some of these organizations, states, and businesses give to military solutions to national and international problems and the ongoing wars, economic inequalities, and neoliberal capitalist exploitative practices evident in many parts of the world, and especially in poor countries.

Conclusions

In this chapter, we have addressed the challenge of analyzing, and indeed opposing, the relations of gendered globalization and violence. To do this, we have translated this challenge through a focus on three transnational examples, all framed in relation to violence and violation: global, international, and transnational violences; interpersonal violence in intimacy; and engaging men and boys in global and local anti-violence initiatives. They point to the range of connections between globalization and diverse forms of violence and highlight the benefits of thinking about globalized violence and local violence in global terms, as well as the constraints and potential pitfalls and dangers in such transnational frameworks. At the same time, we wish to add some caveats to this overview of the range of impacts of globalization and transnationalizations. First, these three examples are not discrete entities but rather overlap with each other, as in the close connections of research and activism and the interrelations of interpersonal violence and collective violence, and also of macro (global), meso (institutional and regional), and micro (local and interpersonal) realms. Second, these three are far from being the only perspectives or the only way of framing gendered globalization and violence we could have chosen. Other perspectives might include those based on international law and treaties on and against violence, such as the Istanbul Convention, the UN Rights of the Child, and UN Resolution 1325, or geographical framings or elaborations in terms of forms of violence such as sexual, physical, or structural.

Similarly, our highlighting of gender in this chapter, as in gendered globalization or gendered transnational patriarchies, certainly does not mean a neglect of class, disability, mobility, nation(alism), racialization, religion, sexuality, and many further intersections, when considering violence or violences. Whilst we have emphasized here that gendered violence is predominantly a matter of men's violence against women, children, and other men, men's violences should not be understood as monolithic, and nor should this be a means to downplay women's and children's agency and their own – if lesser – violence and support for violence. Other important forms and configurations of violence include violence against and by LGBTIQ+ people (lesbian, gay, bisexual, transgender, intersex, queer, further non-normative genders and sexualities), class violence, nationalistic violence, and ethnic and racialized violence.

All of these perspectives, approaches, and formations raise fundamental issues for the theory and practice of social work and related social welfare policies, globally and locally. Social work is often involved in both direct work on violence and against violence and less direct work on the effects and aftermaths of violence, previously or elsewhere. This applies in both individual, family, and small group work, and more generally in large group and community work. Globalizations and transnationalizations make those direct and direct involvements of social work with and against violence all the more familiar, local, and intimate – for social workers, those who do violence, and those violated, who indeed may not always be distinct and separate people.

Notes

1 That is, the compression of time and space across the globe – at least for some people and some aspects of life.
2 In transnational processes the nation can be simultaneously affirmed and deconstructed in several different ways:

- *moving across* or *between* two or more somethings: across national boundaries or between nations, as in migration or policy negotiations between sovereign states;
- *metamorphosing*, problematizing, blurring, hydridizing, transgressing, breaking down, even dissolving something(s), nations or demise of the nation or national boundaries, as in blurrings of boundaries;
- *new configurations*, intensified, transnational, supranational or de-territorialized, de-materialized or virtual entities, the material/virtual sex trade.

3 On the UN Women's work on engaging men, see http://www.unwomen.org/en/news/in-focus/engaging-men
4 On the extensive work of Promundo, see http://promundoglobal.org/
5 On Sonke Gender Justice, see http://www.genderjustice.org.za/
6 On White Ribbon Campaign, see http://www.whiteribbon.ca/who-we-are/
7 See http://www.chsj.org/masvaw.html
8 On MenEngage, see http://menengage.org/about-us/
9 See http://www.whiteribbon.ca/who-we-are/
10 See http://menengage.org/about-us/who-we-are/

References

Acker, J 2004, 'Gender, capitalism and globalization', *Critical Sociology*, vol. 30, no. 2, pp. 17–41.

Airhihenbuwa, CO, Shisana, O, Zungu, N, Belue, R, Makofani, DM, Shefer, T, Smith, E & Simbayi, L 2011, 'Research capacity building: A US-South African partnership', *Global Health Promotion*, vol. 18, no. 2, pp. 27–35.

Bhana, D & Pattman, R 2009, 'Researching South African youth, gender and sexuality within the context of HIV/AIDS', *Development*, vol. 52, no. 1, pp. 68–74.

Black, SE & Brainerd, E 2004, 'Importing equality? The impact of globalization on gender discrimination', *Industrial and Labor Relations Review*, vol. 57, no. 4, pp. 540–559.

Boorstin, R & Nolan, S (eds) 2004, *Iraq in Transition: Post-Conflict Challenges and Opportunities*, [pdf] Open Society Institute and United Nations Foundation. Available at http://www.opensocietyfoundations.org/sites/default/files/iraq_Transition.pdf

Bowen, Jr, SW 2009, *Hard Lessons: The Iraq Reconstruction Experience*, [pdf] Inspector General Draft Document, 2 February 2009. Available at http://s3.amazonaws.com/nyt-docs/docs/319/319.pdf

Brouard, P & Crewe, M 2013, 'Sweetening the deal? Sugar daddies, sugar mummies, sugar babies and HIV in contemporary South Africa', *Agenda*, vol. 26, no. 4, pp. 48–56.

Connell, R 1993, 'The big picture: Masculinities in recent world history', *Theory and Society*, vol. 22, no. 5, pp. 597–623.

Connell, R 1998, 'Masculinities and globalization', *Men and Masculinities*, vol. 1, no. 1, pp. 3–23.

Connell, R 2014, 'Margin becoming centre: For a world-centred rethinking of masculinities', *NORMA: International Journal for Masculinity Studies*, vol. 9, no. 4, pp. 217–231.

The Convention on the Elimination of all forms of Discrimination against Women (CEDAW) 1979, [online] Available at http://www.un.org/womenwatch/daw/cedaw/ [Accessed 12 February 2016].

Cornwall, A & Lindisfarne, N (eds) 1994, *Dislocating Masculinity: Comparative Ethnographies*, Routledge, London.

Cornia, GA 2012, *Inequality Trends and Their Determinants: Latin America Over 1990–2010*. Working Paper No. 2012/09. UNU-WIDER. [pdf] Available at https://www.wider.unu.edu/sites/default/files/wp2012-009.pdf

Donaldson, M, Hibbins, R, Howson, R & Pease, B (eds) 2009, *Migrant Men: Critical Studies of Masculinities and the Migration Experience*, Routledge, New York.

Ehrenreich, B & Hochschild, AR (eds) 2002, *Global Woman: Nannies, Maids, and Sex Workers in the New Economy*, Henry Holt and Company, New York.

Escobar, E 2004, 'Beyond the Third World: Imperial globality, global coloniality and anti-globalisation social movements', *Third World Quarterly*, vol. 25, no. 1, pp. 207–230.

Etienne, M 1995, 'Addressing gender-based violence in an international context', *Harvard Women's Law Journal*, vol. 18, pp. 139–170.

Forces Watch 2013, *The Last Ambush.* [online] Available at http://www.forceswatch.net/content/last-ambush

Fuentes-Nieva, R & Galasso, N 2014, *Working For the Few: Political Capture and Economic Inequality*, Oxfam International, Oxford.

Fundamental Rights Agency (FRA) 2014, Violence Against Women: An EU-Wide Survey, FRA, Vienna. http://fra.europa.eu/sites/default/files/fra-2014-vaw-survey-main-results-apr14_en.pdf

Giddens, A 1990, *The Consequences of Modernity*, Polity, Cambridge.

Grewal, I 2013, 'Outsourcing patriarchy: feminist encounters, transnational mediations and the crime of "|honour killings"', *International Journal of Feminist Politics*, vol. 15, no. 1, pp. 1–19.

Hearn, J 1996, 'Deconstructing the dominant: Making the One(s) the Other(s)', *Organization*, vol. 3, no. 4, pp. 611–626.

Hearn, J 2014, 'International studies on men, masculinities and gender equality', *Men and Masculinities*, vol. 17, no. 5, pp. 455–466.

Hearn, J 2015a, *Men of the World: Genders, Globalizations, Transnational Times*, Sage, London.

Hearn, J 2015b, 'Transnational reflections on transnational research projects on men, boys and gender relations', *NORMA: International Journal for Masculinity Studies*, vol. 10, no. 2, pp. 86–104.

Hearn, J, Blagojević, M & Harrison, K (eds) 2013, *Rethinking Transnational Men: Beyond, Between and Within Nations*, Routledge, New York.

Holter, ØG 2014, '"What's in it for men?" Old question, new data', *Men and Masculinities*, vol. 17, no. 5, pp. 515–548.

Hughes, D 2002, 'The use of new communication and information technologies for the sexual exploitation of women and children', *Hastings Women's Law Journal*, vol. 13 no. 1, pp. 127–146.

IPCC (Intergovernmental Panel on Climate Change) 2001, *Climate Change 2001 Impacts, Adaptation, and Vulnerability.* [online] Available at http://www.ipcc.ch/ipccreports/tar/wg2/index.php?idp=674.

Jones, A (ed) 2006, *Men of the Global South: A Reader*, Zed, London.

Jungar, K & Oinas, E 2004, 'Preventing HIV? Medical discourses and invisible women', in *Re-Thinking Sexualities in Africa*, (ed) S Arnfred, Nordic Africa Institute, Uppsala, pp. 97–114.

Jungar, K & Oinas, E 2010, 'A feminist struggle? South African HIV activism as feminist politics', *Journal of International Women's Studies*, vol. 11, no. 4, pp. 177–191.

Jungar, K & Oinas, E 2011, 'Beyond agency and victimisation: Re-reading HIV and AIDS in African contexts', *Social Dynamics*, vol. 37, no. 2, pp. 248–262.

Kabeer, N & Mahmud, S 2004, 'Globalization, gender and poverty: Bangladeshi women workers in export and local markets', *Journal of International Development*, vol. 16, no. 1, pp. 93–109.

Lash, S & Urry, J 1994, *Economies of Signs and Space*, Sage, London.

Levtov, R, Barker, G, Contreras-Urbina, M, Heilman, B & Verma, R 2014, 'Pathways to gender equitable men: Findings from the International Men and Gender Equality Survey in eight countries', *Men and Masculinities*, vol. 17, no. 5, pp. 467–501.

Lewis, D 2011, 'Representing African sexualities', in *African Sexualities: A Reader*, ed. S Tamala, Fahamu, Fish Hoek, pp. 199–216.

Lugones, M 2007, 'Heterosexualism and the colonial/modern gender system', *Hypatia*, vol. 22, no. 1, pp. 186–209.

Ouzgane, L & Coleman, D 1998, 'Postcolonial masculinities: Introduction', *Jouvert: A Journal of Postcolonial Studies*, vol. 2, no. 1. Available at http://english.chass.ncsu.edu/jouvert/v2i1/CON21.HTM

Oxfam 2016, *An Economy For the 1%*. Oxfam Briefing Paper (18 January 2016). Available at from www.oxfam.org

Pattman R 2007, 'Researching and working with boys and young men in Southern Africa in the context of HIV/AIDS: a radical approach', in *From Boys to Men: Social Constructions of Masculinity in Contemporary Society*, eds T Shefer, K Ratele, A Strebel, N Shabalala & R Buikema, UCT Press, Cape Town, pp. 33–49.

Patton, C 1997, 'Inventing 'African AIDS'', in *The Gender/Sexuality Reader: Culture, History, Political Economy*, eds R Lancaster & M di Leonardo, Routledge, New York, pp. 387–405.

Ratele, K 2014, 'Currents against gender transformation of South African men: Relocating marginality to the centre of research and theory of masculinities', *NORMA: International Journal for Masculinity Studies*, vol. 9, no. 1, pp. 30–44.

Ratele, K 2015, 'Location, location, location: Reckoning with margins and centres of masculinities research and theory in an inter/trans-national South Africa–Finland project on youth', *NORMA: International Journal for Masculinity Studies*, vol. 10, no. 2, pp. 105–116.

Ratele, K & Shefer, T 2013, 'Desire, fear and entitlement: sexualising race and racialising sexuality in (re)membering apartheid', in *Race, Memory and the Apartheid Archive: Towards a Transformative Psychosocial Praxis*, eds G Stevens, N Duncan & D Hook, Palgrave Macmillan, Houndmills, pp. 188–207.

Ratele, K, Shefer, T & Botha, M 2011, 'Navigating past 'the white man's agenda' in South Africa: organizing men for gendered transformation of society', in *Men and Masculinities Around the World*, eds E Ruspini, J Hearn, B Pease & K Pringle, Palgrave Macmillan, New York, pp. 247–260.

Reddy, V, Meyer, S, Shefer, T & Meyiwa, T 2014, 'Towards a critical theory of care', in *Care In Context: Transnational Gender Perspectives*, eds V. Reddy, S. Meyer, T. Shefer & T. Meyiwa, HSRC Press, Cape Town, pp. 1–27.

Ritzer, G. (ed.) 2007, *The Blackwell Companion to Globalization*, Blackwell, Malden, MA.

Robertson, R 1995, 'Glocalization: time-space and homogeneity-heterogeneity', in *Global Modernities*, eds M Featherstone, S Lash & R Robertson, Sage, London, pp. 25–44.

Robertson, R & Khondker, HH 1998, 'Discourses of globalization: Preliminary considerations', *International Sociology*, vol. 13, no. 1, pp. 25–40.

Ruspini, E, Hearn, J, Pease, B & Pringle, K (eds) 2011, *Men and Masculinities Around the World*, Palgrave Macmillan, Houndmills.

Safa, HI 2002, 'Questioning globalization: Gender and export processing in the Dominican Republic', *Journal of Developing Societies*, vol. 18, no 2–3, pp. 11–31.

Shefer, T 2016, 'Resisting the binarism of victim and agent: Critical reflections on 20 years of scholarship on young women and heterosexual practices in South African contexts', *Global Public Health: An International Journal for Research, Policy and Practice*, vol. 11, nos. 1–2, 211–223. doi:10.1080/17441692.2015.1029959.

Shefer, T & Strebel, A 2013, 'Deconstructing the "sugar daddy": A critical review of the constructions of men in intergenerational sexual relationships in South Africa', *Agenda*, vol. 26, no. 4, pp. 57–63.

Shefer, T, Stevens, G & Clowes, L 2010, 'Men in Africa: Masculinities, materiality and meaning', *Journal of Psychology in Africa*, vol. 20, no. 4, pp. 511–518.

Shefer, T, Hearn, J & Ratele, K 2015, 'North-South dialogues: Reflecting on working transnationally on young men, masculinities and gender justice', *NORMA: International Journal for Masculinity Studies*, vol. 10, no. 2, pp. 164–178.

SIDA 2013, *SIDA's Portfolio Within Gender Equality 2012*, SIDA, Stockholm. Available at http://www.sida.se/English/publications/Publication_database/publications-by-year1/2013/november/sida8217s-portfolio-within-gender-equality-2012/

SIDA 2014, Development Trends: Increasing Engagement of Men and Boys for Gender Equality, SIDA, Stockholm. Available at http://www.sida.se/English/publications/ Publication_database/publications-by-year1/2014/october/development-trends-increasing-engagement-of-men-and-boys-for-gender-equality/

SIPRI 2012, *SIPRI Yearbook 2012*, Oxford: Oxford University Press.

Stiglitz, J & Bilmes, L 2008, *The Three Trillion Dollar War: The True Cost of the Iraq Conflict*, WW Norton, New York.

Turner, BS 2007, 'The futures of globalization', in *The Blackwell Companion to Globalization*, ed G Ritzer, Blackwell, Malden, MA, pp. 675–692.

van der Gaag, N 2014, *Feminism & Men*, Zed, London.

Walby, S 2009, *Globalizations and Inequalities*, Sage, London.

Waters, M 1995, *Globalization*, Routledge, London.

World Health Organization 2007, *Engaging Men and Boys in Changing Gender-Based Inequity in Health: Evidence From Programme Interventions*, World Health Organization, Geneva. http://www.who.int/gender/documents/Engaging_men_boys.pdf

World Health Organization 2010, *Policy Approaches to Engaging Men and Boys in Achieving Gender Equality and Health Equity*, World Health Organization, Geneva. http://apps.who.int/iris/bitstream/10665/44402/1/9789241500128_eng.pdf

4 Globalisation and Glocalised Responses to Asylum Seekers

A Comparative Analysis of Australia and the United Kingdom

Shepard Masocha

Introduction

The unfolding refugee crisis represents the worst humanitarian crisis and largest movement of asylum seekers since the Second World War. The United Nations High Commissioner for Refugees (UNHCR) estimates that between January 2015 and February 2016 over one million migrants and refugees arrived by sea in Greece, Italy, Malta and Spain (UNHCR, 2016). Governments of developed western countries have responded in very different ways to the increased presence of asylum seekers. These responses exist on a continuum that ranges from Germany's 'open door' policy of welcoming the new arrivals to Hungary's frosty reception evinced by the erection of the controversial razor wire fence along the Hungarian-Serbian border, which evokes memories of the Iron Curtain. Much of the media attention has focused on the public's attitudes and responses to the plight of new arrivals in Europe, particularly the public displays of compassion and generosity. However, rarely has the unfolding crisis been articulated within the media and political debates in the context of globalisation, yet this nexus is crucial in understanding the crisis. The unfolding crisis and the western countries' responses need to be understood within the wider context of these nation states' existing global capitalist relationships with poor countries.

As signatories of the 1951 UN Convention Relating to the Status of Refugees, both Australia and the United Kingdom are committed in principle to the protection of refugees. Article 1(A)2 of the Convention defines a refugee as a person who

> ... owing to a well-founded fear of being persecuted for reasons of race, religion, nationality, membership of a particular social group or political opinion, is outside of the country of his [sic] nationality and is unable or, owing to such fear, is unwilling to avail himself of the protection of that country; or who, not having a nationality and being outside the country of his former habitual residence as a result of such events, is unable, or, owing to such fear, is unwilling to return to it.

At face value, Australia and the United Kingdom appear to have responded in distinctly different ways to the presence of asylum seekers within their respective national borders. Although Australia has abandoned its blatantly racist White Australia immigration policy of the 1950s, the government still insists that the country has the sovereign right to 'decide who comes to Australia and the circumstances in which they come' (Parliament of Australia, 2001). Australia has a highly controlled and rigid system for processing refugee applications to which a fixed quota of visas is made available annually. In the 2014–15 financial year, there were 13,750 visas made available, of which 6,000 were for refugees resettled with the assistance of the UNHCR (Karlsen, 2015). Humanitarian entrants were allocated 5,000 visas under the Special Humanitarian programme, and the remaining 2,750 were available for onshore protection visas (Karlsen, 2015). Since 1991, Australia has been operating a policy of mandatory detention of asylum seekers who arrive by boat without a valid visa. As part of the Pacific Solution, asylum seekers who arrive by boat are transferred and detained in offshore processing centres in Papa New Guinea and Nauru with no prospects of being resettled in Australia (Phillips, 2014). In contrast, in the United Kingdom, most of the asylum applications are lodged in the country and very limited numbers of refugees enter through the UNHCR resettlement programme. In ways not very dissimilar to Australia, the United Kingdom has also set up barriers to prevent people from exercising the right to seek protection from persecution and has a well-established infrastructure for the internment of this group of unwanted 'Others'. For instance, only a small percentage of applications for asylum are recognised. Of the 24,914 applications that were received in 2014, 59 per cent were rejected (Blinder, 2015). The detention and deportation of asylum seekers are also integral parts of the UK asylum system (Bloch and Schuster, 2005). The United Kingdom has one of the largest immigration detention infrastructures in Europe, with a capacity of 3,500 on any given day (Silverman and Hajela, 2015).

Drawing on the concept of glocalisation (Robertson, 1995), this chapter illustrates that the asylum-seeking policies adopted by Australia and the United Kingdom are fundamentally similar as they are informed by a protectionist discourse. It is argued that a global discourse of control and deterrence permeates through and undergirds Australian and UK responses, resulting in the liminal and marginalised positions of asylum claimants irrespective of which part of the developed world asylum seekers are located in. The chapter also uses the concepts of governmentality and neoliberalism as frameworks to illustrate how the asylum policies are similar. It also draws attention to the similarities in the discourses which legitimate and result in practices that marginalise, constrict and exclude asylum seekers in both countries.

Globalisation, Migration and Asylum Seekers

The process of globalisation in its neoliberal form provides a wider context within which the increased presence of asylum seekers and refugees in western countries can be understood. For Mittleman (2004, p. 220), globalisation 'encompasses an historical transformation in the interactions among market forces, political authority and the life ways embodied in societies, as they encounter and join with local conditions'. The term captures 'the transforming dynamics of social, cultural, economic, and political relations between different combinations of national, sub-, multi-, and trans-national actions and institutions that constitute multi intra-, inter-, and trans-border flows and movements' (Morrell, 2008, p. 9). Within this chapter, globalisation is accepted as 'not simply a market driven economic phenomenon. It is also – and very much – a political and ideological phenomenon' (Mishra, 1999, p. 7) that is observable across the globe and impacts on everyday lives. Globalisation is characterised by the establishment of transnational networks which facilitate greater mobility of capital investment, production processes, labour and new forms of communication, particularly information technology.

A contradiction exists in that globalisation is predicated on the unfettered movement of goods, highly skilled labour, information and services, yet stringent measures have also been instituted to restrict the transnational movement of people, especially those from poor countries. Boswell (2003) also points to this tension that exists between, on the one hand, the freedom of movement that is afforded by globalisation and its associated economic liberalisation, and on the other hand, the protectionist political discourse on migration across the developed western countries. The governmentality of immigration has become a major preoccupation of western governments, leading to walls being erected around the west (Fassin, 2011). These walls have taken the form of tightened internal and external border policing as a direct response to the global movements of people from the poor South. The notion of 'Fortress Europe' is associated with the ways in which 'high walls are being built around the wealthy cores of the Global North to keep out millions of people who are forced to leave their home countries to survive' (Euskirchen *et al.*, 2007). Paradoxically, globalisation has also facilitated the movement of migrants and asylum seekers by linking poor countries with developed countries through complex economic, cultural and social networks and increased connectivity. Castles (2003) notes how globalisation has also resulted in social transformations: social connections that transcend national borders as well as transnational social capital and human agency. As such, the increased presence of refugees and asylum seekers within developed western countries is not simply the result of 'a string of unconnected emergencies but rather an integral part of the North-South relationships' (Castles, 2003, p. 17). For example, the endemic inequalities in the North-South relationships have further entrenched the existing income and wealth disparities across the world. Such inequalities, when combined with local factors, contribute to the sociopolitical conflicts that result in forced migration. This link between processes of globalisation and the increased presence of asylum seekers within developed western countries has not been the subject of extensive social work research.

The concept of glocalisation provides a useful framework for understanding the ways in which individual nation states have responded to the global movements of asylum seekers. Robertson (1995) argues that glocalisation is a much more useful and precise term for globalisation as it recognises the mediating role played by local factors in shaping processes. The term glocalisation was coined to denote the synthesis and immanent intertwining between the local and the global. It refers to the interconnection between processes of globalisation and local particularities. The term, popularised by Roland Robertson but having its roots in Japanese economics, draws attention to the ways in which global phenomena are influenced and even at times subverted by local conditions, applications, interpretations and adaptations.

Asylum-seeking policies are an example of glocalisation. Triggered by processes of globalisation, forced migration has significant and specific local consequences for the host countries. Asylum seekers' presence in western countries represents an intrusion of global issues into everyday lives at the local level. It can be argued that this intrusion illustrates the extent to which the local/global bifurcation is, in fact, an artificial one that obfuscates an otherwise complex relationship. Although it may be a global issue in terms of its origins, the issue of asylum is often transmuted and articulated as a local and/or national issue. In this respect, the asylum policies adopted by Australia and the United Kingdom should be seen as the products of 'the interpenetration of the global and the local, resulting in unique outcomes in different geographic areas' (Ritzer, 2004, p. 193). As such, the asylum policies exist in a dialectical relationship with the processes of globalisation which result in forced migration. Thus, the global and the local 'are not separate containers but mutually constitutive social processes' (Smith, 2001, p. 182) that are virtually bound in an inextricable and irreversible dynamic relationship. Such a perspective challenges the tendency within existing social work research to view the two countries' asylum systems as being distinctly different and unconnected.

Visibilising 'The Global' in Asylum Policies

Within the field of social work, there is a paucity of research that offers a comparative analysis of Australia and the United Kingdom's asylum-seeking systems. Notable exceptions to this are studies by Cemlyn and Briskman (2003), Barrie and Mendes (2011) and Robinson (2014), which offer a comparative view of the Australian and UK policy contexts and their implications for social work practice. Focusing on the experiences of asylum-seeking children, Cemlyn and Briskman (2003) highlight the ways in which both policies are built on racist foundations and how the asylum systems are geared towards restricting and deterring people from exercising an internationally enshrined right to seek protection from persecution. They note that although there are 'numerous differences between the two countries related to their geopolitical situation, and to their treatment of asylum seeking children … there are also unnerving parallels which are currently drawing closer' (Cemlyn and Briskman, 2003, p. 163). They argue that the nature of these systems has significant implications for the realisation of human rights-based social work. Barrie and Mendes (2011) provide a literature review in which they compare and contrast the experiences of unaccompanied asylum-seeking children in and leaving out-of-home care in Australia and the United Kingdom, and draw attention to how such experiences are impacted by the prevailing policies and legislation which govern welfare provision for this service user group. Robinson (2011, 2014) explores the significant challenges encountered by frontline social workers who work with asylum seekers in non-governmental organisations (NGOs) in Australia and the United Kingdom. She illustrates how the ethical dilemmas encountered by practitioners are linked to asylum policies which promote the marginalisation and exclusion of asylum seekers. However, although this body of research provides important comparative insights, it does not focus on the nexus between processes of globalisation, the discourse of deterrence and the glocalised legislative and policy responses to the presence of asylum seekers within the two countries.

Regulating transnational mobilities has become a key concern for contemporary asylum and immigration policies in Australia and the United Kingdom as well as in other developed countries. The asylum regimes that have been established by these western governments can be seen as part of the efforts to deal with the 'darker side of globalisation' (Urray, 2002, p. 57). These efforts have taken the form of specific surveillance and control technologies that are aimed at curbing the ability of people from poor countries to seek asylum in these two developed countries. Unlike the roles that Australia and the United Kingdom have assumed in the technological and economic domains, the two nation states have assumed a particularly vigorous role in the governmentality of immigration. In his characterisation of asylum seekers as the 'human waste' of modernity, Bauman (2007, p. 42) aptly sums up these two countries', and indeed all other wealthy western nation states', responses and attitudes towards this group of immigrants:

> ... all measures have been taken to assure the permanence of their exclusion ... Wherever they go they are unwanted and left in no doubt that they are ... The statesmen of the European Union deploy most of their time and brain capacity in designing ever more sophisticated ways of fortifying borders and most expedient procedures for getting rid of seekers after bread and shelter who have managed to cross borders nevertheless.

Therefore, there is a particular concern across western nations to deter asylum seekers. The only difference between the nation states is in the particularities of the systems they have adopted; otherwise, the basis and spirit of the policies are essentially the same.

A raft of measures has been instituted in both countries which has effectively taken asylum seekers out of mainstream welfare provision as well as limiting their work rights (Neumann, 2004, Sales, 2007). In both countries, these policies are meant to act as deterrents and are part of a wider strategy to discourage people from coming to these countries to seek asylum. It can be argued that, driven partly by media-generated panic about the dangers that asylum seekers pose, both the governments of Australia and the United Kingdom have decisively shifted towards deterrence and protectionism (Zetter *et al.*, 2005, pp. 9–10). As a whole, the discourses relating to asylum seekers in both countries have decisively shifted away from human rights to a focus on belonging to and membership of the nation state. This has largely been made possible by the ways in which asylum seekers have been demonised in the media and politicians' discourses in both countries. Asylum seekers now represent the inverted image of the 'good citizen' (Bigo, 2002). In the case of the United Kingdom, as Capdevila and Callaghan (2008) note, there is an entrenched discourse that constructs asylum seekers as *not like us* and therefore a danger to the British way of life. Research by Every and Augoustinos (2008a, 2008b) notes how asylum seekers are represented in similar ways in Australia. Sarah Ahmed, in her book *The Cultural Politics of Emotion*, discusses the relationship between politics and fear. She illustrates that affective politics of fear, such as those relating to asylum seekers, legitimate the containment and denial of rights of groups that are categorised as the Other (Ahmed, 2004). One of the outcomes of such affective politics of fear is that, in both Australia and the United Kingdom, issues of human rights and social justice are no longer considered of paramount importance in asylum-seeking debates, making it possible to marginalise and exclude this group from mainstream society.

Foucault's ideas on governmentality provide a useful framework for understanding the extent to which asylum-seeking policies in Australia and the United Kingdom are similar in terms of how they are used to exercise sovereignty over this population group and how this is legitimated. The eighteenth century saw the emergence of a new way of governing populations, which saw governments increasingly deploying strategies that enabled them 'to govern at a distance' (Rose, 1996, p. 42). Governmentality can be understood as the

> ... ensemble performed by institutions, procedures, analyses and reflections, the calculations and tactics that allow the exercises of this very specific and albeit form of power, which has as its target population ... and as its essential technical means apparatuses.
>
> (Foucault, 1991)

The concept of governmentality helps in understanding the ways in which power in its various permutations is exercised to govern and control asylum seekers in more or less similar ways in Australia and the United Kingdom. The concept draws attention to the strategies, procedures and tactics deployed and the specific ways such treatments are legitimated. As already illustrated, both countries have put in place an elaborate 'surveillance apparatus of frontiers and territories, regimes of exception for the detention and deportation' (Fassin, 2011, p. 213) with negative effects on people's rights to claim asylum.

The governmentality risk thesis (Rose, 2000, Garland, 2003, O'Malley, 2008) enables an understanding of the ways in which advanced liberal governments conceptualise, articulate and manage risk in relation to asylum seekers. Research studies have illustrated how asylum seekers in both countries are portrayed as posing a credible threat to national security (for a detailed analysis of these negative representations see; Masocha and Simpson, 2011, Lynn and Lea, 2003, Every and Augoustinos, 2008a, Pickering, 2001, Gabrielatos and Baker, 2008, Klocker and Dunn, 2003). Within western countries such as the United Kingdom, Australia and the United States, the notion of asylum seekers as a threat has become particularly entrenched in public discourse in the post 9/11 era with links being made between asylum seekers and terrorism. The tragic events in Paris in November 2015 clearly illustrate this point as links were instantly established between the act of terrorism and the currently unfolding refugee crisis. Framing asylum seekers as the threatening Other serves the important ideological function of rationalising and rendering understandable the deployment of specific technologies of governmentality, containment and securitisation.

The responses of the United Kingdom and Australian governments, as well as other western countries such as the United States, has been to focus on the threats that asylum seekers present to national security as well as other areas such as welfare and the labour market. For instance, the 'war on terror' is characterised by an intensification of border controls and increased state surveillance (Aas, 2007). Borders have become increasingly militarised and the language deployed to articulate asylum policies has also become militarised. An example is how, in both Australia and the United Kingdom, immigration service departments have been renamed 'Australian Border Force' and 'UK Border Force', respectively. The activities of these departments are increasingly being framed in military terms. For example, Operation Sovereign Borders in Australia is headed by a lieutenant-brigadier, giving the impression that the country is engaged in a military conflict (Doherty, 2015). This nomenclature of war/conflict serves an important ideological purpose in the governmentality of asylum in these two countries. Doherty (2015, p. 26) argues that

> ... in times of war or national crises, other competing interests such as concern for individual rights, can be overridden by the need for decisive government action. The language of war gives the government the imprimatur, indeed the obligation, to respond to the threats enlivened by its rhetoric.

It renders understandable and acceptable the harsh treatment that is then meted out to asylum seekers.

Furthermore, constructing asylum seekers as a risk places them outside the moral order, which provides justification for their segregation, marginalisation, exclusion and banishment within neoliberal democracies like Australia and the United Kingdom. A core aspect of neoliberalism is the affirmation of people's freedoms, but one that is a 'well-regulated and "responsibilized" liberty' (Barry *et al.*, 1996, p. 8). However, illiberal and contradictory practices exist within liberal regimes. According to Christie and Sidhu (2006, p. 451), 'what distinguishes liberal from despotic regimes is the forms of rationality justifying illiberal action'. Liberal governments have long histories of subjecting sections of their society to 'all sorts of disciplinary, biopolitical and even sovereign interventions' (Dean, 1999, p. 134). As Dean (2002, p. 39) cogently argues, 'governing liberally does not entail governing through freedoms or even governing in a manner that respects liberty'. As such, the harsh treatment that asylum seekers receive in these countries is not necessarily incompatible with neoliberal governmentality. In both the United Kingdom and Australia, detention centres where asylum seekers are held have become 'sites of exception, where regimes of police prevail over regimes of rights' (Fassin, 2011, p. 219) as evidenced by the prevalence of concerns and reports of human rights abuses within these institutions. In fact, especially when understood in the context of the deterrence, such treatments are important practices for managing those who are deemed as falling outside the realm of mainstream society and on whom neoliberal governmentality strategies of self-responsibility, accountability and prudentialism are difficult to apply. The constitution of asylum seekers as a risk and the institution of restrictive legislative regimes that result in asylum seekers' human rights being undermined are, as Rose (2000, p. 330) argues, part of the strategies instituted 'to manage these anti-citizens' and the marginal spaces they occupy 'through measures which seek to neutralize the dangers they pose'. Within Australia and the United Kingdom, asylum seekers are seen as 'the repository for fears not simply about risk but about the breakdown of social order and the need to maintain social boundaries and divisions' (Tulloch and Lupton, 2003, p. 7). It is on this basis that the harsh treatment of asylum seekers in both Australia and the United Kingdom is legitimated, and in any case, both governments are clear that these constrictive measures are an essential part of the deterrence framework that underpins their respective asylum policies.

The analysis, thus far, clearly illustrates the role that nationalism plays in the negative representations and treatment of asylum seekers. Existing research studies also illustrate how nationalist discourses, drawing on nation and nationhood as discursive resources, have been used to legitimate the denial of asylum seekers' human rights (for Australia, see Every and Augoustinos, 2007, O'Doherty and Lecouteur, 2007, Pickering, 2001; and for the United Kingdom, see Khosravinik, 2010, Masocha, 2015). However, there is also a need to understand the economic dimensions of the issue of asylum in the context of globalisation in its neoliberal form. The development towards national economies that are open to trade and capital inflows entails a retracted and diminished role of the nation state within the economic and technological domains. The role that economic considerations play in the negative formulations of asylum seekers and the repressive practices that have been instituted has received minimal attention within social work research, yet there is 'an interesting interplay whereby neoliberal and nationalist discourses come together to legitimate the exclusion of asylum seekers' (Lueck *et al.*, 2015, p. 609). The asylum systems in Australia and the United Kingdom are a good example of how the boundaries between state and private enterprise are becoming increasingly blurred within a neoliberal environment. Although one of the key arguments for restricting asylum in both countries has been framed around the cost to the public purse, the policies that have been instituted have led to the development of a multi-billion dollar 'asylum market'. Multinational companies such as Serco and G4S, which run detention centres in both countries, have dominated this market (Gammeltoft-Hansen, 2015). In the United Kingdom, G4S is also a major player in the provision of accommodation for asylum seekers who are not detained but are dispersed across local authorities whilst their applications are under consideration. Therefore, the detention and management of asylum seekers needs to be understood as part of the larger ideological shift towards neoliberalism, and in particular the specific ways in which the current asylum regimes service the interests of private enterprise. Such an understanding provides a strong moral basis for transnational social work advocacy and political activism against current legislative and policy frameworks that regulate asylum seeking.

Conclusion

The comparative analysis that has been presented here serves as a proxy for understanding, in other national contexts, the link between asylum seeking, globalisation, governmentality and individual nation states' glocalised legislative and policy frameworks. The chapter highlights that, whilst a humanitarian discourse based on both international conventions and national laws exists which recognises the need to protect those fleeing persecution, there are also dominant economic, political and ideological forces that actively seek to deter, limit, control and contain the global movements of asylum seekers. When viewed in the context of globalisation and governmentality, Australia and the United Kingdom share striking similarities as well as differences in terms of the ways that they have responded to asylum seekers. However, such an appreciation of the impact of 'the global' in shaping the responses to asylum seekers should not be at the expense of understanding the influences of local contextual factors. Blommaert (2010) cautions against overlooking the resilience of the local in the face of the global given the influence that the local criteria and norms exerts on the processes of change. Although this chapter has focused on the macro-positioned discourses, ideologies and practices that shape the (negative) treatment of asylum seekers, it is important to note that these responses to asylum seekers are also shaped by the local conditions that are specific to each of these countries. For instance, it has been noted in this chapter that media discourses and national politics are influential in shaping each country's responses to asylum seekers, which in turn produce the differentiated particularities of Australia and the United Kingdom's asylum policy regimes. As such, asylum policies of these two countries should be understood as a complex interplay between 'the local' and the 'the global' (Giddens, 1990). This complexity has not been widely appreciated in existing social work research, yet it has fundamental implications for practice.

Understanding the nexus between the global processes and practices and how they impact on situated local practices can lead to significant enhancements in social work deriving from the in-depth and nuanced understanding of the policies and treatment of asylum seekers in western countries. As illustrated, asylum seekers are subject to repressive practices emanating from a globally positioned discourse of control and deterrence. As such, the work that individual practitioners undertake with asylum seekers is shaped and affected by these discourses. In fact, it can be argued that locally situated social work practices with asylum seekers are a microcosmic reflection of these discourses. This has significant implications for social work given the profession's commitment to social justice. Therefore, there is an urgent need for social work to take up a more collective and politically active role in advocating for the individual rights of asylum seekers. This requires going beyond just the local but also focusing on the global. One way social work can achieve this is by taking an international approach in advocating for the plight of asylum seekers and others in need of humanitarian protection. For instance, this can take the form of transnational advocacy in which social workers in one country establish strategic alliances with social workers in other countries specifically to challenge and disrupt the dominant political ideologies and hegemonic identities which negatively impact on asylum seekers (Cox, 2015). Such a strategy has the potential to mobilise international resources and make them available to social work activists engaged in local sociopolitical struggles. Doing this can provide social work with the capacity to be 'agents of globalisation with freedom to resist, accept or modify the unyielding global forces at national, community, and personal levels' (Mendis, 2007, p. 2). As illustrated, the treatment of asylum seekers is strikingly similar despite the different national contexts. This presents opportunities for a social work advocacy that transcends national borders. With a unified voice, the profession can begin to engage at local, community, national and global levels in discursive acts and policy debates that may result in significant changes in the governmentality of asylum. This would promote the development of alternative narratives and practices that pay specific attention to the humanity of asylum seekers and the need for social justice.

References

Aas, K. F. 2007. Analysing a world in motion: Global flows meet 'criminology of the other'. *Theoretical Criminology*, 11, 283–303.

Ahmed, S. 2004. *The Cultural Politics of Emotion*, New York, Routledge.

Barrie, L. & Mendes, P. 2011. The experiences of unaccompanied asylum-seeking children in and leaving the out-of-home care system in the UK and Australia: A critical review of the literature. *International Social Work*, 54, 485–503.

Barry, A., Osborne, T. & Rose, N. 1996. Introduction. *In:* Barry, A., Osborne, T. & Rose, N. (eds.) *Foucault and Political Reason: Liberalism, Neo-Liberalism and Rationalities of Government*, London, Taylor and Francis Group.

Bauman, Z. 2007. *Liquidity Times: Living in an age of uncertainty*, Cambridge, Polity Press.

Bigo, D. 2002. Security and immigration: Towards a critique of the governmentality of unease. *Alternatives*, 27, 63–92.

Blinder, S. 2015. *Migration to the UK: Asylum*, Oxford, The Migration Observatory; available at http://www.migrationobservatory.ox.ac.uk/sites/files/migobs/Briefing - Migration to the UK - Asylum_0.pdf [accessed 10.12.2015].

Bloch, A. & Schuster, L. 2005. At the extremes of exclusion: Deportation, detention and dispersal. *Ethnic and Racial Studies*, 28, 491–512.

Blommaert, J. 2010. *The Sociolinguistics of Globalization*, Cambridge, Cambridge University Press.

Boswell, C. 2003. The 'external dimension' of EU immigration and asylum policy. *International Affairs*, 79, 619–638.

Capdevila, R. & Callaghan, J. E. M. 2008. 'It's not racist. It's common sense'. A critical analysis of political discourse around asylum and immigration in the UK. *Journal of Community & Applied Social Psychology*, 18, 1–16.

Castles, S. 2003. Towards a sociology of forced migration and social transformation. *Sociology*, 37, 13–34.

Cemlyn, S. & Briskman, L. 2003. Asylum, children's rights and social work. *Child and Family Social Work*, 8, 163–178.

Christie, P. & Sidhu, R. 2006. Governmentality and 'fearless speech': Framing the education of asylum seeker and refugee children in Australia. *Oxford Review of Education*, 32, 449–465.

Cox, P. 2015. Transnationalism and social work education. *Transnational Social Review: A Social Work Journal*, 5, 326–331.

Dean, M. 1999. *Governmentality: Power and Rule in Modern Society*, London, Sage.

Dean, M. 2002. Liberal government and authoritarianism. *Economy and Society*, 31, 37–61.

Doherty, B. 2015. *Call Me Illegal: The Semantic Struggle Over Seeking Asylum in Australia*, Oxford, The Centre on Migration, Policy and Society, Working Paper 126.

Euskirchen, M., Lebuhn, H. & Ray, G. 2007. From borderline to borderland: The changing European border regime. *Monthly Review*, 59; available at: http://monthlyreview.org/2007/11/01/from-borderline-to-borderland-the-changing-european-border-regime/ [accessed 12.12.2015].

Every, D. & Augoustinos, M. 2007. Constructions of racism in the Australian parliamentary debates on asylum seekers. *Discourse & Society*, 18, 411.

Every, D. & Augoustinos, M. 2008a. Constructions of Australia in pro- and anti-asylum seeker political discourse. *Nations And Nationalism*, 14, 562.

Every, D. & Augoustinos, M. 2008b. 'Taking advantage' or fleeing persecution? Opposing accounts of asylum seeking. *Journal of Sociolinguistics*, 12, 648–667.

Fassin, D. 2011. Policing borders, producing boundaries. The governmentality of immigration in dark times. *Annual Review of Anthropology*, 40, 213–226.

Foucault, M. 1991. On governmentality. *In:* Burchell, G., Gordon, C. & Miller, P. (eds.) *The Foucault Effect: Studies in Governmentality*. Brighton, Harvester Wheatsheaf.

Gabrielatos, C. & Baker, P. 2008. Fleeing, sneaking, flooding: A corpus analysis of discursive constructions of refugees and asylum seekers in the UK press, 1996–2005. *Journal of English Linguistics*, 36, 5–38.

Gammeltoft-Hansen, T. 2015. Private security and the migration control industry. *In:* Abrahamsen, R. & Leander, A. (eds.) *Routledge Handbook of Private Security Studies*. Abingdon, Routledge.

Garland, D. 2003. The rise of risk *In:* Ericson, R. V. & Doyle, A. (eds.) *Risk and Morality*. Toronto, University of Toronto Press.

Giddens, A. 1990. *The Consequences of Modernity*, Cambridge, Polity.

Karlsen, E. 2015. *Refugee Resettlement to Australia: What are the Facts?* Canberra, Parliament of Australia; available at: http://www.aph.gov.au/About_Parliament/Parliamentary_Departments/Parliamentary_Library/pubs/rp/rp1415/RefugeeResettlement-_Toc410727182 [accessed 25.02.2016].

Khosravinik, M. 2010. The representations of refugees, asylum seekers and immigrants in British newspapers: A critical discourse analysis. *Journal of Language and Politics*, 9, 1–28.

Klocker, N. & Dunn, K. M. 2003. Who's driving the asylum debate? Newspaper and government representations of asylum seekers. *Media International Australia Incorporating Culture and Policy*, 2003, 71.

Lueck, K., Due, C. & Augoustinos, M. 2015. Neoliberalism and nationalism: Representations of asylum seekers in the Australian mainstream news media. *Discourse & Society*, 26, 608–629.

Lynn, N. & Lea, S. 2003. 'A phantom menace and the new apartheid': The social construction of asylum-seekers in the United Kingdom. *Discourse and Society*, 14, 425–452.

Masocha, S. 2015. *Asylum Seekers, Social Work and Racism*, Basingstoke, Palgrave.

Masocha, S. & Simpson, M. K. 2011. Xenoracism: Towards a critical understanding of the construction of asylum seekers and its implications for social work practice. *Practice*, 23, 5–18.

Mendis, P. 2007. *Glocalization: The Human Side of Globalisation as If the Washington Consensus Mattered*, Morrisville, Lulu Press.

Mishra, R. 1999. *Globalisation and the Welfare state*, Cheltenham, Edward Elgar.

Mittleman, J. H. 2004. What is critical globalization studies? *International Studies Perspectives*, 5, 219–230.

Morrell, G. 2008. *Globalisation, Transnationalism and Diaspora*, London, ICAR.

Neumann, K. 2004. *Refuge Australia. Australia's Humanitarian Record*, Sydney, University of New South Wales Press Limited.

O'Doherty, K. & Lecouteur, A. 2007. 'Asylum seekers', 'boat people' and 'illegal immigrants': Social categorisation in the media. *Australian Journal of Psychology*, 59, 1.

O'Malley, P. 2008. Neoliberalism and risk in Criminology. *In:* Anthony, T. & Cunneen, C. (eds.) *The Critical Criminology Companion*. Leichhardt: Federation Press.

Parliament of Australia 2001. *Transcript of the Prime Minister The Hon John Howard MP Address at the Federal Liberal Party Campaign Launch, Sydney*; available at: http://parlinfo.aph.gov.au/parlInfo/search/display/display.w3p;query%3DId%3A%22library%2Fpartypol%2F1178395%22 [accessed 25.02.2016].

Phillips, J. 2014. A Comparison of Coalition and Labor Government Asylum Policies in Australia Since 2001, Parliament of Australia; available at: http://parlinfo.aph.gov.au/parlInfo/download/library/prspub/3024333/upload_binary/3024333.pdf;fileType=application%2Fpdf [accessed 10.12.2015].

Pickering, S. 2001. Common sense and original deviancy: News discourses and asylum seekers in Australia. *Journal of Refugee Studies*, 14, 169–186.

Ritzer, G. 2004. *The Globalization of Nothing*, Thousand Oaks, CA, Sage.

Robertson, R. 1995. Glocalization: Time-space and homogenity-heterogeneity. *In:* Featherstone, M., Lash, S. & Robertson, R. (eds.) *Global Modernities*. London, Sage.

Robinson, K. 2011. *'Helping People Through a Horrendous System'. An Examination of the Roles of Frontline Workers in Refugee Non-Government Organisations in Australia and the United Kingdom. Unpublished PhD.* University of Kent.

Robinson, K. 2014. Voices from the front line: Social work with refugees and asylum seekers in Australia and the UK. *British Journal of Social Work*, 44, 1602–1620.

Rose, N. 1996. Governing 'advanced' liberal democracies. *In:* Barry, A., Osborne, T. & Rose, N. (eds.) *Foucault and Political Reason: Liberalism, Neo-Liberalism and Rationalities of Government.* London, UCL Press.

Rose, N. 2000. Government and control. *British Journal of Criminology*, 40, 321–339.

Sales, R. 2007. *Understanding Immigration and Refugee Policy: Contradictions and Continuities*, Bristol, Policy Press.

Silverman, S. J. & Hajela, R. 2015. *Immigration Detention in the UK*, Oxford, The Migration Observatory.

Smith, M. P. 2001. *Transnational Urbanism*, Oxford, Blackwell.

Tulloch, J. & Lupton, D. 2003. *Risk and Everyday Life*, London, Sage.

UNHCR 2016. *Refugees/Migrants Emergency Response – Mediterranean*; available at: http://data.unhcr.org/mediterranean/regional.php, [accessed 25/02/2016].

Urray, J. 2002. The global complexities of September 11th. *Theory, Culture and Society*, 19, 57–69.

Zetter, R., Griffiths., D. & Sigona, N. 2005. *Refugee Community Organisations and Dispersal: Networks, Resources and Social Capital*, Bristol, Policy Press.

5 'The Humanitarian Gaze', Human Rights Films and Glocalised Social Work

Sonia Tascón

Introduction

This chapter is an attempt to explore how the concept of 'the humanitarian gaze' (Tascón 2015) may help social work educators, practitioners, and activists in their activities to promote social equality through cultural representation in a glocalised world. As moving images are used more and more to communicate and express features of our social world, the profession is now required to become adept at working within this new landscape of 'the social'. Social work scholars and practitioners are increasingly using moving images to illustrate various social issues, and for advocacy and activism. Within the work that social workers perform, the types of moving images used are often of the 'humanitarian' type. As we deploy these sorts of images, it is salient to understand their power, as images both express our social worlds but also co-opt us into their messages in distinctly immersive ways. In this chapter I turn to the discursive power of 'the humanitarian' and also to the practices of looking that emerge from such a discourse. I will argue that humanitarianism has developed as a global discourse reliant on unequal geopolitical relationships and reproduces this via a consistent feed of negative and catastrophic images of 'the other' as frozen in continuous suffering or struggling to become 'like us'; the discourse is then further reproduced through practices of looking that centre on the searching for and finding these figure types. The practices of looking that give rise to the humanitarian gaze can, however, be undone at a local level, and this is where its subversion can take place by social workers. Through a heightened awareness of the power of images social workers can act to make screening decisions that will further a relationship of equality rather than one founded on inequality.

Global-Local: Unequal Forces

Social workers are perfectly positioned to straddle the nexus between the global and the local, or the 'glocal'. This is because social workers are asked, as part of their education, to consistently and simultaneously understand the person in front of them in their private troubles, in relation to broader discourses and structures. In contemporary times, this analysis now needs to take into consideration the global dimensions (Dominelli 2010; Healy 2008). Although the term glocal was originally coined to express an economic possibility, that of permitting global markets to insert local permutations (Hong *et al.* 2010; Maynard 2003), others have applied the concept to social, cultural, and political dimensions (Porto & Belmonte 2014). That is, the term glocal has also come to be used to acknowledge that the realities of our lives are lived primarily through local existences, relationships, and experiences (Bauman 1998) as 'encumbered selves' (Webb 2003) in our physical materialities, bound to localised contexts yet all the while impacted upon by global forces that circulate ideas, goods, and services. In yet other versions of the use of the term, this is taken further to promote the local over the global as a means of overriding the powerful influences of globalising capital (Bauman 1998; de Young & Princen 2012) and its erasure of alternative political-economic models. Those involved in environmental movements are often at the forefront of the latter use of the term (Dryzek 2012), advocating for a greater emphasis on microeconomics, community organisations, and local cooperation for economic exchange and production. In effect, the latter iteration of the term is a politicised resistance of globalising forces, as this has come to be understood as a juggernaut monolithic form of neo-colonisation (Sparke 2003). In social work the tensions and contradictions inherent in local-global, as they refer to the profession, have also been extensively debated (McDonald 2006; Hugman 2010; Gray & Webb 2008; Webb 2003; Healy 2008; Dominelli 2010). Although those debates are in and of themselves significant, and also germane to this chapter, I cannot engage in any great detail in an overview of such here. What is of direct relevance is that some of the social work discussions in this realm raise similar questions to those that underpin this chapter. Namely, that once we interrogate the power dimensions of the local-global (Hugman 2010; Gray & Webb 2008; Webb 2003), we confront a disparate relationship, made manifest in many different guises and often leaving 'the local' at the mercy of the forces that enable 'the global' to be made possible. For this reason, all frameworks and structures – whether discursive or as their material practices – that attempt to construct 'universalised' or 'borderless' visions become suspect or, at the very least, require serious examination. In this chapter I take the view that the global-local relationship, or glocal, does not denote an equal relationship as the infrastructures, epistemologies, and ontological realities that are formulated by global interests are not ahistorical or apolitical, and yet are capable of re-configuring local realities in radical ways and in a variety of ways in which localities have little say. Indeed, the unequal relationship is simultaneously necessary for the continuation of the current economic-political global order and its energy source, and for this reason has been defined as a modern form of colonialism, or neo-colonialism.

In this chapter, I am concerned primarily with the ways in which the unequal power relations in the global-local are being created, circulated, and consumed as images. That is, I am assuming from the start that 'glocal' does not denote an equal relationship between global forces and local realities, as 'the global' has been a vision and a set of material realities made possible primarily through the maintenance of the inequality. For example, for the purposes of this chapter, the global circulation of information via images would not be possible without the communication technologies that could only have been developed as a result of economic and political disparities. Here, I am specifically interested in images of a 'humanitarian' ilk and in understanding how the humanitarian story, as a globalising discourse benefiting some people over others, has been generated, disseminated, and reproduced via moving images. My emphasis is on humanitarianism as a *discourse* and on one of its resultant discursive manifestations, that which configures a particular kind of relationship between image and spectator. Humanitarianism has become a way of entering into other people's spaces under the guise of helping and, as Naomi Klein and others suggest (Klein 2009; Recuber 2013), is a means of reshaping a region within the scope of a disaster in the vision of the helper. Indeed, the notion of disaster has played a key role in the procreation of the humanitarian discourse. Humanitarian images have, hence, developed certain 'watching' traditions or 'relations of looking' (Gaines 1986); what I came to term 'the humanitarian gaze' in recent research (Tascón 2015). These images reproduce a relationship that is unequal via the *assumption*, not merely the [re]presentation, of an unequal relationship between gazer-gazed (or spectator and film subject), mediated by distinct figure-types, perhaps to be considered as archetypes. But the relationship can be undone, resisted, or shifted, largely through local actions. So, here, I am proposing a type of glocal work for social workers that considers the global-local as unequal and seeks to realign it. That is, while I would always wish to acknowledge that our lived realities now incorporate many significant dimensions of the global, I also wish to propose a new politicised vision that shifts the emphasis to the local. I do this by proposing that social workers can resist the dominant global story reproduced by the humanitarian gaze, through local decisions. Social workers have the greatest opportunity to do so if they are prepared to become more knowledgeable about the power of visual images and of the dominance of visual culture in modern life.

Humanitarianism: From Discourse to Images

Humanitarianism has been, and continues to be, a powerful global discourse, largely surrounding practices of intervention in others' troubles. Much of that intervention is informed by unequal power relationships between giver and receiver, based on both economic and political factors, and premised on a form of relief that emerges from 'suffering' in conditions of immediacy and emergency (Middleton & O'Keefe 1997; Lischer 2005). Humanitarianism as an institutionalised undertaking has a lengthy history but it has mostly been associated with aid from wealthier nations or international organisations funded by wealthier nations, in times of crises as a result of natural disasters or 'man made' violence such as civil unrest, genocide, war, famine, and so on (Barnett 2011). This already begins to draw out some of the primary elements in humanitarian images; that is, the making visible of abrupt events that result in catastrophic dislocations, violence, conflict, and immense tragedy, and which can be responded to quickly, immediately, and unquestioningly. Additionally, these images are not simply of anywhere, but often of 'poor … parts of the world' (Sontag 2004, p. 65). This reinforces a perception that some regions are problem-saturated while others have 'no such problems' (Laber 2002, p. 100).[1] This view then 'cannot help but nourish the belief in the inevitability of tragedy in the benighted or backward – that is, poor – parts of the world' (Sontag 2004, p. 65).

As human troubles are disseminated worldwide as images, they tend to arrive as news items. Michael Barnett (2011), tracing the history of humanitarianism, draws the direct connection between the growth in humanitarianism as a profession, and news. These images are distributed

> by twenty-four hour news agencies, the world could now watch the horrific spectacles of state failure and civil war, ethnic cleansing and genocide, the use of children as soldiers capable of committing war crimes, and the flight of people from all forms of violence, only to find "safety" in city-sized refugee camps without adequate food, shelter or medical care
>
> (Barnett 2011, p. 2).

Human troubles 'elsewhere' are then equated with images of violence or disaster; emergencies or catastrophic situations of deprivation and displacement; war, unrest, and genocide; but also longer-standing social evils such as sex trafficking. While sex trafficking represents a set of social ills that are not immediate emergencies, the moral panic with which it is often greeted adds it to the list of 'horrific' spectacles. News items tend to be reliant on the easy and quick consumption of events; their immediacy, drama, and conflict is their stock of trade. As two social work scholars state:

> News reports play a large role in our lives. Stories of crime and deviant behaviour, in particular, provide a significant part of those news reports. Grabosky and Wilson (1989) suggest that issues of crime and criminal justice attract so much attention because such reporting is full of drama, involves life and property, and the frightening power to deprive a person of liberty
>
> (Goddard & Saunders 2001, p. 14).

News stories are immediate and constant, fast-paced bits of information, and thus rely on their ready association with and consumption of dominant discourses for their effect. This often produces information that is unidimensional and unnuanced, often reducing events to readily consumable 'bites', reliant on stereotypes and easy labels. Films, in contrast to news items, enable greater complexity to emerge, even while also reliant on dominant discourses for their meanings and interpretations. Films can more fully 'flesh' out complexity and ambiguity. For example, film portrayals of social workers can be kinder and more multifaceted than those of news stories (Henderson & Franklin 2007). And yet, social work scholars writing in this area (of visual representation) continue to feel under attack, even when discussing film representations of social workers (Valentine & Freeman 2002; Freeman & Valentine 2004; Edmonson & King 2016), something that I seriously question (Tascón, unpublished). Part of the reason may simply be that social workers have not developed a close understanding of the diversity of media and how each operates. But it is also very likely due to the overemphasis on news media as the primary source for the profession to evaluate its own public status (Aldridge 1990; Franklin & Parton 1991; Ayre 2001; Mendes 2001; Reid & Misener 2001; Cree *et al.* 2013; Barns 2016; Brindle 2016). News media are not kind to any profession, if complexity is being sought to measure 'kindness'. Understanding these differences in media may help social work practitioners recognise that the oft-expressed complaint that the profession is not well represented in the media (Barns 2016) is not altogether well founded.

Much of the humanitarian discourse has been developed with, and through, images to illustrate and cement its power. And these images have been, largely, of disaster-laden peoples, frozen in their tragedies, on whom the assumed relatively affluent, comfortable, and privileged viewer will act. In what follows, I want to very briefly glean some key aspects of what I came to term 'the humanitarian gaze' (Tascón 2015, 2016), as I studied human rights film festivals (HRFFs). The humanitarian gaze outlines a set of features/figures that either appear on screen, or are expected to appear, and help to explain the inequality of global-local in the relations of looking that have developed through and with humanitarian images.

The Humanitarian Gaze: Key Figures

The concept of 'the gaze'[2] in images was originally coined by Laura Mulvey as 'the male gaze' (Mulvey 1975), to propose that the production of images and their reception are primarily filtered by an assumed male spectator that co-opts non-male viewers into its scope. When we discuss images about other people's troubles, however, a slightly different, while related, set of dynamics requires consideration. In this realm it is not simply gender that informs the humanitarian gaze as a *practice* of looking (Sturken & Cartwright 2009) but also global power relations as they have been shaped by various historical and contemporary forces. The humanitarian gaze positions some to look at others' troubles, with the expectation that the gaze will not be returned, at least not in the same manner. It is not a reciprocal gaze.

The humanitarian gaze is a surveilling gaze (Foucault 1978). It is one that seeks to retain the unequal relationship between gazer and gazed, and binds them in a continuous loop of inequality. It performs this function primarily as a panoptical effect (Foucault 1977), in which unrestricted access is given to the gazer over the gazed while reducing the gazed's possibilities to a set of limited behaviours. This is made manifest at every stage in the production, selection, and reception of humanitarian films,[3] but primarily via two distinct mechanisms: by producing a limited representational scope for those who are being gazed at (the film subject, but also usually 'the other' of the audience), and permitting greater agency to the gazer. What I mean by 'gazer' is not necessarily the immediate audience, but an *assumed* spectator. In the case of humanitarian films, the assumed audience is often the powerful, affluent Westerner. That is, the surveilling humanitarian gaze will produce and reproduce an unequal relationship between assumed gazer and gazed, often by reducing the film subject to a humanitarian object while simultaneously conferring unequal agency to the assumed viewer/gazer.[4] In this relationship, it is an assumed privileged viewer that is being addressed and needs to be included in the very act of creating the images.

The reduction in the representational register for the film subject, transforming them into a humanitarian *object* – here I call them humanitarian archetypes – is carried out through a manoeuvre that limits them to two primary possibilities: abject victim and/or freedom fighter. These two figures exist, furthermore, largely to regulate the complexity of 'the other's' portrayal while simultaneously conferring, furthering, and cementing the authority of the gazer or the intended spectators of the humanitarian object.

The 'victim' archetype is primarily silent and/or is spoken about and for through either the filmmaker – in voice-over, for example – or given little voice and presence in the film itself. This film subject is often limited to the tragedy that motivates the filmmaker to make the film in the first instance, and is often portrayed as either paralysed in their plight or purely a function of that trouble. Their subjectivity is thus reduced to a unidimensional field of vision, of tragedy, coupled with limited or paralysed agency.[5] In this representational figure there is the highest possibility for the assumed viewer to 'act for'. The 'freedom fighter' is one that is permitted a greater range of agency, although still almost entirely bound to the tragedy that motivates them to fight. This figure is, however, still subsumed within the discursive field of the humanitarian gaze by virtue of needing to have the struggle filtered for its assumed viewer. In this sense, the freedom that is being fought for needs to be one that the [assumed] viewer will recognise as valid. There are a number of examples of such films from research I carried out on HRFFs (Tascón 2015, 2016), including Pamela Yates' *Granito: How to Nail a Dictator* (2011), but the best one that illustrates this phenomenon was the screening of Iranian filmmaker Tanaz Eshaghian's *Love Crimes of Kabul* (2011) at the Human Rights Watch International Film Festival in 2011. Although I have closely described and analysed this film elsewhere, briefly how I became aware of this archetype was by what took place at the festival. At that time, the festival applied the figure of the freedom fighter in its description of the film, clearly to appeal to its audiences, and yet the film resembled that description in very few ways. Instead of 'banding together' as 'fighters for freedom' and 'self-determination' (Film Society Lincoln Centre online), as the festival described, the film subjects were on display as full of agency and cunning in their 'criminal' acts, in most cases having committed them knowingly or for their own gain and in one case having manipulated the arrests (of herself and the boy by whom she was pregnant) to put pressure on others to gain what she wanted. The individuals on the screen were shown as devious, ambiguous, and fraught individuals who did not band together other than in brief friendship as they were thrown together in prison. That dynamic led the audience to be disconcerted and to interrogate the filmmaker as to her 'intent'; this is when I became aware of this dimension of the humanitarian gaze. This figure's primary function is to permit greater agency to the 'other' on the screen, but only insofar as it is drawing closer to the norms and values of the assumed viewer. The description worked through a cultural framework that assumes the *individual* as an ideal subjectivity ('self-determination'), whose morality is organised individually rather than collectively but whose political agency is to be collective in order to overturn their 'society's norms'; this, in order for the individuals to reach a new moral goal, one resembling the assumed viewer's moral world.

Concurrently, the assumed privileged viewer is bestowed with an unequalled range of possibilities, and this has been expressed by the associated discussions of 'distant suffering' (Boltanski 1999; Chouliaraki 2006; Borer 2012) and 'compassion fatigue' (Moeller 1999); both of these discussions signal that the assumed viewer of the humanitarian spectacle has the possibility to enter and withdraw from the scene of pain at will (Sontag 2004; Hesford 2011; Chouliaraki 2006, 2013), or is to be mobilized through coercive or manipulative means to act (Keenan 2004). That is, the entire realm of discussions that the term 'distant suffering' refers to has named the relationship of which I write above as occurring between a 'suffering' screen subject and a 'distant' viewer. The distance occurs not only as a result of the mediated nature of the relationship (through a screen), but also because the mediation is always already sociocultural. The discussions on 'compassion fatigue' assumes a privileged viewer whose attention will be sought and exhausted; a very real effect, but one that does not alter the relationship on which this analysis relies. Although these analyses have been extremely useful in outlining the unequal relationship in gazer/gazed, I do seriously question the terms of the discourse as, by naming the relationship this way, they paralyse the film subject in 'suffering', with the privileged gazer at their distance. My critique of this is based on the fact that there is a third figure that appears in humanitarian films, and within this one is the seeds of hope for a different relationship, one that can be used by social work educators and practitioners as they make their film selections.

Although largely confined to film subjects from the filmmakers' own (broadly-defined) cultural and social world, the third figure that appears in humanitarian films tends to portray greater complexity and active agency and would appear to stand outside the logic of the humanitarian discursive contract. This is mostly because the relationship that is created between assumed viewer and film subject in these sorts of films is of a [more] equal recognition, one that plays to the complexity of the film subjects, even if this means portrayals of ambiguously positioned characters on the moral scale. These characters are usually activists, whose methods may sometimes be questioned, but not their motives. I recall one film, in particular, *Better This World* (2011), at the New York HRFF in 2011, about a couple of eco-activists living in the United States who are incited and then entrapped into a set of dangerous activities by a 'planted' member of the group, who then uses the evidence to have them convicted of terrorist acts. The film was described as a 'story of idealism, loyalty and betrayal' by the festival (Human Rights Watch International Film Festival online). There are many other examples of films that were screened at either the New York Human Rights Watch International Film Festival or the Buenos Aires' Festival Internacional de Cine de Derechos Humanos of films of this ilk. Outstanding in this category were *The Yes*

Men (2005) and the sequel *The Yes Men Fix the World* (2009), about hacktivists in the United States whose humorous and outrageous antics in penetrating large corporations and organisations led to much attention to the organisations' violations. At the Buenos Aires festival, this category of films forms the bulk of their programming, as they rely mostly on local and regional cinemas but particularly Argentine productions (Argentine cinema is one of the most significant and vibrant in South America, but other nations also produce a small number of their own films). The best example of such films at the Buenos Aires festival was the large number of Pino Solanas films screened there. Solanas was one of the founders of the political cinematic movement Third Cinema in the 1970s, one that went on to have global influence (Pine & Willemen 1989). This movement sought to emphasise local cinemas, in opposition to large and powerful 'global' cinemas such as Hollywood and European avant-garde cinemas, to facilitate local stories that reflect their peoples' lived experiences and issues.

The active, complex figure is not necessarily a standalone one, and can easily appear in co-existence with the other two in humanitarian films. This will often occur where the powerful Western activist is given prominence as the active agent, and poor 'others' are given subsidiary roles or appear largely in order to give substance and status to the main Western protagonist. The best example of this film was *The Day After Peace* (2008),[6] a film that we screened at the 2007 Australian Human Rights Arts and Film Festival. But there are many others, such as *Granito: How to Nail a Dictator* (2011), as mentioned above.

Undoing the Global Disparity: Local Social Work Practices

How do we, as social work educationists and practitioners, avoid reproducing the unequal global relationship promulgated by humanitarianism and the gaze that accompanies it? I believe that it will require a much more nuanced knowledge of visual communication by the profession than we currently possess. This will enable us to tap into debates and issues that have been part of media and film studies for a significant time, especially in relation to the reception of images (Staiger 2005). Something that social workers already have is an interest in human relationships, and in this chapter I have been asking the profession to consider the [power] relationship extant in the discourse of humanitarianism and the images it has given rise to. I believe that this unequal global relationship can be 'undone' on the basis of programming alone.[7] That is, we can make a significant contribution to subverting the humanitarian gaze by maintaining a critically analytical stance when making film/visual image selections to those that shift the relationship towards greater equality and respect between assumed viewer and film subject. We can do this by considering our selections along four different planes.

Fair Programming: Glocal Social Work

In order to construct an alternative path for the global power relations extant in the humanitarian gaze, local action needs to be given prominence. For social workers/researchers, educators, and professionals in social work this means a heightened awareness of the fact that images encode cultural power as much as any other form of communication, written or oral, and that humanitarian images enact a particular type of power. Although many films reproduce this power, appealing to a powerful spectator by further entrenching that privilege, there are also many films that enact the relationship differently. In this section, I outline four dimensions for glocal social work educators/practitioners/activists to consider in their selections of films/visual images, but also one in relation to the context of viewing.

The Film Subject

Within this theme, social workers need to ask themselves who the subject on the screen is and what is intended for their presence on that screen. What kind of subject is being presented to you? Is it a 'suffering' subject, with little resources of their own to enact change? This may be for good reasons, but are you being given this unidimensionality in order to harness your pity? And does this unidimensionality also then co-exist with the presentation of them as 'noble'? One of the most common pitfalls for social workers and activists is to think that we need subjects that are absolutely helpless as well as perfect in their helplessness before we can move in to assist. This is akin to the application and continuation of the 'deserving' and 'undeserving' categories. Can we not still assist someone who is flawed, imperfect, and with complex dimensions, but who still requires our helpful solidarity? Do we need to have helplessness reflected to us on the screen in order to harness our solidarity? Also, do they need to be fighting for 'our things', or things we believe in? Or is it possible to select films that display things that we can learn from them? *Love Crimes of Kabul* (2011) was a film that showed the resilience and strength of some women in Afghanistan and stood as a corrective to the many films that draw the figure of the oppressed Muslim Woman, as part of an Orientalist discourse (Said 1978), in order to show Occidental Woman her superiority. Could we select films to admire, join with, or support those who may, for example, wish to draw on us for assistance with issues that are important to them but not necessarily to us? For example: Not to promote a day of international peace, but to expulse foreign corporations in their region? For example: To help local women to continue to wear the shador in Western countries as a reassertion of their distinct identity? Are we prepared to select films that show the strength, audacity, and innovation of 'others', and that show the locals mobilising; to show what is already being done, for example, and how the audience can assist, but on the terms of those on the screen? How prepared are we to also submit ourselves to the analysis of the privilege we possess? That is, can we, and will we, select films that both implicate our localities within the global power structures that dispossess others and, further, promote their strengths, resiliences, and cleverness above our own? In effect, what I search for is that we eventually seek only images that promote equality between film subject and assumed viewer – in a stance of solidarity – and that where images show us the inequality, we do not use this for our own advantage and further our privilege.

The Intended Audience

As part of this dimension, we need to ask about the production process. That is, who produced the film? Who directed it, and what is the intended audience? A usual indication of this will be the language in which the film is made, or the language that is predominantly used. This will give us a great deal of information about the intended audience, although it is not the full picture, of course. Undoing the globally powerful humanitarian gaze requires giving conscious consideration and emphasis to local productions, as films and visual images are cultural products and stories that are 'encumbered' (Webb 2003) within particular locations geographically, culturally, temporally, politically, and economically. Within this theme I would ask that social workers – whether they be social work scholars, in research, education and/or in professional activities or activism – where possible, search for and select images produced by people that live that experience. While this is not to suggest that filmmakers from 'outside' an issue/lived experience have nothing to say, we need to be fostering and furthering the storytelling from 'within'. As I noted above, it is often those films made by those 'within' (*The Yes Men*, 2005; *Love Crimes of Kabul*, 2011; *The Day After Peace*, 2008), but also selected for consumption by the same group, that will permit the greatest range of complex behaviours to be displayed and understood. Clearly this speaks to social workers to find film narratives from within the localities in which they are screening. In Australia, for example, this means selecting from the ever-growing number of productions by excellent Indigenous filmmakers such as Warwick Thornton, whose evocative film *Samson and Delilah* (2009), his first feature film, won the prestigious Cannes Festival Camera D'Or in the same year. There are also many other examples of the same excellence within every nation's indigenous and local groups.

Relationship Between Viewer and Film Subject

In this area, we need to then put the two above topics together and consider the 'unsaid'. That is, every film/image has been constructed with a particular relationship in mind, whether it be commercial or, in the cases I have been considering, a humanitarian one to show us other people's troubles to harness our helping impulse. Embedded within the image is also a set of power relationships that are already part of our sociocultural worlds; images deploy these knowledges in order to make meaning available to you, and with images they do so easily, quickly, and readily. As social workers concerned with social justice and human rights, we need to watch and select images/films that are less about trying to 'plead' to an affluent viewer to intervene on grounds that are familiar to that viewer's terms of reference and are more based on Hannah Arendt's politics of justice. That pleading cements the privilege of the intended viewer, while a film that asserts a human right, as a claim to our very humanity, is a claim made on the grounds of justice. Now, I am aware that, in apparent contradiction to the discussion above, where I ask for local storytelling to be given prominence, notions of justice that appeal to a global humanity transcend localities. And perhaps this is where the new glocal needs to be built, through notions of justice that truly equally distribute, recognise, capacitate, and share resources, wealth, stories, and privilege (Schlosberg 2007). I believe that the current collection of environmental films is beginning to show us the way in overcoming the globally unequal relationship embedded in images. I am specifically thinking about films screened recently at the Australian HRFF, particularly one at the 2016 festival called *Land Grabbing* (2015). In this film, produced by an Austrian filmmaker, a situation in which we are all made complicit – the displacement of indigenous peoples for the mass production of foods for the affluent world – is exposed, as well as the mobilisation of local peoples to claim their rights; in one case, at least, successfully. Films about the environment have begun to depict the wisdom and strength of Indigenous peoples throughout the globe and the suspect role of the privileged West's economic system in bringing about its troubles. These films transgress the usual social and global hierarchies and crisscross the power of the humanitarian gaze by positioning a traditional 'other' as holding the solutions and the powerful West as complicit in this looming catastrophe. Films about environmental activism need to form part of social work education more centrally, both for their creation of a new type of gazing, but also as a topic that is truly a glocal issue.

Context of Screening

I introduce this fourth aspect here, although I have given it scant attention above, because it is actually quite important in this context. The possibility of the subversion of the humanitarian gaze is heightened in a context of viewing that enables further conversations. For example, activist film festivals are renowned for their difference to other festivals for the traditional, and often mandatory, inclusion of post-screening panel discussions. These discussions enrich the images through further thought and elaboration of the meanings of the images. Media scholars dealing with the 'spectacle of suffering' in news coverage, where much of the theoretical discussion of 'distant suffering' has taken place, have, since Boltanski's (1999) investigation, complexified the field by exploring various contextual and viewing factors and how these change spectators' perspectives and responses (Scott 2014; Ong 2014; Cameron & Seu 2012). One study in particular noted that the length of time given to a topic produces greater audience responsiveness (Scott 2014), for example, documentary films versus time-limited news coverage. This demonstrates that time and space of reception have an effect on the way that spectators absorb the material with which they are confronted. This has clear relevance for social work, but not necessarily that festivals be organised every time in order to provide sufficient time for the discussion and exploration of issues. More saliently, this suggests that sufficient time and thought are given to the selection and post-screening discussions of the visual material used. I would go further and plead that the profession acquires a level of expertise and sophistication in reading visual images, especially as these are becoming more and more part of our social worlds. If we continue to treat visual images instrumentally, reducing them to raw tools for the demonstration of social issues, we fail to note their power to both express the hierarchies present in our social worlds but also to reproduce the hierarchies across the globe as they navigate and cross political and cultural borders.

Concluding Comments

Armed with this knowledge, social work practitioners, scholars, or activists, using films or other visual images for their teaching, illustrations, and activism, can make more informed and thoughtful selections. We seek, after all, to promote the interests of the very figures that are often portrayed in humanitarian films. When doing so, purposely selecting films that will not use the abject victim is vital, as well as purposely seeking the third figure of actor with mobilising agency, even when acknowledging their troubles. This is to construct a new relationship at the local level, overlaying it on one that has been built up over a long time through catastrophic news stories and a global relationship of power that has been severely unequal. What we need to do is rebuild the relationships both globally and locally, but possibly more productively through local film selections that acknowledge global power inequalities. This is to reconstruct the relationship of gazer and gazed built on solidarity and equality. That is, to make selections of films or other images where we ask ourselves, before the selection, what it is we are attempting to do with the screening: whose interests, whose needs and how are they represented; whose strengths and weaknesses; what response we are hoping for, and so on; but also to enable sufficient discussion to take place after the screenings.

We need to become much more sophisticated in the reading of images than we have been in research, education, and activism, and as a profession, in order to do this respectfully. Those film subjects are people, after all, and not mere objects for our needs. Yes, they are images, and in the powerful West we have become used to those images equating to entertainment, performance, and mediated distance, which leads to the belief that we can walk in and out of those stories and human lives as into and out of the cinema. In many other cinematic traditions, visual images are understood as encoding political action and interaction. For example, in Latin American cinema and particularly Argentine cinema, politics and social issues are never distant from the screen production, even when intended to entertain; politics and entertainment are inextricably part of each other (Lusnich & Piedras 2009). And in Third Cinema, which originated in Latin America (Getino & Solanas 1969) but went on to influence many other cinematic traditions worldwide (Pine & Willemen 1989), there is a requirement that films be constructed to enable discussion and interaction. Films are powerful, but we need to fully understand their power and political potential to be part of the global-local as we are permeated more and more by visual culture.

Notes

1 This was a comment made by an early founder of Human Rights Watch about the United States, as they set out to monitor the USSR's fulfilment of the Helsinki Accords of 1975.

2 The concept actually emerges from Lacan's (1988) notion of the gaze, but is applied for the first time by Mulvey to images.
3 Much of this discussion emerged from empirical research carried out in relation to human rights films and film festivals, and is fully fleshed out by Tascón (2015).
4 These two terms are not the same, as 'gazer' encompasses the power dimension within it much more than the term 'viewer' does. I have decided to use them interchangeably here, purely for convenience's sake, as in broader usage the two can be seen as the same.
5 Although there are a number of examples from films for this abject victim, the clearest is Jeremy Gilley's 2007 *Peace One Day*, about which I say more below. I have also written about this film elsewhere and I turn the reader to that, if interested (Tascón 2012, 2015, 2016).
6 I have had much to say about this film elsewhere, as it was the one that set me off on my current film research. I turn the reader's attention to those extensive analyses, if interested: Tascón 2012, 2015, 2016.
7 This is, actually, in keeping with my findings in the human rights film festivals I studied, where almost no films that present the abject victim figure were screened; one of the few exceptions was *The Day After Peace* (2008). I believe this to have been a deliberate decision by the festivals, although there was a wavering between the 'freedom fighter' and 'the active, complex agent'.

References

Aldridge, M 1990, 'Social work and the news media: A hopeless case?', *British Journal of Social Work*, vol. 20, no. 6, pp. 611–625.
Ayre, P 2001, 'Child protection and the media: Lessons from the last three decades', *The British Journal of Social Work*, vol. 31, pp. 887–901.
Barns, J 2016, 'Social workers need a voice to champion the vital work that we do', *The Guardian* 16 March 2016. Available from: <http://www.theguardian.com/social-care-network/social-life-blog/2016/mar/16/social-workers-need-voice-community-group>. [20 May 2016].
Barnett, M 2011, *Empire of Humanity: A History of Humanitarianism*, Cornell University Press, New York.
Bauman, Z 1998, *Globalisation: The Human Consequences*, Columbia University Press, New York.
Better This World 2011, (DVD), Public Broadcasting Service, United States.
Boltanski, L 1999, *Distant Suffering: Morality, Media, and Politics*, Cambridge University Press, Cambridge.
Borer, TA 2012, *Media, Mobilization, and Human Rights: Mediating Suffering*, Zed Books., London, New York.
Brindle, D 2016, 'The state of social work: Unity and leadership are needed', *The Guardian* 16 March 2016. Available from: <http://www.theguardian.com/social-care-network/2016/mar/15/social-work-leadership-is-needed>. [20 May 2016].
Cameron, L & Seu, B 2012, 'Landscapes of empathy: Spatial scenarios, metaphors and metonymies in responses to distant suffering', *Talk Text*, vol. 32, no. 3, pp. 281–305.
Chouliaraki, L 2006, *The Spectatorship of Suffering*, Sage, London.
Chouliaraki, L 2013, *The Ironic Spectator: Solidarity in an Age of Post-Humanitarianism*, Wiley Publishing, New Jersey.
Cree, VE, Clapton, G & Smith, M 2013, 'Moral panics and social work: Towards a sceptical view of UK child protection', *Critical Social Policy*, vol. 33, no. 2, pp. 197–217.

De Young, R & Princen, T (eds) 2012, *The Localization Reader: Adapting to the Coming Downshift*, MIT Press, Cambridge, London.

Dominelli, L 2010, 'Globalization, contemporary challenges and social work practice', *International Social Work*, vol. 53, no. 5, pp. 599–612.

Dryzek, JS 2012, 'Ecological Democracy', in *The Localization Reader: Adapting to the Coming Downshift*, eds R de Young & T Princen, MIT Press, Cambridge, London, pp. 243–256.

Edmondson, D & King, M 2016, 'The childcatchers: An exploration of the representations and discourses of social work in UK film and television drama from the 1960s to the present day', *Journal of Social Work*, vol. 16, no. 6, pp. 1–18.

Love Crimes of Kabul 2011, (DVD), Home Box Office, United States.

Film Society Lincoln Centre 2011, 'Human Rights Watch Film Festival 2011: Love Crimes of Kabul', Available from: <https://www.filmlinc.org/films/love-crimes-of-kabul/>. [13 June 2016].

Franklin, B & Parton, N 1991, *Social Work, the Media and Public Relations*, Routledge, London.

Freeman, ML & Valentine, DP 2004, 'Through the eyes of Hollywood: Images of social workers in film', *Social Work*, vol. 49, no. 2, pp. 151–161.

Foucault, M 1977, *Discipline and Punish: The Birth of the Prison*, Pantheon, New York

Foucault, M 1978, *The History of Sexuality*, Random House, New York.

Gaines, J 1986, 'White privilege and looking relations: Race and gender in feminist film theory', *Cultural Critique*, vol. 4, pp. 59–79.

Getino, O & Solanas, F 1969, 'Toward a third cinema', *Tricontinental*, no. 14, pp. 107–132,

Goddard, C & Saunders, BJ 2001, 'Child abuse and the media', *NCPC Issues Australian Institute of Family Studies*, no. 14, pp. 1–24. Available from: <https://aifs.gov.au/cfca/publications/child-abuse-and-media>. [19 May 2016].

Granito: How to Nail a Dictator 2011, (DVD), Public Broadcasting Service, United States.

Gray, M & Webb, S 2008, 'The myth of global social work: Double standards and the local-global divide', *Journal of Progressive Human Services*, vol. 19, no. 1, pp. 61–66.

Healy, L 2008, 'Exploring the history of social work as a human rights profession', *International Social Work*, vol. 51, no. 6, pp. 735–748.

Henderson, L & Franklin, B 2007, 'Sad not bad: Images of social care professionals in popular UK television drama, *Journal of Social Work*, vol. 7, no. 2, pp. 133–153

Hesford, W 2011, *Spectacular Rhetorics: Human Rights Visions, Recognitions, Feminisms*, Duke University Press, North Carolina.

Hong, P, Young, P & Song, IH 2010, 'Glocalization of social work practice: Global and local responses to globalization', *International Social Work*, vol. 53, no. 5, pp. 656–670.

Hugman, R 2010, 'Towards a borderless social work: Reconsidering notions of international social work', *International Social Work*, vol 53, no. 5, pp. 629–643.

Human Rights Watch International Film Festival 'The 2011 Human Rights Watch Film Festival', Available from: <https://www.hrw.org/news/2011/05/13/2011-human-rights-watch-film-festival>. [13 May 2016].

Keenan, T 2004, 'Mobilizing shame', *South Atlantic Quarterly*, vol. 103, no. 2–3, pp. 435–449.

Klein, N 2009, *The Shock Doctrine: The Rise of Disaster Capitalism*, Knopf, Canada.

Laber, J 2002, *The Courage of Strangers: Coming of Age With the Human Rights Movement*, Public Affairs, New York.

Lacan, J 1988, *The Seminar. Book II. The Ego in Freud's Theory and in the Technique of Psychoanalysis*, trans. S Tomaselli, Cambridge University Press, Cambridge.

Land Grabbing 2015, (DVD), Outlook Filmsales, Austria.

Lischer, SK 2005, *Dangerous Sanctuaries: Refugee Camps, Civil War and the Dilemmas of Humanitarian Aid*, Cornell University Press, New York.

Lusnich, AL & Piedras, P 2009, *Una Historia del Cine Político y Social en Argentina. Formas, Estilos y Registros (1896–1969)*, Nueva Librería, Buenos Aires.

McDonald, C 2006, *Challenging Social Work: Institutional Contexts of Practice*, Palgrave Macmillan, Basingstoke.

Maynard, ML 2003, 'From global to local: How Gillette's sensor excel accommodates to Japan', *Keio Communucation Review*, vol. 25, pp. 57–75.

Mendes, P 2001, 'Blaming the messenger', *Australian Social Work*, vol. 54, pp. 27–36.

Middleton, N & O'Keefe, P 1997, *Disaster and Development: The Politics of Humanitarian Aid*, Pluto Press, London.

Moeller, S 1999, *Compassion Fatigue: How the Media Sell Disease, Famine, War and Death*, Routledge, New York.

Mulvey, L 1975, 'Visual pleasure and narrative cinema', *Screen*, vol. 16, pp. 6–18.

Ong, JC 2014, '"Witnessing" or "mediating" distant suffering? Ethical questions across moments of text, production and reception', *Television & New Media*, vol. 15, no. 3, pp. 179–196.

Pine, J & Willemen, P 1989, *Questions of Third Cinema*, BFI Publications, London.

Porto, MD & Belmonte, IA 2014, 'From local to global: Visual strategies of glocalisation in digital storytelling', *Language & Communication*, vol. 39, pp. 14–23.

Recuber, T 2013, 'Disaster Porn!', *Contexts*, vol. 12, no. 2, pp. 20–33.

Reid WJ, & Misener E 2001, 'Social work in the press: A crossnational study', *International Journal of Social Welfare*, vol. 10, pp. 194–201

Samson and Delilah 2009, (DVD), Madman Entertainment, Australia.

Said, E 1978, *Orientalism*, Pantheon, United States.

Schlosberg, D 2007, *Defining Environmental Justice*, Oxford University Press, New York.

Scott, M 2014, 'The mediation of distant suffering: An empirical contribution beyond television news texts', *Media, Culture & Society*, vol. 36, no. 1, pp. 3–19.

Sontag, S 2004, *Regarding the Pain of Others*, Picador, United Kingdom.

Sparke, M 2003, 'American empire and globalisation: Postcolonial speculations on neocolonial enframing', *Singapore Journal of Tropical Geography*, vol. 24, iss. 3, pp. 373–389.

Staiger, J 2005, *Media Reception Studies*, New York University Press, New York.

Sturken, M & Cartwright, L 2009, *Practices of Looking: An Introduction to Visual Culture*, Oxford University Press, Oxford.

Tascón, SM 2012, 'Considering human rights films, representation, and ethics: Whose face?', *Human Rights Quarterly*, vol. 34, no. 3, pp. 864–883.

Tascón, SM 2015, *Human Rights Film Festivals: Activism in Context*, Palgrave Macmillan, United Kingdom.

Tascón, SM 2017, 'Watching others' troubles: Revisiting "The Film Act", and spectatorship in activist film festivals', in *Activist Film Festivals: Towards a Political Subject*, Intellect, United Kingdom.

Tascón, SM (unpublished), 'Looking at social work: Nuancing understandings of portrayals of the profession in news and films'.

The Day After Peace 2008, (DVD), Warner Music, United States.

The Yes Men 2005, (DVD), Home Box Office, United States.

The Yes Men Fix the World 2009, (DVD) Home Box Office, United States.

Valentine, DP & Freeman, ML 2002, 'Film portrayals of social workers doing child welfare work', *Child and Adolescent Social Work Journal*, vol. 19, no. 6, pp. 455–470.

Webb, S 2003, 'Local orders and global chaos in social work'. *European Journal of Social Work*, vol. 6, no. 2, pp. 191–204.

Part II

Methodological Re-Shaping and Spatial Transgression in Glocalised Social Work

6 'What We Learn How to See'

A Politics of Location and Situated Writing in Glocalised Social Work

Mona Livholts

Feminist objectivity is about limited location and situated knowledge [...] It allows us to become answerable for what we learn how to see. [...] The eyes made available in modern technological vision science shatter any idea of passive visions; these prosthetic devices [sic] show us that all eyes, including our own organic ones, are active perceptual systems, building on translation and specific *ways* of seeing, that is, *ways* of life.

(Haraway 1988, p. 583)

Feministisk objektivitet innebär en begränsad platsspecifik position och situerad kunskap. [...] Den lär oss att bli ansvariga för vad vi lär oss att se. [...] De ögon som gjorts tillgängliga med hjälp av den moderna teknologiska vetenskapen omöjliggör varje idé om ett passivt synfält; dessa protetiska uppfinningar visar oss att alla ögon, inkluderat våra egna organiska, är aktiva system för vår uppfattningsförmåga som bygger på översättning och specifika <u>sätt</u> att se, det vill säga, <u>sätt</u> att leva.

(My translation from English to Swedish: Haraway 1988, p. 583. Underlining corresponds to the italics in the original text)

Some windows allow more sight than others. Her grandmother's window was designed as a triangle, bravely sticking out from the brick body of the house. In her early teenage years she spent a lot of time in her grandmother's flat and would often sit by the window and watch [...]

Watching silence.

There was not much to see, yet sameness seems to be a very good starting point for imagination.

This is how I describe a location from which I could see 'the world' as a young girl (Livholts 2010b, p. 105). The story is intended as much to account for the architecture of the house as it is for people, sounds, objects, (day)dreams and imagination. Indeed, seeing and seeing again are rarely the same thing, and this continues throughout a lifetime. In this chapter, I make use of the metaphorical expression 'what we learn how to see' as a point of departure to think and re-think, shape and re-shape, locate and re-locate ourselves and our knowledge base for glocalised social work. In her influential essay from the late 1980s, Haraway argues that researchers need to become accountable for 'what we learn how to see', '*vad vi lär oss att se*'[1] (Haraway 1988, p. 583). Learning to see is actively created through a politics of location '*politisk lokalisering*', an embodied and spatial process by which seeing is shaped and re-shaped through translation, '*översättning*'. Haraway suggests that specific ways of seeing are equivalent to 'ways of life', '*sätt att leva*'. Thus, epistemological questions such as: Who can know? What is it possible to know? What counts as legitimate knowledge? Who can write? What is it possible to write? What counts as legitimate writing? can be understood as processes of negotiating personal and intellectual positions in historical and geopolitical contexts (see, for example, hooks 1989; Richardson 1997; Mohanty 2003; Livholts 2012).

In the introduction to this volume, we (the editors, Livholts & Bryant) have argued that one of the aims of the book is to extend the reach of social work to understand lives which are increasingly subject to glocal influences, and that glocalisation is useful as a theoretical and methodological framework for social work. Taking these questions further in this chapter, I argue that the glocalisation of social issues and the responses from social work call for a politics of location in social work research, education and professional practice. De los Reyes (2011, p. 33) employs the expression 'the power to remain ignorant', '*makten att vara okunnig*', to describe a position occupied by privileged selves, and refers to the need to problematise such a position of power. This means taking into consideration forms of knowledge that question established images of the world and challenge categorisations, stereotypes and fixed understandings of people and locations. De los Reyes (2011, p. 33) talks about 'epistemological disobedience', '*epistemologisk olydnad*', as a way to seek an alternative consciousness. I argue that such a critical stance is central for social work to create a knowledge base that promotes accountability and theoretical lenses and methodological tools that promote social equality and social justice. I would like to situate myself through a set of overlapping ideas that are central to shaping the content of this chapter, inspired by my previous work on the politics of location (Livholts 2015a). Firstly, I suggest that a politics of location in glocalised social work is geopolitically and historically grounded and contextualised in (post)colonial relations of power. Secondly, that a glocalised methodology makes use of intersectional analysis to bring into focus the 'unseen', the tensions and dynamics between oppression and privilege. The researcher's position too is characterised by shifting and multiple locations and knowledges in time and space; therefore, thirdly, I include the often-overlooked issue of writing '*skrivande*' as an epistemological, embodied, geopolitically and spatially situated practice imbued with relations of power that shape knowledge.

Historical and Geopolitical Locations: Re-Creating Epistemological Spaces

Feminist and postcolonial scholars remind us that epistemological questions are bound to particular locations within a global perspective and intimately intertwined with institutional relations of power, local practice and self and othering. Loomba's (1998) analysis of colonialism and knowledge shows how, historically, dominant ideologies of race and gender have denied subordinated groups the status of subjects of knowledge conducted by a science that claimed neutrality and objectivity. Connell (2007) addresses social science as an embodied practice which is organised through colonial power. The production of knowledge is focused on particular groups, people and institutional settings in rich countries. From a global perspective, Connell (2007, p. ix) states that 'data-gathering and application happen in the colony, while theorising happens in the metropole'. Rose (1997, p. 315) emphasises how institutional practices are shaped through particular cultural practices in academic life. Doing research is a process of becoming through a number of choices about questions, theoretical framing and methods. Writing, supervision, publishing and seminar audiences create social relations and structures of knowledge which actively contribute to creating gender, class, race and sexuality. A glocalised methodology for social work strives to decolonise knowledge and take into account the spatialities of the researcher, the research subject and the academic university culture. Central to the creation of such a culture is the critique and transformation of the internationalisation of research and it is essential to move away from a methodological nationalism that focuses on limited and specific dominant methodologies. Gobo (2011) points towards an emerging need to develop postcolonial methodologies that are culturally flexible and value diverse forms of knowledges. Dominant contemporary methodologies were developed in the United States and Europe and carry the legacy of colonialism. For example, the survey, which was developed in the United States during the 1930s, gained influence in Asian and African countries, replacing local methodologies, and was seen to represent progress and modernisation. In a historical and geopolitical context, Gobo (2011, p. 419) shows how this development was intimately intertwined with the growth of the English language, which dominated 'in communicating scientific results, findings, and theories just as Latin did until the 1700s'. As a result, Gobo (2011, p. 420) contends that 'local (Anglo-American culture) became international and universal', an issue to which I will return later, in the section 'A Politics of Translation'.

Appadurai (2013, p. 270) argues that ideas about what research is have not been sufficiently discussed, but are often taken for granted. He introduces a rights-based definition of research, which, he argues, should also include everyone in poor countries:

> By this I mean the rights to the tools through which any citizen can systematically increase the stock of knowledge that they consider most vital to their survival as human beings and to their claims as citizens.

Appadurai (2013) discusses the challenges faced by researchers attempting to gain knowledge about the as yet unknown, the collective features of research and the importance of democratising the right to research. This analysis is underpinned by the problematisation of the gap between the 'globalization of knowledge and the knowledge of globalization' (ibid., p. 281), which has increased the gap between the struggle for jobs, educational mergers and collaborations on a global scale, while traditional university education, particularly in the social sciences and humanities, is shrinking. Against this background, there is a need to create new institutions for research. For the purpose of democratising research, Appadurai (2013, p. 279) argues that we need to create frameworks for 'creative action, artistic action and political action' within which academics and non-academics with an interest in the research collaborate and create this new space. The creating of such equal, respectful and creative spaces is vital for glocalised social work (see Gordon's and Alfred & Åberg's chapters in this volume). Thus, methodological spaces that include a relationship between social research, creative writing and art are of particular importance for glocalised social work.

The metaphor 'what we learn how to see' can be used to actualise critical theoretical lenses of importance for glocalised social work. As researchers, educators and practitioners, we need to acknowledge the risk that established viewpoints based on taken-for-granted 'truths' can be an obstacle to asking new questions and creating new knowledge. Ranta-Tyrkkö (2011) provides an example in social work, where issues of colonisation have to a large extent been silenced. Her study focuses on colonialism and social work, geopolitically in the contexts of colonial India, Finland and other Nordic countries, cases that represent diverse places often considered to have strong or weak colonial legacies. As Ranta-Tyrkkö discusses the impact of the colonial past and postcolonial present, she argues that there is a need to ask critical questions about the impact of colonisation and to resist the silence about this question in social work, but also to make use of concrete examples. She shows that the colonial past and postcolonial present of the Nordic countries is often not discussed in social research, although a historical perspective reveals both occupation of land in other parts of the world and 'distant' colonialism through missionary work. She warns against the risk of theorising in a universalising way and emphasises the importance of specifically taking into account historical and geopolitical contexts:

> Like any other theory, postcolonial theory can also be used in a [...] universalizing way, to produce predetermined results. Yet no matter how universal knowledge is claimed, it remains always only partial, related to particular historical and geo-political contexts. (p. 37)

Chambon (2012, p. 1) brings into focus how borders shift and change in the discipline of social work and how these border crossings are related to other disciplines historically. The historical period she looks at in her study covers from the beginning of the nineteenth century until today and includes North America, Canada and the United States, with links to Britain. Her analysis shows that shifts occur as a result of changes both within disciplinary boundaries and from other scholarship, and also that they 'are very much shaped by economic, social, and political conditions of societies [...]', which 'shape the many responses to these changed conditions' (Chambon 2012, p. 1). This question of the inter/disciplinarity of social work is not new, but the kind of knowledge base, epistemological and methodological, that social work needs in order to respond to societal changes, emergent social issues and problems varies historically and geopolitically. Contemporary social problems such as migration, conflict, war and environmental destruction all require the boundaries of the discipline to be extended into less acknowledged areas such as glocal, postcolonial and intersectionality studies, cultural geography, creative writing and art.

In an overview of the emerging field of glocal studies, Roudometof (2015) identified that continental Europe and Asia had developed the conceptualisation of glocalisation and glocal studies to a greater extent than North America and/or the United Kingdom. Roudometof (2015, p. 783) refers to a 'silent glocal turn at the dawn at the twenty first century', noting that centres and institutions that explicitly address glocalisation have mainly been established in Italy, Japan, Israel and Scandinavia, primarily in media, urban and community studies. For contemporary glocalised social work, the continuous work of establishing a voice for the discipline and the profession is visualised, among others, in *The Global Definition of Social Work* (2014), in which questions about interdisciplinarity, the concept of knowledge and indigenisation are brought up in the commentary on the definition (n.p.):

> Social work is both interdisciplinary and transdisciplinary, and draws on a wide array of scientific theories and research. 'Science' is understood in this context in its most basic meaning as 'knowledge'. [...] Part of the legacy of colonialism is that Western theories and knowledges have been exclusively valorised, and indigenous knowledges have been devalued, discounted, and hegemonised by Western theories and knowledge. The proposed definition attempts to halt and reverse that process by acknowledging that Indigenous peoples in each region, country or area carry their own values, ways of knowing, ways of transmitting their knowledges, and have made invaluable contributions to science. Social work seeks to redress historic Western scientific colonialism and hegemony by listening to and learning from Indigenous peoples around the world.

The challenge to 'halt and reverse' the devaluation of knowledges other than Western theories is a core issue for a politics of location in social work, which is intimately intertwined with decolonising methodologies (for a critical discussion, see Pease's chapter in this volume). Given the structural conditions of knowledge production, under which university settings, publishers and journals make use of internationalisation as a key dimension, questions about glocalising knowledge contribute a critical and reflexive lens to aid in changing 'what we learn how to see' (Haraway, 1988, p. 183). Gobo (2011) argues that a glocalised methodology challenges the well-known expression 'think global and act local', since understanding knowledge as situated means that it is based on thinking that is saturated by specific contexts, which are local in their character rather than global. This, I argue, is important for social work and calls for a methodological framework that recognises the becoming of embodied selves, '*förkroppsligade jag*', and ways of seeing and knowing theoretically and methodologically, taking into account the history and geopolitics of knowledge.

Situated Intersectionality: Storytelling, Critical Consciousness and Social Change

> I can see him as if it were today. Standing there beside the car, waiting for me to come and drive him to the train station. It was one of our weekends together, one of his visits. He was surprised that it was raining and looked up only to see blue sky. It was however the effect of the wind and the lake which threw rain at our faces. He looked surprised. He was soon leaving on the train and I missed him already. Every time he came to visit he would send an SMS to say how far away he was at a particular moment. Every time he left he would send an SMS to say that he misses me already.

> In the age of speechlessness.
> A letter arrives.
> Untimely message.
> In the age of speechlessness.
> Dear Mother,
> cannot come, so sorry.
>   (Livholts 2013, p. 183)

An increasing number of people live transnational lives (Baldassar & Merla 2014). Families, kin and friends who live in such relationships do so in both real and imagined spaces. The situations and contexts for transnational lives vary extensively across diverse national borders, shaped by the reasons for leaving, the conditions in the new local communities upon arrival and the conditions under which a 'new home' can be created. At the same time, many workers who leave their local communities to work abroad to support their families are subjected to exploitation and live under inhuman conditions (see also Chapter 12 in this volume). The short memory section that introduces this section illustrates a situation from my own transnational family life, which is historically and geopolitically shaped by the Swedish-Finnish relationship. The history and geopolitics between Finland and Sweden and Finland's geographical and political relationship with the former Soviet Union have consequences for individual lives and families. Sweden colonised Finland, which was 'lost' to the Soviet Union, and Finland first declared itself free in 1917 after the revolution in the Soviet Union. The Second World War involved Finland in the fighting on two occasions, and the great-grandfather of two of my children was killed during the Second World War. During the 1960s, many Finnish immigrants came to Sweden to work in the industries. In terms of inequality, ethnicity played a role in discrimination. For example, having a Finnish name could make it difficult to find housing in Sweden or could lead to the experience of negative treatment from professionals in healthcare and the social sector. Thus, aspects such as geographical origin, language and socioeconomic and health conditions are interwined in people's lives' the following words 'and constantly change. In 2017 Finland celebrates the centenary of its independence, looking back and towards its future becoming.

There is an increasing awareness in research and practice in social work that intersectional analysis is important in understanding the complexity of diverse lives and structural conditions contextually (e.g. Crenshaw 1991; Hill Collins 2000; Mohanty 2003; Dill & Zambrana 2009). In social work, intersectional analysis focusing on the tensions and interconnections between gender, ethnicity, racialisation, class, sexuality, able-bodiedness and age is expanding (Mattsson 2014; Mehrotra 2010; Pease 2010; Sewpaul 2013). The Council on Social Work Education's (CSWE) (2008) *Educational Policy and Accreditation Standards* has established that understanding issues of oppression and diversity is a core competence for all social workers:

> The dimensions of diversity are understood as the intersectionality of multiple factors including age, class, color, culture, disability, ethnicity, gender, gender identity and expression, immigration status, political ideology, race, religion, sex, and sexual orientation. Social workers appreciate that, as a consequence of difference, a person's life experiences may include oppression, poverty, marginalization, and alienation as well as privilege, power, and acclaim.
>
> (p. 5)

In the following, I draw on two studies that I think are helpful for intersectionality analysis in glocalised social work: Yuval-Davis' (2015) framework for situated intersectionality, which includes spatiality, and Sewpaul's (2013) intersectional analysis, which makes use of storytelling and critical reflection.

Yuval-Davis (2015) develops four points of departure for what she names a situated intersectionality. The first is that intersectional analysis should make use of critical race theory to include all people, not focusing solely on marginalised and racialised women, but also analysing the privileged lives of white heterosexual women. This aspect is important because it emphasises that all people, although in different ways, live their lives in intersections of privilege and oppression. For social work, 'what we learn how to see' in terms of intersectionality requires us to continuously take into account the dynamics and changeable situations and processes involved in diverse and interconnected lives (Pease 2010). Yuval-Davis' (2015) second point is to make use of Haraway's critique that seeing from nowhere is ethically irresponsible and that there is a need to account for the social positioning of both researcher and researched. Although this insight is not new and can be considered self-evident in qualitative studies, I argue that it is challenging and risks ending up in a confession rather than practice. It is necessary to build ways of creating such dialogical practice into the research design, which can be achieved in various ways in different kinds of studies. As one example, Eliassi (2012) makes use of episodes to situate and re-situate his locations in relation to the subject of the study, the research participants and locations. Yuval-Davis' (2015) third approach is to work with sensitivity linked to geographical, social and temporal locations in a translocal and transcalar manner. Translocal means to be aware of how diverse categories of social divisions regain different meaning, impacted by the different spaces within which they take shape. The transcalar means that social dimensions of power take on different meanings depending on whether they take place in a household, a neighbourhood, a city, a region or a state. Fourthly, a situated intersectionality also needs to include diverse orders of stratification, such as global, national, regional and local. I argue that the third and fourth aspects are increasingly important for a glocalised methodology in social work. Epistemological questions such as: Who can know? What is it possible to know? and What counts as knowledge? need to take into account understandings of place and space and make use of disciplines such as anthropology, cultural geography and art (see Bryant & Garnham's, Gottzen's and Alfred & Åberg's chapters in this volume).

* * *

> Once while I conducted a leadership training workshop with a group of students from the Students Representative Council of the former Natal Technikon, the students said that they initially thought I was part of the catering team (we had arrived at the same time). Given the nature of the workshop, I introduced myself by my first name, we sat in a circle on the floor and were soon into exercises on race, class, gender, power, leadership, and status. The environment was such that it allowed for the free sharing of ideas and thoughts. Some of the students said that even when we began the session, they were confused; they thought I must be 'the professor's assistant,' and they were still expecting a white, male professor to arrive. They struggled with their own cognitive dissonance. The reflective exercises and my sharing with them some of my assumptions about race and gender constituted powerful forms of praxis. The sessions opened up spaces for the students, who were all African black, to confront stereotypes about race and gender; how these stereotypes might mediate the performance of their leadership roles; and how we can begin to deconstruct dominant thinking and socialized senses of inferiority, believe in ourselves, and develop confidence enough to reach our highest possible standards.
>
> (Sewpaul 2013, p. 28)

The citation above, illustrating how a group of students don't 'see' the professor because she is a black woman, is taken from an article written by Professor Vishiantie Sewpaul, Professor of Social Work, University of KwaZulu Natal, South Africa. Sewpaul's (2013) critical intersectional analysis of gender and race in this study makes use of personal narratives in the form of short memory scenes that are analysed theoretically to better understand how the history of (post) colonial relations discursively shapes and risks sustaining a sense of inferiority. Inspired by emancipatory theorists such as Freire, Giroux and Hall, she argues for a pedagogy that makes change possible by remaining '[...] open to be positioned and situated in different ways, at different moments throughout our existence'

(Hall, cited in Sewpaul 2013, p. 122). I believe that this strategy of situating and re-situating, with its emancipatory potential beyond fixed categories and as a life-long process, is central to social work research, education, practice and activism. Sewpaul's approach to intersectionality analysis is important due to the way in which it situates actors, provides insights into situations in context and highlights the transformative force of stories, as well as for its analytical reflexivity and emancipatory potential (see also Gordon's chapter in this volume and Livholts 2015b). Sewpaul (2013, p. 122) discusses the risk of how gender and racism, and the normalisation of privilege, can be manifested through a lack of understanding of one's own 'structural location'. She writes:

> [...] students who have normalized poverty and inequality and privilege often expect nothing better for users of services [...]. On the basis of the under-standing that there is a relationship between one's understanding of the world and one's structural location in it, I make efforts – through reflective dialogue, debate, drama, students' presentations, reflective assignments (including stu-dents' biographies), and journaling – for students to transform common sense into good sense (Gramsci, 1971), so as to understand and challenge external sources of oppression and to understand and undo sources of privilege.
>
> (Sewpaul 2013, p. 122)

I wish to make use of the idea of situated intersectionality as a storytelling prac-tice that has the potential to create a critical consciousness and agency for social change as a strategy in glocalised social work. Through a critical reflexive discus-sion, Patel and Lynch (2013) advocate 'glocal learning perspectives characterised by dialogue and action as opposed to internationalisation', which they critique for tending to create passive and non-autonomous learning and the ascendancy of dominant cultural knowledges over subjugated knowledges. They wish to promote what they call a 'third culture space' where glocalisation (ibid., p. 225) 'introduces a just and responsible ethics of framework that situates learning and teaching within a respectful, equitable and inclusive learning space'. One of the central strategies in glocalised learning spaces is storytelling that involves critical self-reflection and awareness, to work against ethnocentrism and dominant cultural norms. Freire (1970/2005) argues that dialogue is not merely a technique, but a process that moves beyond the individualistic. It is not based on what I like or do not like about another person, but is characterised by the social in processes of knowing. I wish to emphasise that making use of storytelling and memories as a dialogical practice for creating new epistemological spaces is an activity that combines the personal with the social from an epistemological viewpoint. For glocalised social work, the spheres of research, education and practice are intimately intertwined.

A Politics of Translation, *'Översättningens Politik'*

It is early summer and the greenish light of sunbeams *'solstrålar'* flashing through leaves in the tree crowns *'trädkronorna'* outside my window meets my eyes whenever I look up from the computer space. My bare feet rest on the old worn '*slitna*' wooden floor of my flat. This old concrete building, erected in the 1930s, painted yellow, is located on one of the islands of Stockholm, Sweden. This kitchen table in my flat and the train '*tåget*' are the places where I most often write. Train writing is writing in a mo(ve)ment strictly clocked by the timetable; however, as Dahl (2012, p. 157) expresses so poetically, 'we always write from *somewhere* in time and space – even if the clock in one's body is not that of one's location'. In the present state of writing, in early August 2016, I am struggling to keep the promise I made in the abstract I wrote for this chapter. There are several challenges: the imagined readers, the sense of alienation when I enter into the academic language style, the swirl of words, the many voices and memories. I return several times to read and re-read Spivak's (1993) text, 'A politics of translation'. Within a poststructuralist and postcolonial framework of ideas, translation is an active practice which places languages (words, gestures, expressions) in situations where meaning is created in complex relations of power between dominant groups, across national borders and local sites geographically. Spivak's text (1993) actualises the disciplining that English reinforces, and changes the way in which I see things. Reading this particular text by Spivak (1993) spurs me to read more and different texts than I believe I would have otherwise. It becomes more difficult to keep the focus of the chapter, and I begin to question the Swedish translations I make as I re-read them day by day. My writing increasingly appears to be a series of disconnected stories and I realise, despite what I have said during my academic life since I wrote my PhD dissertation fourteen years ago, about how I felt liberated by writing in English – that I now need to re-think this.

Spivak writes:

> Yet language is not everything. It is only a vital clue to where the self loses its boundaries. [...] The history of the language, the history of the author's moment, the language in-and-as-translation, must figure in the weaving as well.
>
> (Spivak, 1993, pp. 180 and 186)

I write:

> *Ändå är språket inte allt. Det är bara en central ledtråd till den punkt där självet förlorar sina gränser. (...) Språkets historia, historien om författarens ögonblick, språket i-och-som-översättning, måste också få existera i de skapande processerna.*
>
> (My translation from English to Swedish:
> Spivak, 1993, pp. 180 and 186)

As I begin to move between Swedish and English, translating selected words and citations throughout the text, the creation of meaning becomes a creative and reflexive narrator's position, but one that opens up space for doubt because changing language changes the creation of meaning. Indeed, actively taking on the role of 'a translator' takes me away from the writing that the abstract for the chapter stated so clearly. As Gannon (2012, p. 7) suggests, an abstract may be written in a confident tone, while the writing of a paper may be characterised by 'blocks, stoppages, impossibilities'. She introduces the reader to the gap between the confident tone of an abstract and being haunted by a sense of loss.

Gannon writes:

> Despite the confident tone of the abstract, this paper is haunted by a sense of loss, and its writing has been experienced as a series of tiny aporias, blocks, stoppages, impossibilities. Thus this paper is shaped more like a series of curves, a meandering, than the linear rational argument of academic convention. It is not that I eschew academic registers or modes of thinking but rather, this time, I want to incorporate the inchoate and erratic trajectories of desire, longing and, perhaps, of loss that are part of my stories of place.

I write:

> *Trots den självsäkra tonen i abstrakt så plågas/förföljs det här paperet av en känsla av förlust och att skriva det har upplevts som en serie mycket små aporier/motsägelser, blockeringar, stopp, omöjligheter. På så sätt är paperet format mer som en serie av böjningar/kurvor, slingrande, istället för det linjära rationella argument som kännetecknar akademiska konventioner. Det är inte så att jag vill fly undan akademiska upplägg eller sätt att tänka, utan snarare, den här gången vill jag införliva det ofärdiga och oberäkneliga som en väg/bana av lust, längtan och kanske, av förlust som är en del av mina berättelser om plats.*

Situated Writing, Creating Spaces

> In the beginning, writing is always a matter of staging. You put your pen to the white surface of the paper or enter the document-page on your computer, and there you are. [...] The paper, the screen, may also be a door, a window or a newly painted wall to avoid leaning on; a floor for the silenced and a multivocal chorus of voices that urges the author and the audience to listen. [...] The spatiality of writing is always both personal and political, and it is embodied in the way form and content are intertwined. The tightly woven texture of power and privilege, marginalized and subjugated knowledge, ethics and change, are altogether tied to the praxis of style.
>
> (Livholts & Bränström Öhman, 2010, p. 223)

It has always been through experimenting with different forms and genres of writing that I have found it possible to address issues of power in academe, to find a language *'ett språk'* for my critical relationship with mainstream social work, which I have found to be built on defining 'the other' as a basis for its existence (Scheffer Kumpula[2] 2000). Inspired by postcolonial and postmodern feminists (e.g. Collins 2000; hooks 1989; Lorde 1984; Richardson 1997), I made use of writing to situate myself as an author and researcher in relation to the research questions, contexts and ways of life that saturated my seeing. This was vital for me to retain a sense of self that was critical, creative and reflexive – to develop a consciousness and theoretical framework for social justice. There was an intimate interconnectivity between my life experiences as a white woman growing up in rural areas of Sweden, which were considered spaces for the less intellectual, the patriarchal rule in my family of origin, and later the creation of a family with a partner of Finnish background that shaped my transnational family life in a Nordic postcolonial context (Livholts 2001/2011, 2010a, 2010b, 2013). Difference was also a matter of textual shaping and this disturbing of the normalisation of the dominant form and sound of academic writing. In this chapter, I argue that the ways in which we write as academics enable or prevent the methodological creativity and reflexivity that are important for glocalising methodologies in social work.

In my earlier work on the politics of location (Livholts 2015a, p. 194), I introduce situated writing as a 'methodological strategy that combines feminist theorising of situated knowledges (Haraway 1988) and writing as a methodological tool (Livholts 2012)'. Following up on Haraway's critique of reflexivity as representing only more of the same, I (Livholts 2015a, pp. 144–147) developed ideas on situated writing as a position that can allow an exploration of our subjective locations as 'diffracted', that should challenge us, create doubts and spark unexpected insights. As Haraway (1988, p. 590) argues, we don't need 'partiality for its own sake but, rather, for the sake of the connections and unexpected openings situated knowledges make possible'. Beginning with writing with the purpose of learning more about our situatedness, and guided by Haraway's optical metaphor of diffraction, this means to both '*sight*' *and* '*site*' *ourselves*. Rendell's 'site writing' (2007, p. 151) develops from the critique that a large majority of scholarship still takes place 'at a distance'. She promotes the relational, situated and dialogical: '"site-writing" is what happens when [...] spatial qualities of writing become as important in conveying meaning as the content of the criticism' (ibid.).

What can we learn by looking at our own sites as writing locations? What are the spaces where we write – the desk, or the bed, the sofa, the train, the park etc.? In what way do they matter if we look at them as discursive storyworlds, which we inhabit? (Livholts 2015a, p. 145). In *The Auto/Biographical I* (1995), Stanley situates the biographer as 'a socially-located person, one who is sexed, raced, classed, aged' and states that 'any biographer's view is a socially located and necessarily partial one' (Stanley 1995, p. 7). She makes use of photography to examine how the autobiographer's desk represents authoring through multiple stories in which artefacts, memories and imagination are intertwined (ibid.: 50–52). A photograph of Stanley's desk is used to illustrate and discuss questions of truth and lies, and how a dominant image of the intellectual life of the biographer influences the placement of artefacts 'to create a pleasing fiction, a romance about the auto/biographer's desk which daily surrounds me as I work' (ibid.: 52). A close reading of the photograph opens up space for locating the discourse of the author, the many stories through the memories on the desk. In an interview with Connell, I asked about the creating of a writing space and she tells this story:

> Most of my career, I had a desk in the bedroom, which in Sydney was and is a fairly dark room with an opening towards an urban view. I created a kind of cocoon I suppose, a close space in which I could concentrate deeply. In the last few years, as a result of changes in my family, I've acquired a study.
>
> I now write in a brightly lit room, which has windows on the north side, which in Australia is the sunny side [...] I have a fairly bare room, I don't like clutter. People comment that my room at the University is amazingly tidy, and I say that's just because I keep the chaos well hidden. But I do have places for the books, places for the papers, places for this and that. So it's a biggish room, brightly lit, with a desk on a side wall so the light comes over my shoulder, good ergonomic stuff. And a computer around to the right facing away from the window, on a sit/stand desk, which is ergonomically good so that I can type some work standing up and some sitting down.
>
> [...] So that's my physical space of writing at the moment, and it's a *lovely* space, it's glorious. On the wall over my computer I have the original painting by an Aboriginal artist, Peggy Patrick, which is on the cover of *Southern Theory*. On the wall above my desk I have a poster that was made by an artist in Melbourne, a colorful screen-printed poster that was made out of a quotation from one of my articles about the democratisation of culture. So that's up there to urge me on in the democratic project of creating knowledge. And on the back wall, pictures of my mother and my partner and my daughter; and a painting by another Australian artist, which I inherited from my parents. So it's both an open space and a very personal place, in which I have an emotional connection with everything in the room. Including a big fern on the mantelpiece in the middle of the north wall, which has the maidenhair fern that belonged to my partner before she died, which I have managed to keep alive for about thirteen years. There you go. That's my space.
>
> (Livholts 2010c, p. 276–277)

To be situated as a writer involves a complex entanglement of the personal and the political in the context of history and geopolitics. The embodied self, the collection of objects, items, images, memories, indoor and outdoor spaces and landscapes are all part of the shaping of writing. For glocalised social work, situated writing is a practice that considers ways of disrupting dominant forms of writing knowledge and thus the dominant 'sound' of scientific storytelling (Hau'ofa 2008). Witkin (2007) problematises the literary/science divide that took place during the seventeenth century, creating a distinction between art, culture and humanities – areas that took an interest in the expression and shaping of language and knowledge – and scientific writing as 'a vehicle for recording the regularities of nature' (p. 389). As I have previously argued, all writing, including the mainstream forms that propose a universalising claim to knowledge, actively participate in the subjective re-presentation of knowledge (Livholts 2012). If writing is part of the methodological strategy, then form and style in writing are central to what can be known. De-hegemonising and decolonising writing in glocalised social work aims to disrupt the hegemonic forms of writing knowledge and the dominant 'sound' of the scientific languages of storytelling (see also Hau'ofa 2008), bridging the theory-practice gap and the evaluation of different kinds of materials and demonstrating that writing is an emotional and embodied practice situated within the complex dimensions of power in people's lives in homes, institutions and society. Witkin (2007) suggests a number of alternatives to mainstream writing for social work, such as the personal essay, memoir and autoethnography (see also Witkin 2014). I wish to emphasise the interdisciplinary features that enable social work to push the boundaries to re-shape knowledge in times of glocalisation and argue that glocalised social work scholarship needs to make use of situated writing as a methodological tool where the contexts of the author – personally, theoretically and empirically – design a shape for knowledge that generates accountability for 'what we learn how to see'.

Concluding Reflections: In Mo(ve)ment, Through Mo(ve)ment

In this chapter, I have discussed how a politics of location and the epistemological practice of situating and re-situating in glocalised social work is enriched by making use of postcolonial and situated intersectional theoretical lenses to better understand diversity and inequality, self/other relationships and tensions between privilege and subordination. To conclude, I wish to propose mo(ve)ment as an analytical term to extend the social reach of social work, enabling us to understand how lives are affected by glocal influences and promoting glocalising methodologies in social work. I suggest that this can be taken further in glocalised social work by making use of the idea of being 'in movement, through movement' '*i rörelse genom rörelse*' as Chambon (2005, p. 2) suggests. She proposes that, through telling, we create movement and questions if there can ever be neutral places. She writes (Chambon 2005, p. 5): 'Moving from the desk, moving outward, moving towards knowledge: what do I want to know? What do I not want to know? What am I moving away from?' The questions that Chambon (2005) asks are written to contextualise social work practices employing art, to create movement towards safe and creative spaces for education and research. By asking critical and new questions related to 'what we learn how to see', we can question what we think we already know. Curricula, course lists, teachers and students all create lenses through which to see the world, continuously situating and re-situating their knowledges. The ways in which we can see the interconnectivity of localities create movement; location in terms of the transcalar situates the researcher in movement between households, neighbourhoods, cities and regions in the world. A situated geopolitics of location is translocally shaped, which means that we need to translate the ways in which the diverse dimensions of power that structurally frame people's lives, researcher and researched, as well as objects and items, are affected by the places and spaces in which they are located. Language, words and writing create movement. Writing is a methodological tool that nourishes a transformative agency in glocalised social work. A politics of location is also a politics of translation that allows us to include stories of place, to move between languages and to create spaces for writing that make it possible to see, and see again, to acknowledge the moment and create mo(ve)ments.

Notes

1 In this chapter, I translate short sections and words from English to Swedish, inspired by 'The politics of translation' (Spivak 1993), which critiques the hegemony and textual representation of the English language (see also Dahl 2012; Livholts 2012a).
2 Scheffer Kumpula was my surname until the year 2000, when I changed it to Livholts.

References

Appadurai, A 2013, *The Future as Cultural Fact: Essays on the Global Condition*, Verso, London and New York.

Baldassar, L & Merla, L (eds) 2014, *Transnational Families, Migration and the Circulation of Care*, Taylor & Francis, New York.

Chambon, A 2005, 'Social work practices of art', *Critical Social Work*, vol. 6, no. 1, pp. 1–11.

Chambon, A 2012, 'Disciplinary borders and borrowings: Social work knowledge and its social reach, a historical perspective', *Social Work & Society*, vol. 10, no. 2, pp. 1–12.

CSWE, Council on Social Work Education 2008, Educational Policy and Accreditation Standards. VA, Alexandria, pp. 1–16.

Collins, PH 2000, *Black Feminist Thought: Knowledge, Consciousness, and the Politics of Empowerment*, Routledge, New York.

Connell, R 2007, *Southern Theory: The Global Dynamics of Knowledge in Social Science*, Polity Press, Cambridge.

Crenshaw, K 1991, 'Mapping the margins: Intersectionality, identity politics, and violence against women of color', *Stanford Law Review*, vol. 43, no. 6, pp. 1241–1299.

Dahl, U 2012, 'The road to writing: An ethno (bio) graphic memoir' in *Emergent Writing Methodologies in Feminist Studies*, ed. M Livholts, Routledge, London, pp. 148–165.

De los Reyes, P 2011, 'Postkolonial feminism: Anteckningar om ett fält i rörelse' in *Postkolonial Feminism*, ed. M de los Reyes, Hägersten, Tankekraft förlag, pp. 11–41.

Dill BT & Zambrana RE (eds) 2009, *Emerging intersections. Race, class and gender in theory, policy and practice*, Rutgers University Press, New Brunswick and New Jersey.

Eliassi, B 2012, 'Political terrains of writing belonging, memory and homeland' in *Emergent Writing Methodologies in Feminist Studies*, ed. M Livholts, Routledge, London, pp. 83–97.

Gannon, S 2012, 'From the curve of the snake, and the scene of the crocodile: Musings on learning and losing space, place and body', *Reconceptualizing Educational Research Methodology*, vol. 3, no. 2, pp. 7–15.

Gobo, G 2011, 'Glocalizing methodology? The encounter between local methodologies', *International Journal of Social Research Methodology*, vol. 14, no. 6, pp. 417–437.

Haraway, D 1988, 'Situated knowledges: The science question in feminism and the privilege of partial perspective', *Feminist Studies*, vol. 14, no. 3, pp. 575–599.

Hau'ofa, E 2008, *We Are the Ocean: Selected Works*, Verso Classics, London.

Hooks, B 1989, *Talking Back. Thinking Feminist, Thinking Black*, South End Press, Boston.

Hill Collins, P 1990, *Black Feminist Thought. Knowledge, Consciousness and the Politics of Empowerment*, Routledge, New York and London.

IFSW (International Federation of Social Workers) 2014, Global definition of social work. Available online at http://ifsw.org/get-involved/global-definition-of-social-work/

Livholts, M 2010a, 'The professor's chair: An untimely academic novella', *Life Writing*, vol. 7, no. 2, pp. 155–168.

Livholts, M 2010b, 'The snow angel and other imprints: An untimely academic novella', *International Review of Qualitative Research*, vol. 3, no. 1, pp. 103–124.

Livholts, M 2010c, 'Writing masculinities, gender and the politics of change: A publicly staged interview with Raewyn Connell', *NORA: Nordic Journal of Feminist and Gender Research*, vol. 18, no. 2, pp. 246–266.

Livholts, M 2012, 'Introduction: Contemporary untimely post/academic writings – transforming the shape of knowledge in feminist studies' in *Emergent Writing Methodologies in Feminist Studies*, ed. M Livholts, Routledge, New York, pp. 1–25.

Livholts, M 2013, 'Writing water: An untimely academic novella' in *Documents of Life Revisited: Narrative and Biographical Methods for a 21st Century of Critical humanism*, ed. L Stanley, Ashgate, Farnham, pp. 177–191.

Livholts, M 2015a, 'A politics of location in discourse and narrative studies' in *Discourse and Narrative Methods: Theoretical Departures, Analytical Strategies and Situated Writing*, M Livholts & M Tamboukou, Routledge, London, pp. 137–148.

Livholts, M 2015b, 'Working with memories and images' in *Discourse and Narrative Methods: Theoretical Departures, Analytical Strategies and Situated Writing*, M Livholts & M Tamboukou, Routledge, London, pp. 162–176.

Livholts, M & Bränström Öhman, A 2010, 'Writing change? Challenges for feminist and gender studies', *NORA: Nordic Journal of Feminist and Gender Research*, vol. 18, no. 4, pp. 223–225.

Loomba, A 1998, *Colonialism/Postcolonialism*, Routledge, New York.

Lorde, A 1984, *Sister Outsider: Essays and Speeches*, The Crossing Press Feminist Series, Marshall.

Mattsson, T 2014, 'Intersectionality as a useful tool for anti-oppressive social work and critical reflection', *Affilia: Journal of Women and Social Work*, vol. 29, no. 1, pp. 8–17.

Mehrotra, G 2010, 'Toward a continuum of intersectionality theorizing for feminist social work scholarship', *Affilia: Journal of Women and Social Work*, vol. 25, no. 4, pp. 417–430.

Mohanty, CT 2003, *Feminism Without Borders: Decolonising Theory, Practicing Solidarity*, Duke University Press, Durham and London.

Patel, F & Lynch, H 2013, 'Glocalization as an alternative to internationalization in higher education: Embedding positive glocal learning perspectives', *International Journal of Teaching and Learning in Higher Education*, vol. 25, no. 2, pp. 223–230.

Pease, B 2010, *Undoing Privilege: Unearned Advantage in a Divided World*, Zed Books, London.

Ranta-Tyrkkö, S 2011, 'High time for postcolonial analysis in social work', *Nordic Social Work Research*, vol. 1, no. 1, pp. 25–41.

Rendell, J 2007, *Site Writing: The Architecture of Art Criticism*, in *Critical Architecture*, eds. J Rendell, J Hill, M Fraser & M Dorrian, Routledge, London, New York, pp. 150–162.

Richardson, 1997, *Fields of Play. Constructing an Academic Life*. Rutgers University Press, Brunswick.

Rose, G 1997, 'Situating knowledges: Positionality, reflexivities and other tactics', *Progress in Human Geography*, vol. 21, no. 3, pp. 305–320.

Roudometof, V 2015, 'The glocal and global studies', *Globalisations*, vol. 12, no. 5, pp. 774–787.

Scheffer Kumpula, M 2000 '"Utan dem fanns vi inte..." Socialt arbete, utsatta kategorier och emancipatorisk kunskap', *Häften för Kritiska Studier*, 4, pp. 34-66.

Sewpaul, V 2013, 'Inscribed in our blood: Challenging the ideology of sexism and racism', *Affilia: Journal of Women and Social Work*, vol. 28, no. 2, pp. 116–125.

Spivak, GC 1993, 'The politics of translation' in *Outside in the Teaching Machine*, ed. GC Spivak, Routledge, New York, pp. 179–200.

Stanley, L 1995, *The Auto/biographical I: The Theory and Practice of Feminist Auto/biography*, Manchester University Press, Manchester.

Witkin, S & Chambon, A 2007, 'New voices in social work: Writing forms and knowledge production', *Qualitative Social Work*, vol. 6, no. 4, pp. 387–395.

Witkin, SL (ed.) 2014, *Narrating Social Work Through Autoethnography*, Columbia University Press, New York.

Yuval-Davis, N 2015, 'Situated intersectionality and social inequality', *Raisons Politiques*, no. 2, pp. 91–100.

7 Geographies of Anger and Fear

Exploring the Affective Atmospheres of Men's 'Domestic' Violence

Lucas Gottzén

What is an atmosphere? Literally, it refers to the envelope of gases surrounding a planet. Think of the atmospheric strata around the Earth. Figuratively speaking, atmospheres often represent the tones and moods that envelop different places. When walking into a room, its atmosphere may have a particular character. It might be hostile or welcoming. A workplace atmosphere may be bad or dysfunctional. We may experience a park as unsafe and dangerous and thus avoid it out of fear. A political demonstration might exhibit a variety of moods, including anger, indignation and hope. Expressions such as 'you could cut the atmosphere with a knife' highlight how we understand and experience the affective qualities of certain places and events. These examples also suggest that feelings are not necessarily something that individuals 'have' or possess. We experience them and are affected in our bodies, but they are at the same time outside ourselves, as rather being a relation between bodies. While other contributions in this book (e.g. Chapter 3) explore global issues of violence against women, in this chapter I will zoom in to the local, or rather, different localities of men's 'domestic' violence – such as cities, houses, cafés and women's shelters –and the ways in which atmospheres, in a figurative sense, can refer to the tones and moods that surround such places.

When talking about domestic violence, however, we tend to place emotions within individuals as something they possess. A perpetrator may be aggressive or feel anger and therefore assault his partner, who may have provoked his anger. She is scared. Her children are scared. They all may be ashamed of what others will think of it all. This is also evident in scientific discourse, where some social researchers see aggression as a consequence of being exposed to violence in childhood and developing a disorganised attachment (cf. Ray 2011). Others theorise that the individual's suppression of shame may lead to aggressive and violent behaviour, particularly for men. Rather than recognising and accepting shame through withdrawal, men tend to respond to status loss by defending themselves and resorting to aggression and violence (Scheff 2011). This is also apparent in feminist social work research, which has explored how the notion of violence as a 'private' matter reinforces women's isolation and causes them to see their victim position as shameful (e.g. Fiene 1995). But while this important line of research highlights private/public dichotomies and emotions, it recurrently places emotions within the individual victim.

I am not necessarily disagreeing with these arguments, but they are not the whole story. When placing emotions within individuals, we tend to overlook the relational aspects of affect and violence and – in particular – how other bodies and materialities contribute to transform and transgress spaces. I will therefore, in this chapter, discuss how we could understand the affectivity of violence as a form of atmosphere, as moods and feelings that are not only experienced by individuals or collectives but also move around and coalesce places. I do not see affect as simply embodied emotional expressions but also as the action potential of human and non-human bodies (Deleuze 1988). The concept of atmosphere, I argue, provides methodological tools to understand key questions in social work, such as domestic violence, and explore how they also include spatial and affective aspects.

In the following, I first present recent theorisations of affect and atmospheres and then analyse two cases that illustrate how they could be a useful tool for exploring men's domestic violence as it highlights relations between affect, violence and materiality. The cases are drawn from two qualitative studies on men's violence against women and children in Sweden. Violence against women is a global phenomenon that, during the last decades, has come to be regarded as a major public health problem and human rights violation on the basis of gender inequality (Watts & Zimmerman 2002). In Sweden, major efforts have been made to combat violence against women and there is today a relative political consensus on this issue and a cultural disapproval – at least at a general, abstract level – that a man should not use physical violence towards his female partner (Gottzén 2016). Despite these efforts and cultural changes, violence against women is still widespread. According to a recent Swedish prevalence study (Heimer *et al.* 2014), 1.4 per cent of all adult women have experienced severe forms of physical violence during the previous year and as many as 10 per cent during their lifetime.

Affective Atmospheres and Violence

The relation between affect and place has been increasingly discussed within cultural studies and gender studies, in what is at times called affect theory or the 'affective turn' (Clough 2007). Within this tradition, and following Deleuze's work (1988) on Spinoza, affect tends to be given two primary meanings. First, it refers to specific emotions and affective states characteristic of everyday life, including anger, shame, hope and fear. Second, affect is seen as something broader than emotions, as a particular manifestation of a body's power of acting, its lived force or the action potential of bodies – its unique capacity to affect, and to be affected by, the bodies and things that it encounters (Clough 2007; Massumi 2002). Emotions, it is argued, are only expressing a small part of our entire registers of embodied experience; when we feel a certain emotion, all other experiences are co-present as potentialities (Massumi 2015). At the same time, affect and bodily capacities are not outside culture but are always already mediated by their history; affect and emotions are therefore difficult to separate in practice (Anderson 2015).

This take on affect has been argued to open up a further understanding of space (Thrift 2008). Cultural geographers emphasise that affects are experienced in bodies but emerge from diverse encounters between bodies, which may be human and non-human materialities of various kinds. They affect one another when encountering each other in space; at the same time, bodies are affected by the place where they meet, and places are themselves accumulations of materialities. As affect involves relations between human and non-human bodies, affects experienced in space are simultaneously involved in the production and reproduction of place (Anderson 2015). Thus, affects refer to the feeling states generated in space as well as the capacities that spatial encounters between bodies enable.

Affect theory has been both praised and criticised by feminist scholars. Thien (2005) and Tolia-Kelly (2006) have argued that, within geography, attention to the virtual and transhuman is universalist and ahistorical, and that it portrays affects as transpersonal experiences. This, it is contended, reproduces a binary that represents feelings as feminine, while distant and transhuman affect are masculinised (Thien 2005). It moves us away from engaging with power geometries, embodied experience and the political materialities formed through emotions (Tolia-Kelly 2006).

In this chapter, I follow recent conceptualisations of atmospheres (Anderson 2009, 2015; Böhme 1993; Bille *et al.* 2015; Edensor & Sumartojo 2015) since I believe they help us to address the political issues that the affective turn has been accused of obscuring. Unlike within philosophy and design studies, the notion of atmosphere has only recently been discussed within the social sciences (Bille *et al.* 2015). The concept could be used to bridge the distinction between affect and emotions since it blurs the boundaries between the two categories (Anderson 2009; Edensor & Sumartojo 2015). As in its colloquial use, atmospheres may denote moods and ambiances that, in one way or another, are collective. Epochs, societies and rooms could all be argued to have atmospheres, which are often unacknowledged and non-representational but are nevertheless experienced. Atmospheres are, however, something more than collective feelings; they are, as Böhme (1993, p. 119) puts it, 'spatial bearers of moods'. Still, it is difficult to pinpoint the affective characteristics of a place and impossible to say where exactly atmospheres are since 'they seem to fill the space with a certain tone of feeling like a haze' (ibid., p. 114).

Atmosphere may seem too vague a concept to be useful in understanding such a concrete and material practice as men's violence. But as feminist research has for many years demonstrated, physical violence is only a small part of violent encounters and relationships. Rather, women living with violence in everyday life experience the violence as a constant possibility and threat (Kelly 1988). Tiny gestures, a particular look, bodily movements and intonations may go unnoticed by the outsider but may be behaviours that create certain sensations. They could even be strategies for violent men to make their disapproval clear and help produce what we could call an atmosphere of fear in a household or in a relationship.

But the individual violent man is not necessarily the only agent in creating an atmosphere. Other bodies may also be decisive since atmospheres are collective affects that form and deform as bodies encounter each other in space

(Anderson 2009). Following the notion of assemblage (Deleuze & Guattari 1987), affective atmospheres imply that a body's capacity is dependent on the other bodies present: 'all objects have the potential to equally impact or weigh upon an atmosphere' (Anderson & Ash 2015, p. 42). Even though individuals are pivotal, it is not only human bodies that generate atmospheres but also, for instance, the layout of a city or a place could be crucial (Edensor & Sumartojo 2015). Women's fear in the public realm illustrates this. While women may be afraid of being sexually assaulted in public, they are not frightened of all public places, but, for instance, secluded parks and desolate streets hold more fear than other urban locales. Moreover, a public place does not necessarily always hold fear; the city centre may also be a place of excitement and fun (Pain 2001). This suggests that places do not possess a single tone but may be characterised by different atmospheres depending on a number of factors. For instance, lighting, thickets, seclusion and time of day could be crucial to the atmosphere of a public place being described in terms of excitement or fear.

Atmospheres are, in other words, somewhat elusive while also enveloping places. They are contingent and, by being intermediate between environment and individual experience, people may discern a place differently due to their embodied histories. As Ahmed (2010, p. 41) has argued, an 'atmosphere is always angled; it is always felt from a specific point'. But atmospheres simultaneously seem 'anchored' in a place. As placed assemblages, atmospheres could be more or less set in a particular place, more or less territorialised (Deleuze & Guattari 1987). Certain places seem to evoke particular sensorial qualities. A place filled with familiar things, recognisable smells and intimate friends will most probably be experienced as more homely than a strange place with an assortment of new fragrances, unknown people and undefinable objects. All these different spatial and sensorial materialities may act as 'hinges' for atmospheres while never defining once and for all the tone of a place as they are themselves dependent on the passing human bodies. In this way, materialities are central to how atmospheres emerge and transform while not determining the affective capacities in a place. Following this, I explore atmospheres in relation to violence, particularly how they emerge and change, and how such transformations are consequential for domestic violence and responses to such violence.

Fear in the City

My first case is taken from a study with children and young people who have been 'exposed' to domestic violence, which means that they have experienced that one parent, mostly their mothers, has been abused by the other parent or by a new partner.[1]

Gina is 15 years old and lives with her mother, her mother's new boyfriend and her two half-siblings in a small town. Her mother was exposed to violence from a former boyfriend, Klas, whom she lived with since Gina was a toddler until she was about 10 years old. Klas's violence was mainly due to his growing alcoholism and was exacerbated when Gina's mother decided to leave him. With the help of their family, Gina and her mother were able to take refuge in a women's shelter. In her narrative, the safe house emerged as a place of particular importance to Gina.

> It was very nice to feel safe, but I was so young, so I didn't really get why we were there. […] It was a bit scary, anyway. It was just me, mum and two other families, or a woman, so it was very small. But you felt very protected. It was lonely. […] You couldn't see friends for a really long time. And it was during Christmas too. So we celebrated Christmas there.

While Gina and her mum were at the safe house, they learned that Klas had been arrested and put in jail. They, therefore, dared to go out and have a coffee in the city centre with Gina's father.

> At this women's shelter, this was a big thing for me; at the women's shelter, you weren't allowed to go out. You always stayed there, and there was a basement where I was sometimes, with a playroom. And one time my dad came, and we went for coffee with him since Klas was in custody, and as he was locked up, he couldn't get out. And we were like, 'Yeah, we can go have some coffee!' And I was happy that I could finally go out. And then we went out for some coffee. And I remember the whole thing, the very moment. We sat down and had some cake in a café. Then mum's phone rings and she says, 'I have to take this; it's a private number', and we were just like, 'Okay'; it was nothing special. And my dad and I continued talking as usual, how life was going now, about how I was doing, how he was doing. So we started to eat, but mum came back and said, 'It was the police, and they wonder where we are, huh, and, uh, for they just wanted to say that Klas is free' in the same city. And we were like, 'What?!' And then we had to run back to the women's shelter. And it was awful because I had to cancel everything, because I was so happy and then just running back in panic. For it was very close. I had to hurry back, and so we ran to the women's shelter, and I remember that I ran down to the basement and sat there in the playroom and sort of locked myself in. I was so scared 'cause he was in the same city, and I was afraid he'd come and get us. That was a horrible experience.

Atmospheres can coexist in the same place without necessarily affecting one another because the bodies do not, perforce, have relations with each other. For instance, we could imagine a number of other collective moods in a café at the same time: excitement, happiness, tranquillity, stress and boredom. When atmospheres encounter one another, often some form of change takes place. Such external transformation (Anderson 2015) occurs when you are 'seized' by an atmosphere or an atmosphere replaces a previous atmosphere, similar to when a thunderstorm quickly displaces high pressure and clear skies. The new atmosphere is made up of bodies now assembled with the things that existed in the preceding dominant atmosphere. With these atmospheric shifts, the action potential of bodies and the prevailing feelings alter.

In Gina's narrative, we find several atmospheric transformations. First, Gina experienced the women's shelter as a 'safe' and 'protected' place away from Klas. But note that she was rather ambivalent about it: the women's shelter was also lonely and scary and not a proper place to celebrate Christmas, which ideally should be cosy and magical. Second, on learning that Klas is in jail, they felt safer and dared to move freely around the city and do what a 'normal' family does, namely going out and having a cup of coffee together and enjoying each other's company – in contrast to spending Christmas in the lonely safe house. Gina was happy to get away from the women's shelter and to see her father and catch up with him. With Klas safely behind bars, Gina and her mother could walk in the city centre and be in the café, which became a place for familial intimacy and quality time. Third, we find a new atmospheric shift due to a movement of bodies. Back on the outside, Klas's bodily capacity affected Gina and her mother; they were seized by fear, and their movement in the local urban space was obstructed. On learning of his release, the atmosphere of 'their' city centre altered; his body (being out of jail) affected their bodies – what they were able to do (restricted movement, running) and their affective states (panicking, fear). They were once again forced to take shelter. Finally, Gina hid in the playroom as it engendered a sense of safety.

Exploring affective atmospheres furthers our understanding of emotional abuse, which has been defined as a central part of domestic violence and often as hostile verbal and non-verbal behaviours, patterns of harmful interaction not requiring physical contact, and where the motivation to harm is not necessary (Glaser 2002). We have no idea of Klas's thoughts or intentions when he was released. We can only imagine whether he wanted to hurt Gina and her mother or not, or if he even knew where they were. Klas was probably not even aware that he was harming them at that very moment, but due to their previous violent encounters, his bodily movement (inside/outside jail) quickly changed the atmosphere and the feeling of safety for the others. In this case, it is apparent that the issue of motives in emotional abuse is beside the point as it is not simply dependent on an individual's behaviour and intentions but just as much on the perpetrator's encounter with human and non-human bodies, including the layout of a city where the commercial centre, the jail and the women's shelter may be closely located.

Bitter Pill

While the previous case focused on the victims, the following illustrates responses to interpersonal violence from the point of view of the violent man. It draws on material from a larger study of men's intimate partner violence, where I have interviewed men receiving treatment voluntarily for having used physical violence towards their partners.[2]

Forty-three-year-old Jimmy lives in a small town and runs a rather success-ful import business. He posits that he has not used physical violence towards his former girlfriend Erika, except that he pushed her once. However, he willingly admits that he was emotionally abusive and used material violence against her during their separation. One night they had an almighty row about their property settlement, which ended with his leaving her house and going out for some drinks with his friends. Jimmy says that he never becomes violent when drinking, but that this time his beer had been spiked, which made him unusually aggressive.

> Someone had put something in my beer […] I got very, very, very aggressive, uh, well, raging, you could say. And I decided that if I couldn't get half [of the assets], then neither should she. So I called her dad and told him, 'Tell Erika to leave the house 'cause I'm going to burn down the whole house' ((chuckle)). I went there and broke three windows and then went home.

Anger is one of the most powerful affective expressions as it interrupts the situation, 'the flow of meaning that's taking place' (Massumi 2015, p. 8). Here it interrupts the normalised interaction between Jimmy and Erika during their separation. Affect is multi-scalar and not only produced at a global level or in cities but could also be produced on the micro-scale of the body when different materialities encounter each other. Note how, in the narrative, the 'something' (Rohypnol?) in the beer is ascribed the power to affect Jimmy; this non-human body affects the potentiality of his body, what his body is able and prone to do. At this moment of affective excess, anything could happen (Massumi 2002). But the accumulation of different materialities (his body, the beer, the Rohypnol and the house – the symbol of their life together and his material success) is translated into a closure of potentiality, into a single affective state of rage and its subsequent violent eruption. This affective cut is produced by Jimmy's aligning with a cultural script of masculinity where men's violence is argued to be caused by alcohol or drug use. Although he resisted the temptation to burn down the house, he still went there and broke three windows. With this angry and violent disruption, their fight about their assets turns into a violent criminal act.

Catalytic Facebook

After this violent episode, Jimmy was arrested and put into custody for a few days. In the end, he was given a restraining order and was at the time of the interview awaiting sentence for assault. The incident became local news.

> The day after, or when I was detained, the newspapers said that a 43-year-old man had assaulted his partner for several years, and that he had been detained. And it had nothing to do with what I was charged with, or what had happened; what the papers wrote about, both in [city X] and [town Y], and the local TV news as well had nothing to do with reality. Uh, and, of course, everyone sees this and knows that's me, that I had done that. And my ex didn't deny it, but she used it, thought it was more punishment for me. […] Ah, they wrote that a 43-year-old man had for several years been abusing his partner and had been detained, he came from [town Z], and [town Z] is a small town, so the rumours spread; where they stopped, I don't know.

Rumours about what Jimmy sees as false accusations also spread on Facebook and on a blog that one of Erika's friends had set up.

> So they built that up via Facebook, and there was even a website, uh, or a blog where people could well, where they said that I was gay, that I was schizophrenic, that I was a child molester. […] They made a video about this, in revenge; four ladies, Erika's friends, who sent the link to, I have, or had, about 500 friends on Facebook, and [they] sent it to most of them, messages encouraging people to show their disgust by unfriending me on Facebook and [they] gave some information about what I had not done, uh sort of to deter.

The change and transformation of atmospheres may be understood in terms of thresholds and tipping points (Anderson & Ash 2015). The threshold for internal change is defined by the presence and distribution of bodies; tipping points are relational in that an atmosphere stops discharging its particular affects because it is replaced by another atmosphere. From Jimmy's point of view, the atmosphere changed in his small town when increasing news of his arrest spread. Similar to other men in the study (Gottzén 2016), it is important for Jimmy how others perceive him, and he does not want to be seen as 'gay', a 'child molester', 'schizophrenic' or any other deviant masculinity. In particular, he does not recognise himself as a 'woman batterer'; a stigmatised masculine category the men in the study often refer to and distance themselves from. Being singled out as having abused his partner for several years placed him in an unflattering position where he was labelled a monstrous woman batterer. While the responses from Erika's friends may be seen as supporting and protecting her against an abusive ex, Jimmy only regarded them as a continuation of their fight. As a reaction to all this, Jimmy, therefore, tried to slander Erika and degrade her femininity by spreading rumours on Facebook about her being a member of 'various porn clubs' and 'acting strangely in her private life'. Despite these efforts, many turned their backs on Jimmy, and he felt increasingly socially isolated. Online responses illustrate this. He had friends in the restaurant business who sent Facebook invites to their events to him and others. When accepting these invitations, Erika's friends said they would attend as well, which he saw as hostile responses.

> As soon as I notified them that I was coming, I did that since I planned to come, and I knew it was good for their marketing, then all of Erika's family, everyone announced they'd come. I have a restraining order, so I guess it was something psychological; I didn't care that much; they could come if they wanted to, but they never showed up. […], so I started adding comments; when I signed [the reply], I wrote that '[friend] and I and Erika's family will come, but Erika is not allowed since she has a restraining order'. Since everyone was candid about everything, I could just as well terrorise them through the back door.

We can understand the use of Facebook by drawing on Massumi's discussion (2002) of research that has found a correlation between Super Bowl Sunday (the climax of the American football season) and increased domestic violence. Massumi argues that this could be understood in terms of an 'affective transfer' from the televised game to the home, which challenges the gendered relationships between the bodies in the household. The television becomes a catalyst that organises the bodies around the TV set in accordance with their different potentiality as generally ascribed to their gender. Adjacent words and gestures become increasingly intense. At this moment, Massumi contends, anything can happen, not only abuse, but also the male body translates the different parts of the situation into a reflex ready for violence. This is partly due to the fact that the situation is 'rigged' by the man's already-constituted inclination to violence, a gendered historical pattern repeated when he assaults his partner. In this way, the transfer of media images translates events from the potentiality of the game to a gendered potentiality. In Massumi's example, the TV is a catalyst for the events; a catalyst that makes things happen. But this is not to say that it causes violence, and the channelling function is far from given. The TV broadcast constitutes a potentiality to affect, but it is far from obvious that the individuals in the home will be engrossed in the game and it is unsure how they will be affected in the end. The TV is also perhaps only one of many materialities at play (alcohol, for instance, could be another) but is nevertheless performative.

The aim here is not to prove that televised sporting events generate violence. Rather, the point I am trying to make is that affect, in terms of bodily capacities, transcends space. Bodily movement in a place may affect bodies and their potentialities in another. In this, information technology may be a catalyst. In Massumi's case, the catalyst is the television set. For Gina, it is the mobile phone, where her mother learned that Klas had been released. In Jimmy's case, it is the Internet, and in particular a blog and Facebook.

Alone in the Woods

Rather than due to the restraining order, it was thus the affective transfer through Facebook and the growing number of bodies expected to attend the same events as Jimmy, along with the word on the street, that restricted his movements. He felt increasingly lonely and stressed; he argues the pressure also manifested itself physically as he lost weight and suffered from an inflamed rectum and skin diseases on his hands and feet. Exhausted, he finally fled to his summer house to get away from everything, and he started to think about committing suicide: 'my aim was that it would happen if you don't drink or eat'. But something different occurred.

> I was lying in bed alone in the summerhouse for a month or so ((chuckle)) and just slept. Uh, despite everything that had happened, I woke up and found joy, and I didn't really understand why. Why, huh, happy when you've lost everything? [...] It was, after all this, all this stress and all the things I had let go of; I stopped and took care of myself, trying to listen a bit to how I felt [...] so uh, I began to think positively, not about what I had lost, but what I had left ((chuckle)). After all, you've still got something left; you can never lose it all.

Places represent affective possibilities (Anderson 2009) and their materialities may act as hinges for different moods. Isolation is therefore not simply about geographical distance but is also relational and emotional. For Jimmy, his summer house became a place where he could get away from his small town and the online responses and isolate himself from the outside world. One could say that, as the local atmosphere became increasingly hostile, his only solution was to geographically move away from it. Hiding out at the summer house illustrates his bodily movement being more and more restricted by the events as well as generating certain affective states. He was socially isolated, alone and depressed, staying in bed for 'about five days without getting up'. But the isolated summer house also enabled new affective possibilities as he narrates that his moods altered. With this, he realised too that things had to change, and that he could not go on chasing success and wealth in the way he had done since it was this, he thinks, that led him to become violent. Jimmy's narrative could be seen as a form of epiphany or turning-point story, a form of offender narrative where violent men present themselves as self-conscious. By recounting how they have realised that they needed to change and how they have transformed themselves, Jimmy and the other men in the study not only present themselves as reformed but also as aware and conscious of their abusive behaviour (Gottzén, forthcoming). Jimmy's case illuminates how turning-point stories are spatial and affective events; they are movements towards an insight into who you 'are', but also movements away from who you do not want to be. They are means to move away from a deviant and disgraceful masculinity by narrating how you have rejected anger and aggression, to acknowledge having been violent while distancing yourself from being the crazy guy who threatens and abuses his former partner, defames her on Facebook, gets furious because he is about to lose his house and 'everything' and instead become somebody overwhelmed with joy. This does not necessarily mean that Jimmy condones his violence, but that he presents it as the actions of a violent man placed in a historical past, while the man after the turning point is portrayed as essentially non-aggressive.

Conclusion

By way of conclusion, let me point out some of the advantages of the concept of atmospheres as a contribution to research on violence against women as well as to social work research and practice. To start with, exploring the affectivity of violence, in terms of atmospheres, demonstrates that domestic violence is a socio-spatial and multi-scalar matter; it is not only a 'domestic' affair but is played out in many different spaces, including the city centre, the home and the Internet. These may relate to each other through the transmission of affect between human and non-human bodies.

Further, focusing on atmospheres helps us to draw attention to some of the issues that affect theory has been accused of ignoring, particularly embodied experience and political materiality (Tolia-Kelly 2006). The concept highlights how space and materiality simultaneously influence emotions and bodily capacities. Aggression can be intentional and calculating yet also passionate and constitute something of an affective excess. Affect can be seen as an event where everything is possible, where bodies come together in a specific time and place and influence each other. Following this, violence constitutes the closure of potentiality; the very moment when various affective elements are framed into affective states and actions that violate the normal interaction and fixate gendered and embodied experience. The political potential of atmospheres – like all assemblages – lies in that they are not simply positive or negative (Deleuze & Guattari 1987) but may generate a variety of potential trajectories. They can move in a number of directions. Atmospheres can be characterised by aggression and violence, where a victim experiences fear, but they may also affect the perpetrator when human and non-human bodies respond in various ways in different spaces.

Finally, atmosphere has in this chapter been a lens for exploring victimhood and perpetratorhood, but it could also be used as a point of departure for feminist social work research and interventions where, for instance, safe atmospheres are designed for victims of violence. But it is not sufficient to identify, for instance, which places victims experience as safe; instead, we need to explore how safety – as an affective atmosphere – is produced in different locales. For instance, grandparents and other relatives may produce safe atmospheres for children exposed to intimate partner violence in various domestic and non-domestic places through their physical and spatial proximity, but also through developing disclosive relationships and by siding with the victims (Gottzén & Sandberg, forthcoming). In addition, viewing atmospheres as placed assemblages helps us to understand the significance of non-human bodies, which is particularly important since research and interventions tend to focus only on the individual perpetrator or the couple while the importance of movement, space and materiality is largely neglected. It is not sufficient to simply focus on the relationship between violence and the 'glocal' but also on the emotional, multi-scalar spatialities of violence and the affective atmospheres that permeate social problems in general. This calls for social work research and practice that do not simply pay attention to the multi-scalar and spatial aspects of social problems but that also are sensitive to the sensorial and affective potentialities of social problems and social work practice, both on global and local levels.

Notes

1 The study 'Grandparents' responses to intimate partner violence: Children's experiences and perspectives' was conducted with Linn Sandberg and financed by the Children's Welfare Foundation, Sweden. It included ten children aged 12–18 who have lived in families that have experienced physical violence against one parent. All names have been changed.
2 The project 'Men's violence against women in intimate relations: A study of the perpetrators' social networks' was led by Margareta Hydén and financed by the Swedish Council for Working Life and Social Research. In total, 44 men (aged 17–66) participated (Gottzén 2013, 2016, forthcoming).

References

Ahmed, S 2010, *The Promise of Happiness*, Duke University Press, Durham, NC.

Anderson, B 2009, 'Affective atmospheres', *Emotion, Space and Society*, vol. 2, no. 2, pp. 77–81.

Anderson, B 2015, *Encountering Affect: Capacities, Apparatuses, Conditions*, Ashgate, Aldershot.

Anderson, B & Ash, J 2015, 'Atmospheric methods' in *Non-Representational Methods: Re-Envisioning Research*, ed P Vannini, Routledge, London, pp. 34–51.

Bille, M, Bjerregaard, P & Sørensen, TF 2015, 'Staging atmospheres: Materiality, culture, and the texture of the in-between', *Emotion, Space and Society*, vol. 15, no. 1, pp. 31–38.

Böhme, G 1993, 'Atmosphere as the fundamental concept of a new aesthetics', *Thesis Eleven*, vol. 36, no. 1, pp. 113–126.

Clough, P & Halley, J (eds) 2007, *The Affective Turn: Theorizing the Social*, Duke University Press, Durham, NC.

Deleuze, G 1988, *Spinoza: Practical Philosophy*, City Lights Books, San Francisco, CA.

Deleuze, G & Guattari, F 1987, *A Thousand Plateaus: Capitalism and Schizophrenia*, University of Minnesota Press, Minneapolis, MN.

Edensor, T & Sumartojo, S 2015, 'Designing atmospheres: Introduction to special issue', *Visual Communication*, vol. 14, no. 3, pp. 251–265.

Fiene, J 1995, 'Battered women: Keeping the secret', *Affilia*, vol. 10, no. 2, pp. 179–193.

Glaser, D 2002, 'Emotional abuse and neglect (psychological maltreatment): A conceptual framework', *Child Abuse & Neglect*, vol. 26, no. 6, pp. 697–714.

Gottzén, L 2013, 'Encountering violent men: Strange and familiar' in *Men, Masculinities and Methodologies*, eds B Pini & B Pease, Palgrave Macmillan, London, pp. 197–208.

Gottzén, L 2016, 'Displaying shame: Men's violence towards women in a culture of gender equality' in *Response-Based Approaches to the Study of Interpersonal Violence*, eds M Hydén, D Gadd & A Wade, Palgrave Macmillan, London, pp. 156–175.

Gottzén, L forthcoming, 'Violent men's paths to batterer intervention programs: Masculinity, turning points, and narrative selves', *Feminist Criminology*.

Gottzén, L & Sandberg, L forthcoming, 'Creating safe atmospheres? Children's experiences of grandparents' affective and spatial responses to domestic violence', *Children's Geographies*.

Heimer, G, Andersson, T & Lucas, S 2014, *Våld och Hälsa – En Befolkningsundersökning om Kvinnors och Mäns Våldsutsatthet Samt Kopplingen till Hälsa*, National Centre for Knowledge on Men's Violence Against Women, Uppsala.

Kelly, L 1988, *Surviving Sexual Violence*, Polity Press, Cambridge.

Massumi, B 2002, *Parables for the Virtual: Movement, Affect, Sensation*, Duke University Press, Durham, NC.

Massumi, B 2015, *The Politics of Affect*, Polity Press, Cambridge.

Pain, R 2001, 'Gender, race, age and fear in the city', *Urban Studies*, vol. 38, no. 5/6, pp. 899–913.

Ray, L 2011, *Violence and Society*, Sage, London.

Scheff, TJ 2011, 'Social-emotional origins of violence: A theory of multiple killing', *Aggression and Violent Behavior*, vol. 16, no. 6, pp. 453–460.

Thien, D 2005, 'After or beyond feeling? A consideration of affect and emotion in geography', *Area*, vol. 37, no. 4, pp. 450–454.

Thrift, N 2008, *Non-Representational Theory: Space, Politics, Affect*, Routledge, London.

Tolia-Kelly, DP 2006, 'Affect – an ethnocentric encounter? Exploring the "universalist" imperative of emotional/affectual geographies', *Area*, vol. 38, no. 2, pp. 213–217.

Watts, C & Zimmerman, C 2002, 'Violence against women: Global scope and magnitude', *The Lancet*, vol. 359, no. 9313, pp. 1232–1237.

8 Loss and Grief in Global Social Work

Autoethnographic Explorations of the Case of the Tsunami Catastrophe in Northeastern Japan, March 11, 2011

Els-Marie Anbäcken

Prologue

On March 11, 2011 at 14:46, I am in a restaurant close to Tokyo Station, finishing a late lunch meeting with Sayaka, a friend who some years ago studied and worked in the care of older people in Sweden. I have been invited to lecture at the Lutheran college in Tokyo on existential issues in eldercare the following day, and as it is around 500 kilometers from where I live in the Kansai area of Japan, I arrive a day earlier. At the end of our lunch, at 14:46, we experience an unforgettable rustling sound together with a strong and strangely mild shaking. We realize instantly that these sounds and movements are an earthquake. I have lived around 25 years in Japan—I was born here of missionary parents in the 1950s, so I spent childhood years and later came back to work for a few years in Japan. Earthquakes were—and are—not uncommon in Japan, but this one never seems to end; six minutes' duration with a magnitude of 9.0, and after a few minutes that feel eternal, we manage to leave the restaurant and walk down a few stairs to the street, and as we stand on the ground we feel the earth shaking beneath us. People are silent and there is no panicking. Some have gathered at specific meeting places with emergency rucksacks (obeying orders from their workplace). After some time has elapsed we enter a large building where television screens broadcast what has happened some hundreds and more kilometers northeast. What we see is unbelievable—water masses shuffling away cars as if they were toys, and people at a loss watching this right there and then while we watch at a distance in silence and unbelief—yet knowing it is really happening. Several afterquakes continue to shake the ground. We seek shelter for the night in a friendly restaurant that acts as a temporary shelter before I can return home the next day.

During the weeks that follow, daily television broadcasts show the disaster again and again. The terrifying news tells about the thousands of deaths but also about the radiation accident at the Fukushima plant. Mediated information repeatedly announces that the danger was limited, provoking anger and frustration among many people. Some politician appears in front of the television cameras eating farm products from the radioactivity-stricken areas, as if to normalize the situation and declare that "I am eating this so it is alright for anyone to eat"—which was not perceived by people as much of an assurance of safety. My neighboring city, Kobe, which was hit in 1995 by the Great Hanshin Earthquake, is alert with citizens often representing NGOs (Non Governmental Organizations): now it is our turn to offer help. The constant television broadcasting also shows examples of volunteer activities. Volunteers travel to the disaster sites. Social workers, teachers in social work, students, and civil society react with the attitude: if we can do something, we should. Local gyms become housing for hundreds and thousands of homeless people. One of my senior students who volunteered comments that "TV does not show what goes on backstage, that is, the 'sake' cans and bottles that pile up, a way of escaping in shock and grief." The emphasis in the mediated images is on how people unite to manage and how people help each other. One example from television is a graduate student who spent his spring vacation searching for photographs and restoring them as far as possible to their owners. Getting a treasured photo back brought reminders of loved ones now dead, but the photo had a deep meaning, portraying life before, with a partner, children, or grandchildren.

A photo and article in one of the large daily newspapers some days or weeks after March 11 shows a little girl, perhaps around four or five years of age. She is sitting near the shore with her mobile phone, waiting for her father to call, says her grandmother. He used to call her saying he was on his way home from fishing. This glimpse of existential loss has engraved itself in my memory.

Setting the Scene

The theme of this chapter emerged as an important aspect of the class I taught on global and transnational social work, from 2012–2013, at Linköping University, Sweden. Prior to this, from 2008–2012, I held a professorship at Kwansei Gakuin University (KGU) in Japan and thus encountered the tsunami catastrophe within an academic setting, in research as well as in student and faculty life. The way KGU was engaged to send volunteers left an impression on me. I was amazed, upon returning to work when the new academic year began in early April, at the presence of the disaster on campus. For example, one topic was how to make it possible for students to enroll as volunteers without overly affecting studies. Moreover, KGU arranged volunteer buses with teachers and students to go for a volunteer tour. A meeting in one of the larger classrooms informed about volunteering and how people in grief may react to volunteers coming to help. Two social work students from Linköping University who were on field practice also took part in a few days of volunteer work. Upon my return to Sweden and with the new class on global and transnational work at hand, it was natural to bring up (natural) disasters, social work, loss, and grief as an integral part of this. How do social workers encounter these kinds of losses? Moreover, can it be described as not only a global phenomenon but also a transnational one? While I would like to discuss both these aspects, the scope of this chapter does not allow that. I simply mention that transnational migration can be caused by a variety of disasters, including natural ones, and to write on that would need both contextual and theoretical considerations on transnational social work. I do think that lessons learned from going through a disaster, whether natural or manmade, and having to leave loved ones and places may include similarities in terms of how to deal with it in social work. But, again, this will have to be done in another study.

In this chapter, I will elucidate the theme of loss and grief from the specific case of the Great East Japan Earthquake, March 11, 2011. It will be based in my own experience of witnessing the disaster in various ways, both at the time that it happened and afterward. I witnessed through the media, but also experienced how Kwansei Gakuin University, where I was employed, responded, reacted, and acted. The chapter is a contribution to emergent social issues for social work and disasters based on the overall question: In what ways does social work tackle losses that citizens and clients experience in (natural) disasters? In what ways can autoethnography (AE) be a relevant methodological tool to contribute to answering such a question?

The Great East Japan Earthquake

The earthquake of March 11 was the strongest that had hit Japan since the measuring of earthquakes began, and was preliminarily the fifth strongest in the world since the year 1900. Its epicenter was located off the coast of northeast Honshu, some 380 kilometers northeast of Tokyo. Several afterquakes followed, the three largest with magnitudes between 7.0 and 7.4, all within one hour. The first days that followed saw hundreds of afterquakes with a magnitude of 4.5 or more. Four years later (March 10, 2015), the confirmed deaths were 15,893; 2,572 persons were missing and 228,863 people were living either in temporary housing or away from home (National Police Agency of Japan 2015a, 2015b, 2015c; Kobe Shinbun 2015, p. 1).

The earthquake and the tsunami wave destroyed buildings and infrastructure (Buerk 2011; Syed 2011). The nuclear accidents, primarily the level 7 meltdowns at three reactors in the Fukushima Daiichi Nuclear Power Plant complex, affected hundreds of thousands of residents in the associated evacuation zones (CNN 2011a, 2011b). The radiation was a fact which continues to cast shadows of worry for the population living near the plant—but also elsewhere down as far as the Tokyo area—since it was unclear how radiation moved, and the government was criticized for hiding facts.

Autoethnography

While ethnography has been my basic tool in studies of Japanese society so far, especially the participant observations I did in the early 1990s at two homes for the aged in Japan (Anbäcken 1997), my encounter with AE is recent. Already in ethnography the researcher is allowed to be seen—and not be "a fly on the wall" (Emerson et al. 1995, p. 3). In AE, this visibility is taken much further, with the experiences of the researcher in focus. To include the participants or the people we study is nothing new; in participatory action research the role of the partici-pants is central as research actors, subjects, and objects, while AE is described by Wall as "action research for the individual" (Wall 2006, p. 151, citing Ellis & Bochner). With the role of the "I," where the researcher's presentation of thoughts is central, AE gives room for philosophical reflections.

AE can also be related to the emerging of critical theories when new research strategies appeared, and Ellis, cited in Wall (2006, p. 148), states that it is common for feminist writers to start with their own experience in the research they do, which contrasts with the more logical and objective point of view. Wall goes as far as to claim that "Academic writers are beginning to acknowledge the normative value of inquiry". She further draws on the "growing emphasis on the power of research to change the world" and this implies the need for reflections on what we have learned and what it could lead to. Social research can be expanded to have a moral effect (Wall 2006, p. 148). Berry and Patti (2015) take this line of thought further as they describe how autoethnographic storytelling can function as a tool for change on a personal level, when researchers themselves can be "transformed" in processes involving moments of insights. In the AE tradition, it also means that these insights are shared in ways that stir both feelings and actions.

Another matter that Wall brings up is "voice" (2006, p. 148). I see this voice as the "I" which is common in ethnography and also partly in qualitative studies, as opposed to the detached "objective" third person style which is common in quantitative studies but also in genres of qualitative studies. While it is unrefuted that any reader should understand when it is the writer and when it is somebody else's voice which is heard in the text, in AE the "I" is very much the central figure, whose role needs to be discussed as that of any person involved as an informant in a study. Guzik (2013) describes this, quoting Ellis's declaration that the researcher is "both the author and focus of the story" (Ellis in Guzik 2013, p. 271). I am reminded of Moustakas (1961), whose work on existential loneliness has impressed me and, in addition, has bearing on the theme of this chapter. I have felt some ambivalence to his way of writing. I have asked myself: Is it permissible to be so personal and emotional, perhaps even as "normative" as he is? In this chapter, I attempt to use my own "story" but reflect on it from various angles that I find relevant, both empirically and theoretically, within the limitations of time, space, and context. Perhaps more than anything else, I will illustrate more than describe the experiences (cf. Chase, referred to in Guzik 2013). In Witkin's (2014) introduction to his edited volume on AE and social work, dialogue is mentioned as one (of several) important elements in AE. Viewed in relation to social work I find it a nice match since dialogue is an important part of social work practice. Dialogue is also how other authors on ethnography characterize AE, a dialogue between others' findings and one's own—and between author and reader.

Methodological Reflections

I traveled 11 months after March 11 to visit some of the disaster-stricken areas, and during these visits I held conversational interviews that I interweave in my AE. I met several colleagues in Japan who got involved in volunteer work and research work following March 11. Many had similar experiences, also from the volunteer activities and research in the aftermath of the Great Hanshin Earthquake which hit the Kobe area in January 1995. My research colleague and friend, former professor Minemoto Kayoko is one of those to whom I am especially indebted. Not only did she connect me to literature in this field, especially her Ph.D. study (2015) which is about the two disasters in 1995 and 2011 with the focus on the welfare of older people.[1] Her commitment also appeared in an informal interview (personal communication, May 25, 2012) telling that she has continued to visit twice a year, having café-style programs to take the time to just sit and talk over a cup of tea. She also had counseling with those who were left alone. Another aspect she mentioned was the role of *Zenshakyou* (abbreviation for Japan's third-sector organization in social welfare) to create order in the organization of humanitarian aid, including volunteer activities. Another important informant is Nishida Chiyuki, the program and team coordinator of the NPO organization "Lutheran Emergency Relief" for persons living in temporary housing.

Through my university network, I was connected to Sasao Hiroyuki,[2] who I interviewed in May 2015 for around 90 minutes. Prior to this, we had talked about his experience as a volunteer, but now I took notes and wrote them down soon after the interview. His story will be presented as a case in point, which brings up some aspects which will be further discussed in relation to the theme of this chapter.

Some photos from my visit in February 2012 are included in the chapter. They were not taken for research purposes or with any thought of publishing.[3] Therefore, a nuanced discussion on the methodology of photos in research will not be included. However, Rose (2007) delves deeply into interpretations of visual material, providing a rich account of how visual images can be used in research. She emphasizes the importance of taking images seriously by viewing them carefully, addressing cultural practices as well as their meanings and effects, and considering one's way of looking at the images (Rose 2007, p. 12). As I think of the photos, these aimed to reflect "realities" of the glimpses of disaster stories I heard and to remind me of what was told, expressed, and felt as I met the persons and encountered the places. From this mix of material, I would like to elaborate on various aspects of loss and grief, physical, social, emotional, and existential.

From the first lines, I have thus started out autoethnographically with "I was there." Yet, I was not there in the midst of the disaster; I was in Japan, and close enough to feel the quake, but I never suffered any physical or material losses and in this sense, I am a "viewer". In another sense, I did participate, as a citizen living and working in Japan during the time of the disaster and one year thereafter. My personal reflections are thus from this experience of how I perceived March 11.

Visiting the Earthquake and Tsunami-Stricken Areas in Miyagi Prefecture, Northern Honshu, February 5–7, 2012[4]

The first impression was that, 11 months after March 11, many places still looked as if they had been struck by war. I was drawn into the experience told by the guide to our visit, himself being in a leadership position at his firm at that time and having to prompt his staff to run up to the highest floor. He told us that he could rescue all but a handful who were drawn out by the powerful waves. This bugs his mind.

One of the two specific site visits turned out to take the form of a kind of participant observation. We were invited as guest and speakers to an activity center in Ishinomaki town where an NPO (Non-Profit Organization), "Lutheran Emergency Relief," arranged weekly programs for older persons living in temporary housing. The lasting memory of this event was all the input we received from being there, eating and talking with these elderly adults who had experienced immense losses.

Further, through missionaries who lived south of the disaster areas, we were able to visit Kesenuma town, where one of them, Ann-Christine Kullberg, volunteered with music therapy for children. We start our journey here.

Visit to Kesennuma Town

Japan Baptist Kesenuma Church (98 years old) runs a children's nursery, Aikou Kindergarten (100 years old). Aikou seems to be central to this municipality; we were told that the whole municipal leadership went to this children's nursery in their childhood. At the time of our visit, there were 106 children in preschool from age 3 and up. Some of them were from other preschools that were destroyed by the tsunami. Half of the residents of Kesenuma municipality have suffered from the tsunami. More than half of the children have lost their homes. I recall a little girl who talked in a matter-of-fact way about the temporary housing, *kasetsu juutaku*, a word that children of her age would not need to be familiar with had it not been for the disaster.

We visited the town, still under reconstruction. We heard stories such as "The barber saw from his window a car swept away in the water masses, he had eye contact with the driver." We visited temporary shops recently started, including a restaurant where we enjoyed lunch with a sense of awe. To start business again meant to give a sense of normality. We heard of churches as partners in civil society together with numerous other NPOs helping in various ways; for example, the organization CRASH[5] did both hands-on work of cleaning out the houses (which was a common task for most volunteers in the early days following the disaster) and therapeutic work which, by now (2012), had become their core activity. Many older people in particular live alone in temporary prefab housing, in one or two small bedrooms with a kitchen and bathroom, distributed by chance and not following any community or neighborhood principles (even though this had been recommended from the Kobe Earthquake experience). So strangers had to become neighbors (Figure 8.1 and 8.2).

Typical prefab temporary housing. Perhaps the grayish winter day added to the melancholic atmosphere that the photos convey? Looking into the photos, they remind me both visually and emotionally of what I encountered on this specific site visit. But it is also like a sounding board for the mix of visual, oral, and written information obtained during and after the visit as a whole.

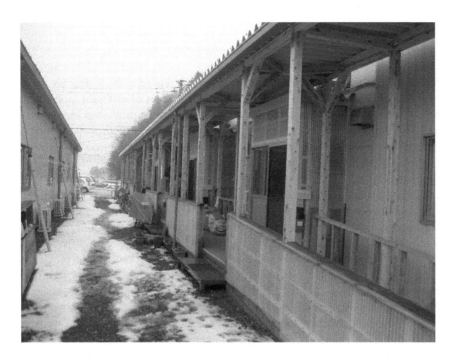

Figures 8.1 Temporary Housing, Ishinomaki, Japan.
Photo: Els-Marie Anbäcken 2012.

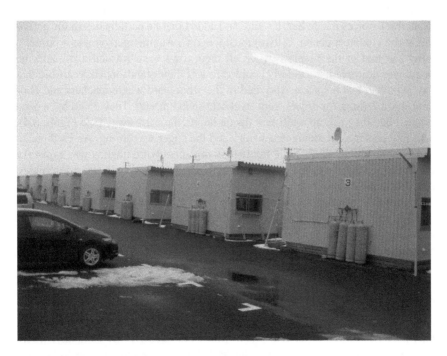

Figures 8.2 Temporary Housing, Ishinomaki, Japan.
Photo: Els-Marie Anbäcken 2012.

Visit to Ishinomaki Town

Ishinomaki was struck very hard by the disaster. There were (at the time of our visit in February 2012) 160 temporary housing sites, each with 30–100 residents. Several volunteer organizations participate in work related to the temporary housing. In each area there is a common house for activities of different kinds, with refreshments, meals, lectures, music, sewing, cooking together, watching movies, and also physical training, to support the residents. We visited one such house called *kasetsu shukaishyo*, "temporary neighborhood meeting place", invited by Nishida Chiyuki from the Lutheran emergency relief.⁶ Welfare in Sweden was the requested theme, and strange as it felt for me to present it, at least it was a "normal" program at activity centers for older people in general in Japan. At the end of the afternoon spent there, some of the ladies went back to their temporary flats and brought their home-made pickles (*otsukemono*) for us to taste. For me, it was a sign of hope, of resilience and coping. Making these pickles shows that something very ordinary in everyday life is recovered. I brought some of the pickles to KGU to a meeting with colleagues, as my *omiage* to them, the obligatory gift to bring after a visit to another part of Japan: "From Ishinomaki with love" suddenly became a real message from my heart, not just a slogan.

We listened to many stories, or glimpses of stories, while we had a Swedish-style lunch (prepared by Chiyuki-san) and later tea and snacks together. The retired school principal told us with a big smile of how he survived and also managed to rescue his wife. He found some air space in his flooded house where he and his wife clung to a sofa that floated on the water. Their house was totally destroyed. They heard others screaming for help but could not do anything. His wife still hears these voices inside her, he said, and added that he participates in the activities at the volunteer center, "(I/we) must live on". Another person was a farmer's wife; she told of the scenario when all their cows were washed away and the house was destroyed. An elderly couple brought their grandson, six years old that day, who had lost his sister who died in the schoolyard where teachers and children stood waiting for orders from an absent schoolmaster. They could have been rescued had they run up a hill less than a hundred meters away (see Figure 8.4). This had become a national news story and the anger was strong. An earthquake and tsunami are no man's fault, but behind this schoolyard tragedy was a mistake by a person, which evoked a lot of strong feelings mixed with the grief, anger, bitterness, and sorrow.

Figure 8.3 shows the memorial at the schoolyard where the majority of the children and teachers died while waiting for orders for what to do. How municipalities can be efficient instead of bureaucratic was emphasized as an issue in the aftermath of the Kobe Earthquake in 1995.

A Volunteer Narrative

At this point, it is time to introduce Sasao Hiroyuki, who became a volunteer and later a social worker. After retirement from work at an electric company, where he worked in the research division, he started to take evening classes to become

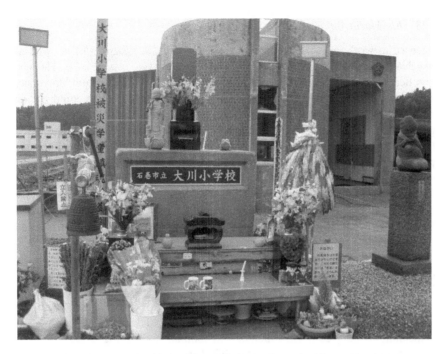

Figure 8.3 Memorial at the Okawa Elementary School Yard, Ishinomaki, Japan.

Photo: Els-Marie Anbäcken 2012.

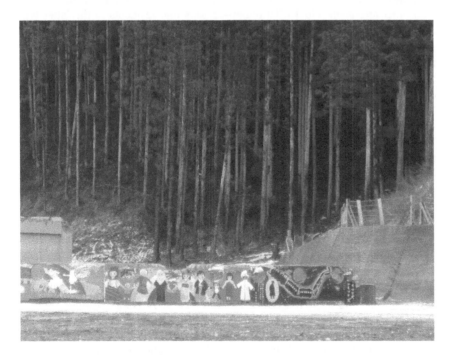

Figure 8.4 The Hill of Possible Rescue at the Okawa Elementary School Yard, Ishinomaki, Japan.

Photo: Els-Marie Anbäcken 2012.

licensed to work in social welfare (社会福祉士, *shakai fukushi shi*)[7] as well as psychiatric care work (精神保健福祉士, *seishin hoken fukushi shi*). He also enrolled as a special student in a social work class at Kwansei Gakuin University for two years. He recalled that when the earthquake hit Kobe he could not do anything, but now he wishes to "give back". A month after the earthquake happened there was a call for volunteers from the Japan Social Worker Association (日本社会福祉士会, *Nihon Shakai Fukushi Shi Kai*). In June he went to Iwate prefecture to help the community support center. There was a need to restore the structures of municipal welfare work—most of the staff had died. After doing volunteer work here and later also organizing the move of people to temporary housing that was being built (in Kobe, many continued to live in such housing for several years), Hiroyuki-san felt that he wanted to work more with people and "connect people". So when he read that they were looking for staff to work in three centers for counseling/mental health care, 心のケア, *kokoro no kea* (literally "the care of the heart," which includes grief care), he applied and stated to work there in early 2013, as *seishin hoken fukushi shi*. He rents a small apartment and visits his wife three or four days a month (and she supports his choice, herself active in welfare research). He communicates with their only grandchild on "FaceTime". It is meaningful and free work, which he will continue until spring 2016.[8]

Hiroyuki-san's daily work now is mainly *kokoro no kea.* It means that he visits people, victims of the disaster, in their homes. There are two kinds of temporary housing for them: prefab housing and apartments paid by the prefecture, mixed with other apartment blocks. Hiroyuki-san says that residents in the latter type express more loneliness. There are 2,000 apartments of each kind in this Miyagi prefecture. His organization performed a health survey with a 60 percent response rate. Common answers were cannot sleep, remembers, worries. Persons are eligible for *kokoro no kea* following certain criteria based on the survey assessment, but the formal decision is made at the *kokoro no kea* centers.

Hiroyuki-san visits up to 100–120 persons, some of them every week, some a few times per year. Some speak a lot, some speak after a while when they have gotten to know each other. These visits can take from ten minutes up to the whole day, but on average last one hour. He does not bring it home anymore, but it took some time to get used to the work. He felt sad when someone refused a visit. He is not the only contact person they meet; one more person visits "his" cases.

What kinds of 心の悩み, *kokoro no nayami* (suffering of heart/emotional suffering), does he encounter? In the beginning it was the losses of family. Now many feel stress about how to live. Now when people have settled down, the need for *kokoro no kea* comes, says Hiroyuki-san. Issues such as how to use one's time are ever-present. Among men in the temporary housing, alcohol consumption or パチンコ, *pachinko* gaming, are common ways to spend time. Many in their forties and fifties have no work. There is a need to find some other ways of enjoying life. Some who also had problems before the disaster used to be in hospital for drug addiction. There was an AA (Alcoholic Anonymous) group, but the AA concept does not suit elderly Japanese so they started another form of AA. "To lose families, some can live with the sadness, some not," Hiroyuki-san summarizes.

Two or three years after the disaster, the numbers of suicides diminished, but now the situation is back to "normal" (high), and Hiroyuki-san thinks that after the disaster people felt strongly that they needed to make efforts together, みんないっしょにガンバロウね (*minna issho ni gambarou ne*), an attitude that helped give focus and energy. Now the lack of work is a problem. This is, in general, a problem for men aged 50 and above in Japan (Yamada et al. 2005), and this double vulnerability of being struck by disaster in middle age makes it a large problem. Some have built new houses to live in, younger families chose uphill locations for safety reasons, and older people will want to live near the sea. In this area of Japan four-generation households were common, but after the disaster many families split, and even if they receive support to build a house to go back to co-living, it is not so easy to live that way again. Building up a new town and community is thus also a process which influences people's lives and feelings. Urban ways of life seem to displace rural lifestyles, where people used to help each other. This view is an ideal cultural memory of the happy multigeneration family (cf. Anbäcken 1997) and the positive image of the good community-mindedness of rural Japan has been used in elder care policy since the aging of Japan began to be highlighted.

The *kokoro no kea* center was planned for five years, but they talk about another five years, learning from the case of Kobe. The sadness of the tsunami is not only the sadness of losses, of family, but losses of another way of living, three or four generations, relatives, neighbors, all along the coast.

What are the needs today? The need for someone who listens remains. Support is reduced now, and Hiroyuki-san is worried about who will support the lives of these people when the system is back to normal. He also describes the different expressions of the loss caused by the disaster; in Fukushima, where the nuclear plant was destroyed, people display feelings of anger. They want to show the nation their anger, but it is people they meet who incur the anger.

Loss and Social Work Responses to Loss in Disasters

Loss and grief are core issues for social work in the globalized condition where disasters have consequences for the lives and well-being of people in local communities, but also for the re-building supported from national and international organizations. My study of loss and grief in social work is from this specific Japanese context and my drawing on it to be applicable more broadly to the knowledge base in globalized social work of relevance to environmental challenges and disasters. What I have come across is a few studies and, in addition, a Japanese (unpublished) literature review (Anzai & Sato 2015), which concludes that few studies in Japan in social work have dealt with loss and grief while other disciplines have, such as psychology and caring sciences. In contrast, an article on a social work intervention after the 2003 earthquake in Bam, Iran, shows that much of the ordinary social work skills can be used in working with survivors (Javadian 2007). This study offers an insightful account of what social workers do, from situational support by being attentive to immediate needs and by listening to confirm the descriptions narrated by the survivors. Support from individual, family and community levels to coordinating services, from intervening on different levels, for example by improving service programs, changing welfare policies and recovery programs to developing volunteer services. This represents a variety of actions from individual counseling approaches to structural societal work including advocacy for change—all which are hallmarks of social work practice. Another study with a more psychiatric perspective and with a family focus considers traumatic loss in natural disasters, emphasizing the need to be involved in early interventions in family or multifamily sessions (Walsh 2007). Quite detailed advice to identify various resources of strength and healing is recounted and the emphasis is on relations in family and community.

Lyons et al. (2006) elaborate on the meaning of loss from many angles in their volume on international social work. They write: "Loss permeates human experience. It is present in any situation encountered by social professionals working with people to improve social functioning and enhance life situation" (Lyons et al. 2006, p. 62). While loss is their core concept, they also provide definitions of grief, bereavement, and mourning, each one related to loss. "Bereavement is the process surrounding the loss of a loved object; *loss* is defined as the harm or suffering caused by losing something or someone; *grief* is the psychological reaction to bereavement; and *mourning* is the public display of grief" (Lyons et al. 2006, p. 64). All these aspects were displayed in the aftermath of March 11, but I shall not go into depth analyzing the different terms; I use only the terms loss and grief. Nevertheless, my introduction touched on the responses of people and organizations to the disaster, thus expressions of mourning. Furthermore, Hiroyuki-san's encounters with persons who had experienced loss (and my own brief encounters) came at a time when they were going through both grief and bereavement.

The need to emphasize the need for knowledge of loss and its meanings as a requirement for social professionals calls for some reflections on the profession. Lyons et al. (2006) chose the label of social professionals, thus encompassing all those who work in the social work field. These may differ in different countries and according to the local geography and circumstances, as the case of Hiroyuki-san shows. Social workers have varying roles. Many aspects need to be understood when working across borders and when working together with different professions. Dominelli (2010), for example, describes and discusses the international social work organizations and their roles in disasters, underlining social workers' various roles in capacity-building initiatives. Examples are the disaster relief initiatives RIPL (Rebuilding People's Lives) for IASSW (International Association of Schools of Social Work) and for IFSW (International Federation of Social Workers) through FAST (Families and Survivors of Tsunami Project). While the authors underline the importance of social professionals working with compassion in their encounters with people experiencing traumatic losses, Lyons et al. (2006, p. 63) also emphasize that

The universal nature and presence of loss and grief in an era of globalization: war, famine, genocide, bombing, torture, natural disasters, and movements of people across borders can all result in loss, sometimes multiplied in unimaginable ways.

They make a point of visual and auditory communications (television, radio, the Internet) which remind of the losses of "identity, home possessions, freedom, childhood" (Lyons et al. 2006, p. 63). The previously mentioned university student who commented after returning from a volunteer activity that, while media show encouraging examples fueling hope from various activities, the "ugly" ways of coping with grief, reflected in piled-up *sake* (alcohol) cans backstage, were not shown. Good ways of coping were focused on by the media, or at least not the stigmatized view of alcohol consumption. I recall a documentary about a family where they toasted the New Year with sake, with tearful eyes, for their lost loved ones.

The loss that is experienced in sudden disasters is first of all very physical. The loved one is gone. There was no time to say goodbye, or to change the last memory of meeting, the last words. There is no chance to repair, an important factor for recovery that Lyons et al. bring up (2006, p. 69). Disasters not only crush things and kill people, but the losses are often traumatic. The loss of all those things that are a part of life, but maybe not thought of in terms of factors that affect one's feelings, is mentioned in relation to disasters: loss of community and how life is organized in the specific community one lives in; loss of routines of daily life—for example, going to school or work, and the many hours spent there which have become substantial parts of one's life. All these and others that are mentioned, including loss of animals (Lyons et al. 2006, p. 69), have appeared in Japan in media coverage, and the latter example was also part of many farmers' experience in the Tohoku area.

The various activities we heard of were about trauma treatment, support in practical matters by and toward municipalities and authorities, gymnastics (simple), handicraft, lectures, sharing experiences, connecting people, etc. Different NGOs/NPOs were allowed different day activity centers or temporary housing to visit (usually once a week). On my visit to the "temporary neighborhood meeting place," a group of policemen participated for the last time in the gymnastics and said farewell to the participants; their term as policemen dispatched from the nearby Tokyo area was over. The character of this activity and meeting center, to support each other to be able to move on, seems to be a common theme in several reports from organizations actually providing humanitarian aid, emotional care, and social activities.[9] Further, Lyons et al. (2006, p. 63) make a point that the awareness of loss is increased, not only for those who experience it but also for those who provide social support and help. Here, one publication will be named as a case in point: 明日への動向―東日本大震災後の地域福祉 (The quickening for tomorrow—Community welfare after the great disaster in east Japan, 2015). It contains reports from many of the municipalities that were hit by the disaster, what actions took place immediately, after two months, nine months, one year, the activities that the communities hosted, and volunteers, both individuals and NPO organizations. The activity of simply being around, spending time with *yorisou katsudo*, seemed important. Feelings of guilt did come up ("Only I survived"), but also different kinds of worries, such as having lost one's job. A theme running through the book is "to move toward independence/autonomy" (*jiritsu ni mukatte*). Behind the lines of the book, the losses shine through but also the strength of doing things together, to move forward "shoulder to shoulder" with other people. This seems to be the essential meaning of the program offered at "temporary neighborhood meeting place" center.

Takahashi (2012) focuses explicitly on grief care as provided by bereavement support groups and how those suffering from the disaster deal with their grief. Some special features include the grief when the body was not found, which was described as ambiguous loss. One specific matter which can be related to this is the sorrow that one cannot fulfill the traditions linked to the family altar, since there are no ashes. Another characteristic of the stress experienced by survivors of the March 11 disaster was described as long-term and also diverse, with many different types of losses, but also survivor's guilt, as well as feelings that others in the community were hit more than oneself—so their grief is greater (Takahashi 2012, p. 67). Different theories were put forward by Takahashi, such as the pendulum model of Stroebe and Shut. Lennéer Axelson (2010) builds on Stroebe and Shut to show that a person in grief moves between loss-oriented and restoration-oriented focus so that, while in loss, emotions take over, and in restoration a person may be able to take action to move on. It may be important to note that if persons in one family or community experience this pendulum at different times, it may be painful (Lennéer Axelson 2010). Grief is sometimes not verbalized but an ever-present reality.

Looking back, the Great Hanshin Earthquake in 1995 triggered research initiatives and the role of volunteer organizations attracted attention. In the next large earthquake in 2004, the Niigata disaster, the need for care management was highlighted. Minemoto (2015) concluded after the third, the March 11 earthquake, that while a lot of reports from the field and several symposia were held, the role of social welfare research should grow from then on. Further, the need to see victims of disasters as simultaneously being socially vulnerable persons was a crucial finding for social work. For example, social class as well as gender mattered. Otani (2014) also saw the need for the municipal authorities to better coordinate their work with community organizations and civil society.

Thus, I interpret it as a need to work within the established structures of social work, for example, the *chiiki houkatsu senta* (community all-inclusive centers), which started to be developed in Japan in 2006. These are crucial in welfare work with older persons, and after March 2011 these were, in fact, one of the facilitators for "activities" in the communities, as Hiroyuki-san also said. Community work continues to be key in welfare work in Japan, both in ordinary and in extraordinary times.

Loss and grief are something that stays with the people who have experienced them, becoming part of their life course. But it does not have to define them altogether, and social work can accompany clients or participants in community activities to move on toward independence and autonomy. In social welfare work with different administrative systems, we can learn from countries such as Japan which, as a (post)modern society, has experienced natural disaster that really has shaken the society and communities and the social welfare system. How to move quickly and cooperate with many volunteer organizations and volunteers is an important lesson to learn more about. Also, how to discern different kinds of loss and grief, such as the anger at the authorities who did not build walls high enough to protect the nuclear plants from being damaged. The anger at what may be seen as fate or may be directed against someone responsible for the catastrophe triggers different feelings and reactions.

The question remains: Why so few studies in social welfare and social work studies on loss and grief? This is a research question to follow up in new studies. Is it so that social work is more focused on providing practical social assistance and leaving grief care to psychologists and therapists? Anzai and Sato (2015) observe that most of the research on grief and loss is found in psychology and nursing science. So a search for *Higashi nihon dai shinsai* (Great East Japan Disaster), together with mental health or psychology (trauma), yields a lot of results. In contrast, very few results were found within social welfare/social work. This is remarkable when we see that a lot of the work to aid the victims was perceived as social welfare in a broad sense. It would be interesting to study more closely whether different professionals and different sectors in public care worked together so that the specific social welfare boundary was blurred. Were health care and psychology (made) more visible due to media coverage? Were the various NPOs/ NGOs seen as the main actors on the scene? Perhaps the municipal formal social welfare work did most of the administrative parts of the work, while the NPOs and NGOs were more out of office, involved directly with people.

From reflections of the autoethnographic memory scenes and conversations with people from the March 11 disaster, it can be concluded that loss (accompanied with grief) is a universal concept that needs to be studied further in social work when encountering people suffering in and from disasters. As social work is increasingly global and transnational, it means that also in countries with little experience of natural disasters, such as Sweden, disaster experience is present and needs to be dealt with.

Epilogue

Back in Japan, and ten days after a research get-together[10] with disaster support as the theme, news broadcasting is interrupted at 21:32 on April 14, 2016: an earthquake of around magnitude 7 has hit Kumamoto, on the southern island of Kyushu. During the days to come the news is filled with reports, and hundreds of afterquakes are mentioned. At around 7 a.m. on Saturday 16, a sound I remember from March 2011 instantly alerts me: a warning in red letters and a special warning sound on television—new earthquakes are expected in Oita prefecture and also in neighboring prefectures … "Please ensure it that you are not near things that may fall down on you." How does this news affect people who once experienced tragedies of losing loved ones, cherished things, and places?

Notes

1 I thank Toyomura Yasushi and Kazumi for their great help in reading and understanding crucial parts of one chapter of Minemoto Kayoko's study and another book in Japanese, to which I refer. Japanese names are commonly written in the order of family name followed by given name.
2 When I tell of Mr. Sasao Hiroyuki later on in "A Volunteer Narrative", I use his given name and add the prefix "-san," which makes it more polite.
3 I have asked Nishida Chiyuki about the use of photos, and since their own photos had been allowed to be publicly displayed, it was concluded that we could use ours.
4 This text is partly translated from Owe Anbäcken's unpublished report, which was written during his work as regional director of Interact Asia. I was interpreting during this site visit while he took he notes and can be defined as "co-author". Rev. Usui Yoshio and his wife were hosts for us at this visit, themselves having experienced the disaster during their last service before entering retirement.
5 CRASH: Christian Relief Assistance Support – HOPE.
6 A note on volunteer organizations in Japan: these are often NPOs/NGOs and of many different kinds. This chapter mentions some which are rooted in Christianity—and these are not uncommon in Japan. Of course there are many more which we did not visit, both those rooted in religion and secular ones. I am deeply thankful to Nishida Chiyuki who has helped me to get an overview of publications in social welfare work, and with a focus on grief care, for this text.
7 Japanese words are written in Japanese characters the first time they appear in this volunteer narrative, together with the translation into English; thereafter the phonetic form is used in the text. The added Japanese language is to strengthen the "voice" of the storyteller. Elsewhere in this chapter, only phonetics and translations appear with one exception: when a book title is cited.
8 Updated information tells that from April 2016 he will continue, but only one week per month.
9 While this was compiled as a book with quite detailed information for the different municipalities, there were other and shorter publications on certain themes, or telling the story and activities of a certain group/NPO.
10 This research group is led by Minemoto Kayoko and focuses community care for older people.

References

Anbäcken, E 1997, *Who Cares? Culture, Structure and Agency in Caring for the Elderly in Japan*. PhD Thesis, Stockholm University.
Anzai, M & Sato, M 2015, *Unpublished Data Base Search*, Hosei University, Japan.
明日への動向―東日本大震災後の地域福祉 *Asu e no doukou – higashi nihon dai shinsai go no chiiki fukushi* [Moving towards tomorrow – community welfare after the East Japan Great Earthquake], 2015, 東北福祉大学地域福祉研究センター、仙台Tohoku Fukushi daigaku chiiki fukushi kenkyu center, Sendai.
Berry, K & Patti, CJ 2015, 'Lost in narration: Applying autoethnography', *Journal of Applied Communication Research*, vol. 43, no. 2, pp. 468–493.

Buerk, R 2011, 'Japan earthquake: Tsunami hits north-east'. BBC [online]. *Archived* from the original on 11 March 2011. [12 March 2011]. www.ktvz.com/news/128143212/detail.html

CNN Wire Staff 2011a, 'Japan: 3 nuclear reactors melted down – news story – KTVZ Bend'. Ktvz.com [online]. Archived from the original on 28 July 2011. [7 September 2011]. www.ktvz.com/news/128143212/detail.html

CNN 2011b, '3 nuclear reactors melted down after quake, Japan confirms'. CNN [online]. Archived from the original on 9 June 2011. [7 June 2011]. www.cnn.com/2011/WORLD/asiapcf/japan.nuclear.meltdown

Dominelli, L 2010. *Social Work in a Globalizing World*. Polity Press, Cambridge and Malden.

Emerson, R, Fretz, R & Linda, S 1995, *Writing Ethnographic Fieldnotes*. The University of Chicago Press, Chicago and London.

Guzik, E 2013, 'Representing ourselves in information science research: A methodological essay of autoethnography', *The Canadian Journal of Information and Library Science (La Revue canadienne des sciences de l'information et de bibliothéconomie)*, vol. 37, no. 4, pp. 268–283.

Javadian, R 2007, 'Social work responses to earthquake disasters: A social work intervention in Bam, Iran', *International Social Work*, vol. 50, no 3, pp. 334–346.

Kobe Shinbun (Kobe newspaper) 2015, "4th Anniversary today" p. 1.

Lennéer Axelson, B 2010, *Förluster: Om Sorg och Livsomställning*, Natur & Kultur, Stockholm.

Lyons, K, Manion, K & Carlsen, M 2006, *International Perspectives on Social Work: Global Conditions and Local Practice*, Palgrave Macmillan, London & New York.

Minemoto, K 2015,「地震災害と高齢者福祉阪神淡路大震災と東日本大震災の経験から Jishin Saigai to Koureisha-Fukushi Hanshin Awaji Daishinsai to Higashi Nihon Daishinsai no Keiken kara (Earthquake Disaster and Social Support for the Elderly Through Experiences from The Great Hanshin-Awaji Earthquake and The Great East Japan Earthquake) 久美 Kumi Publishing, Kyoto.

Moustakas, CE 1961, *Loneliness*, Prentice Hall, Englewood Cliffs, NJ.

National Police Agency of Japan 2015a, 'Damage situation and police countermeasures … 10 September, 2015' [online] (from 'Deaths' template). http://www.npa.go.jp/archive/keibi/biki/higaijokyo_e.pdf

National Police Agency of Japan 2015b, 'Damage situation and police countermeasures … 10 March, 2015' [online] (from 'injured' template). http://www.npa.go.jp/archive/keibi/biki/higaijokyo_e.pdf

National Police Agency of Japan 2015c, 'Damage situation and police countermeasures … 10 September, 2015' [online] (from 'missing' template). http://www.npa.go.jp/archive/keibi/biki/higaijokyo_e.pdf

Otani, J 2010, *Older People in Natural Disasters: The Great Hanshin Earthquake of 1995*, Trans Pacific Press & Kyoto University Press, Melbourne.

Rose, G 2007, *Visual Methodologies: An Introduction to the Interpretation of Visual Materials*, 2nd ed, Sage, London, Thousand Oaks & New Delhi.

Syed, S 2011, 'Japan quake: Infrastructure damage will delay recovery', *BBC News* [online]. Archived 17 March 2011 at WebCite. www.bbc.com/news/business-12756379

Takahashi, S 2012, 'Situation and support of bereaved families in Great East Japan Earthquake', *Japanese Journal of Traumatic Stress*, vol. 10, no. 1, pp. 65–70.

Wall, S 2006, 'An autoethnography on learning about autoethnography', *International Journal of Qualitative Methods*, vol. 5, no. 2, pp. 146–160.

Walsh, F 2007, 'Traumatic loss and major disasters: Strengthening family and community resilience', *Family Process*, vol. 46, no. 2, pp. 207–227.

Witkin, S L 2014, *Narrating Social Work Through Autoethnography*. Columbia University Press, New York.

9 Writing From the Self and the Liberatory Process of Reformulating Identities that Extends to and Beyond the Migratory Experience

Sindi F. Gordon

Introduction

My maternal grandparents were born in the Orkney Islands, Scotland, and after being married for several years they moved to the mainland, to Dundee, and it was here where my mother was born and grew up. I grew up in Leicester, central England, where my mother met my father. My father's grandfather was from the Spanish-speaking Caribbean island, Dominican Republic, although my father was born in the English-speaking Caribbean, in Antigua. I lived for several in the United States, where my son was born; his father is American and my son's paternal grandmother is part Native American. For my 12-year-old son. his multiplicity of identities and ways of being, as well as my own, is our inheritance rooted in migration; a reality aligned to the heterogeneous world so many of us now occupy, which is 'explicitly transcultural and international in nature' (Gilroy, 2009, p. 564).

It is my migratory background that positions me in my research and underlies the discussion for this chapter. The chapter explores the creative processes of writers whose lives have been shaped in various ways by a migratory experience; a transitional experience which often requires people to adjust to new personal, geographical, sociopolitical and cultural realities. For Isabel Hoving, the idea of displacement can bring loss, 'but also the potential for personal transformations' (Hoving, 2001, p. 14), an opportunity for the redefinition of self and for choosing a new way of being and seeing. The migratory space can offer an understanding of the 'tenuous constructions that constitute identity' (Jiménez Muñoz, 1995, p. 116). The notion of shifting between experiencing displacement as a 'loss' to one of 'transformation' and how it captures this liberatory experience in the creative writing process is of significance.

Retelling stories of personal experiences and memories for my parents, as well as for other people of migratory communities, serves as a sustainable thread in the realities of negotiating the concepts of home and displacement. It was here that I became introduced to the necessity of story-making and how stories travelled through memory, generations and play. The stories provide a creative vehicle of memory and imagination 'to navigate the uncharted terrain of a migratory experience' (Grewal *et al.*, 1988, p. 2).

Fictionalising Our Memories: Creative Life Writing for Personal Development

Narratives are crucial to the way we see ourselves and relate to others. I wanted to see whether, by changing the narratives we lived by, we could give new meaning to our past and current experiences and achieve self-growth. This chapter discusses my use of creative life writing as a community-based participatory research method which focuses on writers' experience of fictionalising their memories and examining whether this brings about a change and what that change may be. I am interested in this mindful relationship between memory and imagination which, as feminist theorist and cultural critic bell hooks claims of her own experience of fictionalising her memories, enabled her to look at her 'past from a different perspective and to use this knowledge as a means of self-growth and change in a practical way' (hooks, 1999, p. 86). I was keen to explore hook's reference to 'a practical way', which I interpreted as a transformation that is actively relevant to a writer's life.

My research drew from a body of practice and literature known as 'creative writing for personal development' (CWPD), associated with the work, amongst others, of Gillie Bolton (2004) and Celia Hunt and Fiona Sampson (1998). It could be described as the use of fictional autobiographical writing as a means of self-exploration, whether done on one's own or in a facilitated group in education or health and social care, or in a one-to-one context in some form of psychotherapy (Hunt & Sampson, 1998). In this approach, creative life writing (also called fictional autobiography) is used as a means of self-exploration. It requires that writers give themselves permission to fictionalise their writing, allowing them to explore their memories through feeling and emotion rather than focusing on factual details. Creative life writing (CLW), unlike conventional autobiography or life writing, is where the writer 'may not be aware of the extent to which she is fictionalizing, in fictional autobiography she has given herself permission to fictionalize herself' (Hunt, 2000, p. 12).

The notion behind the exploration of imaginative space(s) for my research is based on the understanding that memory is reconstructed and, therefore, memory is always using imagination. Psychologist Ulric Neisser views memory as a reconstruction of events rather than a recalling of events. We are telling *our* version of experiences, which leaves room for quite a lot of fiction in our memory (Neisser, 1994). Liz Stanley suggests that 'fictions may actually hold more truths about the past than a factual account' (Stanley, 1992, p. 64). The fictionalising of our life story allows us to excavate and explore conscious and unconscious material, memories that have been hidden or previously unavailable; as author Toni Morrison points out: 'the act of imagination is bound up with memory' (Morrison, 1995, p. 98). The research explores how the imagination impacts the telling of memories; stories that 'make sense of our lives'. I refer to memories that appear fixed and prevailing as life-held narratives or, as Neisser calls them, 'life narratives', which he deems critical, as they become significant memories and a 'way of defining ourselves'. CLW requires participants to be more active with their imagination, drawing on the idea that if memory is 'only a reconstructed version', the imagination is always at work in it (Neisser, 1994, pp. 1, 8). Using imagination more actively enables writers to articulate unconscious material, allowing the felt sense to enter the thinking process.

The work of CWPD focuses mainly on individual psychology and does not consider the wider sociopolitical context. By locating the inquiry in a multi-cultural setting I aim to broaden the discussion of CWPD. Recognising the dialogical engagement between an individual's inner psyche and outer realities introduces a psychosocial approach to understanding the makings of identity, and it is this that frames my study theoretically. Thus, I draw from psychodynamics, cultural studies and literature – primarily autobiographical and reflective essays and literary and political writings of the African diaspora – to emphasise the interconnection between self, family, community and society. Research into CWPD shows that participants often discover multiple dimensions of themselves, which enables them to distance themselves from social self-concepts (e.g. Hunt, 2013). I took these ideas and placed them in a more multicultural context where participants were explicitly able to explore difference and multiplicity rather than conforming to fixed hegemonic concepts, and in doing so challenged the notion of a 'multi-ethnic, mono-cultural society' (Hall, 2000). My interest lies in the creative process of writers who require the self to interplay and oscillate between different cultural frameworks. It is this implicit practice of crossing boundaries that, if recognised, can be applied to the creative writing practice. The movement and interaction between the different spaces opens up the possibility of stepping outside existing and limiting conceptual frameworks, as the creative page reveals complex lives and experience of identities that stretch far beyond those inscribed on them.

Community-Based Participatory Research Method in a Hair Salon/Barbershop

The community-based participatory research method looked at the effects on participants of a series of creative life writing workshops I facilitated in the basement of an urban hair salon/barbershop in England. The workshops provide a safe space for people to embark on an exploration of personal memory and experiences as a means to help them engage more reflexively with the narratives within which they are located. The salon serves people of African, Caribbean, Asian and European heritage. It is a microcosm of contemporary urban British society, a setting where boundaries such as gender, culture, ethnicity religion and other signifiers intersect. It is an English community that challenges the deeply held hegemonic claims of Englishness/Britishness, representing a new generation of Europeans. The salon is the 'hub' of the community, a place of collective activities and a natural setting for the telling and sharing of stories.

I was involved in the salon for more than eighteen months, as a client and also as a researcher developing my project. I met regularly with the salon 'steering committee' of staff and clients to discuss the design, developments and objectives for the inquiry. I was led to participatory action research (PAR), particularly a community-based participatory research (CBPR), as it offered a flexible and sustainable framework for an alternative research inquiry that brought together practice, theory and experience. All the participants of the CLW workshops were clients of the salon (including myself as the researcher) and were recruited to the project via flyers or 'word-of-mouth' within the salon. The workshops included men and women of Liberian, Jamaican, Ghanaian, German, Barbadian, Indian, Nigerian, Scottish, English, Brazilian and Chinese cultural heritage. Their ages ranged from early twenties to mid-sixties. The workshops took place in the basement of the salon for two hours every Saturday morning over ten weeks. We sat around a table with snacks and drinks, introducing an element of informality to diminish negative classroom experiences of writing, which many participants referred to, and also to demystify the idea of 'a writer'. My facilitation aimed to install the belief that everyone was equipped to participate fully in the workshop and to become authors of their own stories.

The Role of the Facilitator in the Creative Process

Within the overarching container of the salon lay the contained space of the creative life-writing workshop. Being the facilitator, my aim was to introduce fictional and poetic techniques that would enable people to use their imagination in different ways or at least be more active. This required the participants to let go of their everyday sense of self and open up to a larger sense of internal space which, as poet Audre Lorde suggests, holds 'unexamined emotion and feeling' (Lorde, 1984, p. 37). For Hunt and Sampson, letting go into the creative process requires us to

> ... relinquish, if only temporarily, our reason and to tolerate a state that may seem like a kind of madness or a kind of dreaming whilst awake, with all the potential hazards that involves.
>
> (Hunt & Sampson, 2006, p. 69)

How the participants *felt* in the workshop would help or hinder their personal explorations. It was important that I created a space that, whilst connected, was at the same time independent from the central salon space. The salon represents a public area that has its own prevailing narrative and may have assisted or restricted the participants' own personal journeys. The workshops were held away from the daily activities of business. Creating a space specifically for the workshop helped significantly to develop a group dynamic that was separate from the salon. As the facilitator, I wanted the writers to capture, as psychoanalyst Donald Winnicott says, the 'precariousness of magic itself', when the adult or child experiences letting go into the creative process. For Winnicott 'it is a magic that arises in intimacy, in a relationship that is being found to be reliable' (Winnicott, 1971, p. 64). It was important for me, as the facilitator, that the writers had confidence and trusted my ability to hold the group as they chose the precarious and daring path of self-exploration. The participants spoke: 'It was the trust you had with the tutor; the way you [facilitator] were in the group, I felt I could write anything; you made it fun which really helped'. In Kate Thompson's view, none of the poetic or fictional exercises will work 'without trust between the facilitator and the group' (Thompson, 2006, p. 141).

The Radical Step of Normalcy

Locating my research in a group of British participants with one or both parents from the African and Asian diaspora offered insightful elements, particularly for a research inquiry based around story, self and identity. The participants spoke of the group space as achieving a sense of inclusivity, 'an unspoken understanding because it feels quite rare … we are always in a minority in our current environment because of not being white'; 'when you feel that there is a space created for people like you, you feel more of who you are'. In the course of the research, the participants had to locate themselves, feel comfortable and feel that they belonged in the workshop before they could begin to open themselves up to change.

> Before I enter that space [a university creative writing class], metaphorically, here's my blackness, I put it in there [the participant mimes putting something in the bag]. I have a bad hair day, I put that in the suitcase; I feel depressed, I put that in the suitcase and I lock it tight and I leave it outside, and then I go into that space supposedly to be creative and I have to write my poetry … I am the only black person in the group. I feel they could not cope with it, could not understand and that is why I leave a part of myself outside.
>
> (A workshop participant)

The above comment relates to a writer's experience of attending creative writing courses where she is the 'only black person in the group'. When she spoke about leaving a part of herself in a suitcase outside the class, the powerful metaphor broke through any veils of politeness, constraint or awkwardness in the group, allowing for a burst of emotions and experiences to come forth from the other participants: 'You're never quite comfortable, always trying to fit in'; 'always on the edge and slightly marginalised'; 'I was asked to write about things that I didn't have a deep connection to and I would think how can I trust what I say with you [class teacher] because you probably won't even see it'. The participants spoke of a reality that extended beyond the boundaries of creative writing groups: 'I don't think you ever get used to never being in the majority or never been seen on a daily basis, not noticeable'.

The experience of 'otherness' often restricted and prevented the ability and willingness to write; rather than letting go into the imaginative process, the participants resorted to familiar narratives that offered only shallow representations of themselves. One participant spoke of being 'tired and frustrated' of having to 'over-explain' what she was trying to say. Another writer sympathised and said that she may have walked in as a writer but when she sat down in the class she became a 'black writer'. She said for her the 'space dictates' her writing process, and referred to a prose piece she wrote in the workshop, 'Uncle Ben's car smells like him', as 'reassuring'. It was only when she was rereading her writing to the group that she noticed:

> I was thinking about my uncles but there was no mention of them being black and I did not want to describe them as black ... It wasn't an issue and it is a given, your life is not just a response to slavery and racism, your life is as a human being on earth.
>
> (A workshop participant)

The workshops allowed the participants to feel centred and not in the margins of their experience: 'feeling as an insider is critical for me especially when I want to express or explore things I've not done before'. The group work incorporated poetic and fictional techniques (written and oral) and a wide range of literary texts of poetry and prose including writers of South African, Caribbean, Indian, British and Korean-American origin.

> The books we choose to bring into the classroom say a lot about what we think is important, whose stories get told, whose voices are heard, whose are marginalised.
>
> (Christensen, 2009, p. 6)

The participant who spoke of her experience of leaving part of herself outside the class said that the difference with the workshops in the salon was that 'not only do I bring my suitcase, I open it and all can come out'. Creating a learning environment where *all* participants feel that they belong enables them to engage fully in the process and speak of things that they had not spoken of before in public, and also to feel comfortable using words and mannerisms which they felt they did not have to explain in order to be understood. This contributed to the writers' ability to let go into the creative process and explore beyond familiar grounding.

The research shows the necessity for the participants to see and experience themselves in learning and creative processes and highlighted the power dynamics about whose story is authentic and should be heard and whose stories should not be heard or indeed whose narrative is acceptable or not.

The Creative Life Writing Workshop as a Third Area of Experience

There are a number of key theorists used in the literature on CWPD who I have found particularly helpful in my research. One of these is Winnicott, whose concepts of the 'holding environment' and the 'third area of experience' have very much influenced my approach. The idea of a *holding environment* is central to the conditions needed for creativity and self-growth to happen, which Winnicott believes to be intrinsically connected with each other. Winnicott's notion of a holding framework offers insight into the importance of creating a contained and 'safe-enough' space for the creative process to take place (Winnicott, 1971).

He used the term 'holding' to refer to the supportive environment that a therapist creates for a client. He compares this to the relationship between a mother and her child where the mother is nurturing and caring, which instils the child with a sense of trust and safety. For Winnicott, this relationship is essential for the child to achieve a healthy development; thus, the child feels secure and is therefore able to explore the relationship between his or her inner psychic world and outer realities (Winnicott, 1965). Holding spaces such as the CLW group in the salon allows for feelings and emotions to be explored and expressed safely. Hunt says that for creativity to take place we 'have to find our own particular ways of holding the space for the imagination' (Hunt & Sampson, 2006, p. 70). The holding space therefore enables the writer to enter into an imaginative space.

Winnicott calls the space for the imagination the 'third area of experience', also known as the 'potential space' where 'inner reality and outer life meet' (Winnicott, 1971, p. 3). It is here in the 'third area' that individuals can bring together the multiple dimensions of their lives. He emphasises the idea of fluidity and interconnectedness between spaces which are often perceived as separate. He says this area 'can be looked upon as sacred to the individual', as a place for self-growth (Winnicott, 1971, p. 139). In a Winnicottian context, the third area represents a metaphorical space where the child is gradually able to be alone to explore because the unconscious has become imbued with the presence of the mother. The mother's presence exists particularly in 'transitional objects' such as toys, blankets and teddy bears which have been important parts of the relationship between them. The 'holding environment' is critical; if the child does not feel safe, the experience of exploration can be frightening and chaotic. Winnicott's ideas are located in a therapeutic context but they are still pertinent to a group learning environment.

When I presented an exercise of 'introducing yourself through a favourite item of clothes', participants included their favourite boots, necklaces and a charm bracelet. Most of them were wearing their chosen item in the workshop, and some of the items continued to be worn throughout the series. The reasons offered included 'it's my favourite'; 'it makes me feel good'; 'I wear it for good luck'. It was here that I began to see Winnicott's transitional objects in a different context. The participants had brought into the workshop their own transitional objects, which enabled them to feel safe enough to explore their personal experiences and memories. From there I also began to see the collective identity like a transitional object, something that members of the group brought into the workshop; their shared identity of 'otherness' and difference as well as their 'client' identity installed a collective sense of safety and belonging. In the early stages of the workshop the shared narrative between the participants provided a key component in their ability to let go in the creative process.

The Third Area of Experience in a Sociocultural Context

In the context of my research, Winnicott's idea of the 'third area of experience', which he describes as 'expand[ing] into creative living and into the whole cultural life of man [and woman]' (Winnicott, 1971, p. 38), resonated strongly for me as there were aspects which echoed similarities with the sociocultural conversation of a 'thirdspace', which is also portrayed as a 'location of radical openness and possibilities' (hooks, 1991, p. 153):

> We are transformed, individually, collectively, as we make radical creative space which affirms and sustains our subjectivity, which gives us a new location from which to articulate our sense of the world.
>
> (ibid.)

It was this unified notion of the 'third area' and 'thirdspace' representing space dedicated to exploration and expansion that offered a new understanding to the CLW workshops held in the salon. Urban theorist Edward Soja describes the thirdspace simply as a place where everything comes together: 'a fully lived space, a simultaneously real-and-imagined, actual-and-virtual locus of structured individuality and collective experience and agency' (Soja, 1996, p. 11). I began to recognize the group work and the writings of the participants as potentially a new radical site of transformation, a 'safe-enough' meeting place where the participants could bring everything together; a space which mirrored the complexity and contradictions of their own lives. One of the participants spoke candidly about the difficulties of being of dual heritage growing up in a working class community and living in a care home. She saw her writing practice as allowing her to take 'ownership' of her life: 'I discovered that I was meant to be a bridge between all these different worlds that I was to inhabit'.

Soja says that the aim of the thirdspace is to build further, to move on, 'to continuously expand the production of knowledge beyond what is presently known' (ibid.). Similarly to 'a third area', it was these notions of opening dialogical space which focused on nurturing and inspiring expansion of knowledge that articulated the underlined objectives of the workshop.

The Conviviality of Third Cultural Space

> ... the fact that in Britain 'race' has become ordinary. Crossracial sex is now no more or less meaningful than multiracial football. White kids routinely speak patois and borrow strategically from Punjabi.
>
> (Gilroy, 2005, p. 131)

In my research, I move away from social concepts of centre and margins, showing a new site for radical openness, a reality where people oscillate and interplay between multiple spaces, crossing a myriad of frontiers, compatible with a contemporary world of constant change. A multicultural site, which Paul Gilroy suggests, has become the 'ordinary feature' of contemporary urban Britain and in 'postcolonial cities elsewhere (Gilroy, 2005, p. xv). Gilroy's concept of a 'convivial culture' which describes the daily interaction of different cultures and ethnicities offers a helpful sociopolitical lens to explore the workshop phenomenon taking place in an urban salon. His notion of conviviality is similar to the current notion of the 'third cultural space', as the interactions of different cultures negotiate, intersect and transform into meaningful social relations (Patel and Lynch, 2013). For Gilroy, 'conviviality' revives terms such as 'multiculturalism', which he suggests has become a fixed fixture that is unrealistic in a contemporary reality; conviviality continues from 'where "multiculturalism" broke down' (Gilroy, 2005, p. xv). Although he cites the youth culture as increasingly exhibiting and experiencing fluidity as it oscillates between its multicultural world, his concerns continue to lie with the rest of the population with the issue of race in his view becoming more prevalent, especially in relation to the instigated fear of 'Muslim terrorists' and the fear of migrant and asylum seekers.

He contends that the residue of the colonial past still exists in Britain and continues to impact the way we see race, gender and class within a hierarchal framework and his contention with terms such as 'multiculturalism' suggests a denial or ignoring of the past. Gilroy's notion of conviviality suggests the emerging of a 'third cultural space' which challenges us to understand relationships beyond the confines of fixed racial classification and ordering; to identify diversity and difference without the need to cement it in a place.

> We need to know what sorts of insight and reflection might actually help increasingly differentiated societies and anxious individuals to cope successfully with the challenges involved in dwelling comfortably in proximity to the unfamiliar without becoming fearful and hostile.
>
> (Gilroy, 2005, p. 3)

Creative Life Writing Workshop as a Holding Framework for a Space of Conviviality

The workshops in the salon had not set out to discuss race as a starting point but from the beginning it became evident from the participants that it could not be ignored. As Gilroy (2005) points out, the racial remnants continue to exist from the colonial past; the key is not to be cemented by it. The workshops in the salon provided a safe and reliable environment (Winnicott, 1971) for the participants to engage with group work and a creative process that enabled them to unseat fixed social-political discourses and explore unknown territories of the self which, ultimately, allowed them to increasingly engage 'comfortably in proximity to the unfamiliar without becoming fearful (Gilroy, 2005, p. 3). Gilroy's concept of conviviality is a useful way of thinking about my research. I see the workshops as a space of openness and fluidity, where people are at ease with themselves and others, but also into that space often comes things which are difficult, such as grief, loss, pain, regret or beating oneself up for not having achieved this or that, or for not being a good person. The space is important but not necessarily easy and that's why the concept of the 'holding framework' (Winnicott, 1971) is instrumental.

The highlights the role of the facilitator to hold the space, and to implement tools which hold it, such as the writing and the group work, thus creating a safe enough space to hold people in their process of personal exploration. The salon workshops provided a learning experience, a third area/space which revealed lives that were multifaceted, complex, changing, fearful, liberating and inspiring.

Whilst I was involved in the research I visited my family. It was one of those rare occasions when I was asked about my study – 'What are you doin' again?' I cannot remember exactly what prompted what was to follow but the partner of one of my family members confessed that he had, in the last elections, voted for a far-right political party, the BNP (British National Party). He said that although he regretted doing so he felt that he had been abandoned by the other political parties, being 'white male, working class and unemployed'. A gulf opened up in my aunt's living room between my family and a man whom we had come to love, and because of this (love), a conversation began that we were not prepared for but had to participate in. This is an example of the complexity of crossing borders and confronting them in ordinary lives and relationships.

The writing process offered a space for the participants to be creative with their personal memories and experiences which had not been spoken about before in public; confronting and engaging with differences that interrupt and intervene in alliances and assumptions; replacing the known with the unknown.

One of the participants, in her creative life writing, began to reflect on her life by pulling together the different strands of her biracial African-European identity which felt disconnected: 'She is a sister black and beautiful' and she is reminded of her Germanness when asked if she speaks German, 'Spreken Zi Deutsch?' When her objectified self-character in her story spoke German it connected her to a self that she had denied and kept hidden: 'it came as a shock to feel it so deeply'. She realized at this point the importance of accepting the complexity of her identity and history: 'she almost eradicated her German accent, almost fooled her to be what she wasn't'. Through her creative life writing this participant was able to bring together two worlds of herself that before she did not think could coexist.

The creative writing process opened a dialogical space where the writers, through engaging with multiple objectified self-characters on the page, were able to connect to the many different dimensions of themselves. There was something in this process that was not always easy but it was liberating. By engaging with a multifaceted self the writers were able to experience and authorise a sense of self beyond constructed labels that had been inherited or devised. The writers at times engendered their characters to act and speak in circumstances that in real life they may have found difficult to do, and as a result the participants entered a new terrain of the self that they had not dared to explore before.

In my research I drew from the common thread that runs through the various notions of the third-area cultural space(s); a place which embodies change, multiplicity and fluidity. A meeting point bringing together the inner psyche with outer realities; the unconscious with the conscious; the amicable and the feared. Revealing a new site for radical openness – imagined and real – crossing a myriad of frontiers, and therefore more compatible with the globalised world we share.

The Role of Embodiment and Emotion in Self and Identity

My study is located within a decolonization process, as it explores how we can emancipate ourselves by gaining a fluid relationship to historical and sociopolitical constructs which shape our identities and sense of self. For this purpose it brings ideas of embodiment and emotion into relation with ideas of social construction. My research understands that we are socially constructed because we are born into a language society that frames the world in particular ways, but it also recognises that we are not *only* text. Even cultural theorist Stuart Hall's constructionist ideas of identity recognise that our concepts of self and identity are themselves 'grounded on the huge unknowns of our psychic lives' and that to have a more authentic understanding of ourselves we cannot depend purely on discourse; we have to find ways 'to reach through the barrier of the unconscious' (Hall, 1989, p. 22). Identity politics, since its conception in the 1960s, has broadened its parameters, redirecting our attention not only to how we think about ourselves but possibly more importantly how we *feel* about ourselves. Previously the study of feeling and emotion was marginalised and associated with qualitative and interpretive approaches and so-called 'soft' science, but in the last 30 years has expanded rapidly across a range of academic disciplines including cultural studies, political science, history, sociology and psychology. Margaret Wetherell refers to the term 'psychosocial' as a means to 'expand the scope of social investigation', as it allows for 'a focus on embodiment, to attempt to understand how people are moved, and what attracts them, to an emphasis on repetitions, pains and pleasures, feelings and memories' (Wetherell, 2012, p. 2).

Embodiment is a centrally important concept for my research, as I see the creative life-writing process as helping us to move away from dominant narratives and self-conceptions that mould identity (Hunt, 2004) by engaging with the body and listening to how we feel and our perceptions of what is going on in the world. The creative process enables us to access knowledge previously not available to us within our own stories by connecting to a bodily sense of self which extends outside of the text of social constructions.

> We learn more and more to cherish our feelings, and to respect those hidden source of power from where true knowledge and, therefore, lasting action comes.
>
> (Lorde, 1984, p. 37)

All the different elements of the workshop – the exercises and the group work and the holding environment – generate frames for thinking and feeling, where participants can experience a fuller, more embodied knowledge of self. I have begun to understand embodiment as a holding space; a holding space which is not the shape of the physical body but more of a felt sense, the emotional and bodily felt dimension of thinking processes. It is this engagement with bodily feelings and emotions which allow for a more dialogical relationship between different parts of the self, our different identities; we are multiple rather than fragmented, and if we are loosely multiple we can move between these different dimensions of ourselves. It is this perceptual-emotional dimension that brings inner and outer worlds together and helps us gravitate towards a feeling of wholeness.

Jerome Bruner refers to the fluid nature of life narratives: 'we constantly construct and reconstruct ourselves to meet the needs of the situation we encounter' (Bruner, 2003, p. 64). Acknowledging the loosening of life narratives does not, however, suggest that our stories are arbitrary and that we can just pick and choose the ones we want. Eugene Gendlin says that 'We are not bound by the forms of the past but we cannot construct just any narrative that we like' (Gendlin, 1996, p. 2). According to Gendlin, to gain an understanding of who we are we have to turn our attention to bodily sensed knowledge. He refers to a *bodily felt sense*, a physical feeling that carries deep embodied knowledge and can bring personal meaning. He sees this bodily felt sense as those feelings that are often not given much attention, a 'gut feeling', a sensation that 'begins in the body and occurs in the zone between the conscious and the unconscious' (Gendlin, 1996, p. 1). The felt sense 'is not about words and thoughts but the attention in the body' (ibid., p. 19). He points out that at first the feeling can be 'unclear, murky, puzzling, not fully recognizable' (ibid., p. 26), but in time it can reveal experiences and memories that would otherwise be missed.

Zora Neale Hurston and Gendlin's Bodily Felt Sense of Self

A key element to my research is the notion of crossing borders and exploring new and unfamiliar terrain; one of the ways I explore this is by bringing together writers, theorists, artists, philosophers and cultural thinkers whose ideas had never before engaged with each other. By doing this I was able to open the conversation around identity, embodiment and story. As I read the literature related to the 'affective' or 'corporeal turn', I increasingly began to see connections with the ideas that I had previously read in reflective and literary essays by writers of the African diaspora.

An example of the interconnectivity between the different disciplines is evident between novelist and anthropologist Zora Neale Hurston and phenomenological philosopher Eugene Gendlin. Hurston wrote an essay in 1928, 'How it *feels* to be colored me', which explores the relationship between a felt sense and a sociopolitical construction of identity. I read this essay before I knew anything about the *bodily felt sense* but I was drawn to the title; she wrote about how she *felt* about herself as being intrinsic to her identity.

Although Hurston's essay was written in the early twentieth century, it continues to offer insight to the experience of the participants in the workshop and indeed my own. This ground-breaking essay broadens and endorses an understanding of self, as Hurston explores her own constructed and embodied senses of being 'colored':

> When I disembarked from the river-boat at Jacksonville, she was no more. It seemed that I had suffered a sea change. I was not Zora of Orange country

any more. I was now a little colored girl. I found it out in certain ways. In my heart as well as in the mirror.

(Hurston, 1928/1979, p. 153)

Hurston writes about leaving home for the first time, 'exclusively a coloured town', and moving to a city that included white residents, introducing her to another identity 'that was not Zora'. Psychiatrist Frantz Fanon says: 'as long as the black man [woman or child] is among his own, he will have no occasion, except in minor internal conflicts, to experience his being through others' (Fanon, 2000, p. 326). Civil rights activist WEB Dubois's (1903) concept of a 'double consciousness' could be applied to Hurston's newly emerged identity: the Zora that she knew and the 'colored girl' she had become. Similarly, Stuart Hall writes of his own experience of becoming 'black' in the seventies. 'Black [in the context of Hurston 'coloured'] is an identity which had to be learned' (Hall, 1987, p. 45), an identity comprised of the acknowledgment of self through *difference* (Hall, 1987).

In the essay, Hurston expresses a bodily felt experience of self when listening to music in a jazz club. For her, the music connected to a personal narrative that transcended time and space. She trusted bodily feeling, which is a more fluid process and not so reliant on the fixity of social concepts. She felt liberated from the confinements of social constructs, which she says 'made me American' (Hurston, 1928, p. 153). Hurston wrote how her body responded to the music: 'It constricts the thorax and splits the heart with its tempo' (ibid., p. 154), allowing Hurston to feel connected to a freer, more complex sense of self: 'I dance wildly inside myself' (ibid.), an experience that Gendlin says can only take place 'unmistakably in the body' (Gendlin, 1996, p. 20). Gendlin states that these sensations are not experienced on the periphery of the body: 'It is sensed in the viscera or the chest or the throat, some specific place usually in the middle of the body' (ibid., p.18), a description that fits remarkably well with Hurston's experience. He says that to achieve the fullness of the felt sense the person has to enter inside the body, which Hurston did; it is as if she surrendered her whole being to the feeling that emerged from the dance. Gendlin believes that it is something that the person feels, and when the right word or activity – such as writing or dancing – is found, it creates a 'relief as if the body is grateful for being allowed to form its way of being as a whole' (ibid.).

Similar to Hurston, as the participants in the CLW workshops began to pay attention to their feelings and emotions, they experienced a sense of self that felt more complex and whole. The writers spoke of their writing process as being 'immersed in what's going on rather than slightly holding back'; 'feeling relaxed is what I feel certainly has led me to my breakthrough'; 'a bit like going into a trance and going quite deep'. The writing process connected them to a process which allowed them to 'envision or experience identities beyond those inscribed on them' (Walker, 1995, p. xxxvii).

Moving Towards an Embodied Sense of Self

The workshop participants spoke about the surprises their writing produced, as the creative process unearthed some of the 'many layers of his or her own truth'

(Chandler, 1990, p. 25). One participant felt a 'release' when her stories revealed 'how funny [her mother] was. I completely forgot. I've been angry with her for so long'; without warning her words gave light to a relationship darkened by sorrow and pain. This echoes Jill Kel Conway's experience of recollecting her memories: 'I found that my memory was all the painful things. But in the process of telling that story I rediscovered so much that was beautiful about my child-hood' (Conway, 1995, p. 172). Similarly, the participants' writing process was also at times able to give 'back the good things that [they] had forgotten' (ibid., p. 173). Elbow refers to 'lucky or achieved moments' when writers 'manage to find words which seem to capture the rich complexity of the unconscious' (Elbow, 2000, p. 206).

The practice of CLW enabled the writers at the salon and myself in my own writing to 'access and objectify' our personal material (Hunt, 2001), an invalu-able process of being able, on the one hand, to gain closer access to their deeply felt personal material and, on the other hand, to gain sufficient creative distance from it to transform it into creative writing. As one participant says of her writing process, 'It's like looking at the same thing but twisting it a bit in the light and being able to see it differently'. It is the creative distancing through fiction that helps the insight into the self. We recognise that it is us but by standing outside we view our memories from a distance and in doing so create a space for personal memories and experiences to be seen from a different perspective, which allows a new story to emerge.

> When [she] is able to transform [her] personal crisis into a work of art the writer has taken possession of the thing that has threatened to possess [her].
>
> (Chandler, 1990, p. 23)

The more the participants trusted the creative process, the more organically the stories came forth. Ultimately this meant that they began to trust and authorize the voice from within, which connected them to a deep source of creativity. Through the group work the participants began to recognise how tightly woven into their psyche were the external narratives that had become integral to their identity. The writing practice created a space where they were able to stop thinking for a while and pay attention to things that were more subtle and needed to be articulated. By mindfully fictionalising their memories and experiences, the participants moved towards a more embodied sense of self and found that these embodied memories felt more authentic. As they redirected their attention away from factual details towards the feelings and emotions that were attached to their memories, they began to pay attention and 'listen' to how they were feeling. The participants experienced that 'there is a power in the word', not any old word but the word that *fits*. One participant says: 'I keep going with the words and playing with the words until it fits right, until it describes feeling of what I am trying to convey'. The writing process allows the individual 'to find words which seem to capture the rich complexity of the unconscious'. Elbow suggests that the voice that *resonates* is the voice that is closest to a 'whole person' (Elbow, 2000, p. 206). Through facilitation, group work and fictional and poetic exercises writers learnt to hold a space for the imagination. This involves becoming grounded in the body, in bodily feeling, and trusting bodily feeling as the core of themselves. Being grounded in the body means that identity becomes a fluid process open to change rather than relying on identities rooted in social narratives or self-concepts.

Conclusion

> The ability to change, to respond flexibly to life's circumstances in adaptive and creative ways …
>
> (Leiper and Maltby, 2004, pp. 3–4)

One of the most liberating aspects of the participants' creative life-writing process was the very simple recognition and acceptance that their lives did not fit into a tidy box. What emerged on the page was not a 'single story' – 'a definitive story' (Adiche, 2009) – but an essential space for people to map and redefine their complex and multidimensional lives, challenging single identities and hegemonic notions. The CLW workshops provided a unique opportunity for the participants to not distance themselves from the legacy of migration but to draw from it, recognising movement not always as displacement and loss but as an opportunity of redefining self, past experiences and memories and thus choosing to see things from a different perspective.

The British experience of the participants does not seem to be one that is placed on the margins but is more of a coexistence, a fluidity between multiple spaces that extends to and beyond race. It is an experience that 'lends itself to the notion of fluidity, multiple identities', generating a 'cross cultural, transnational, translocal, diasporic perspective redefine[ing] identity away from exclusion and marginality' (Davis, 1994, pp. 8, 4). It is this 'consciousness of expansiveness' which informs my research; starting from the point of liberation that is not *despite* but *because of* our diasporic and migratory inheritance. This study shows how creative life writing located in a cultural context presents the possibilities of enabling people to become agentic in their own emancipatory processes; introducing the necessity for

> new analyses, new questions and new understandings [as we] unlock some of the narrow terms of the discourses in which we are inscribed.
>
> (Davis, 1994, p. 5)

The CLW workshops provided an opportunity for the participants to put their personal experiences out onto the page, as if putting themselves onto the page. I recognised that it was the things we carry inside of us, usually all muddled up together, that can be brought out and expressed through the creative writing process, as the participants found: 'there is something very powerful to be able to express oneself'; 'It's a good way to examine different aspects of yourself'. It was not so much that they were coming to the workshop with a singular sense of identity, but with an unexplored 'mishmash' of things. The workshop provided a space for people to 'unpack' their identities, as it were, to put an array of personal experience on the page, separate these things out, rearrange and renew them and then put them back in again so that they might work together a little bit better.

The fictional poetic exercises helped the writers to fictionalise their memories and see their story from different points of view, through the eyes of the characters on the page. Using the voices of other characters unearthed emotions and characteristics of themselves previously concealed. Author Annie Lamott (1995, p. 198) says: 'We write to expose the unexposed'. The group work enabled participants to trust their creative process, allowing them to abandon their need for certainty and security and find out what they have to say in the course of the writing itself. Through the creative writing practice the participants recognised the importance of objectifying themselves, as they got in touch more with their felt sense.

Working in the field of CWPD drew my attention to the possibilities of actively fictionalising memories as a move towards a more embodied sense of self; engaging with embodied memories which felt more authentic. This approach highlights the idea that the only way we can truly come to know ourselves as full, complex human beings is by engaging with the unconscious, which echoes Elbow's notion that 'the body shows far more of ourselves than the conscious mind does' (Elbow, 2000, p. 208). The participants in the workshop engaged in a writing process which opened up the space for the imagination; creating generative space in the psyche where language, conscious and unconscious material could come together. This allowed writers to increasingly trust bodily feeling as the core of who they are, and therefore identity becomes a fluid process as they become less reliant on identities embedded in social discourses.

I show the relevance of the process of creative life writing in and for modern multicultural societies in relation to negotiating identities and self-concepts that "[live] with and through, not despite difference' (Hall, 1990, p. 235). The research provides a critical conversation for understanding the world that continues to bear the consequence of the persistence of colonial ways of thinking and impedes the progress of multiculturalism. By drawing from, and interrelating, the works of writers and theorists from the fields of psychodynamics and cultural and literary theory, I have been able to investigate the intersectionality of the imagination and the sociopolitical. It is the pursuit of this union which has allowed me to alter and redefine boundaries and open the conversation between identity and embodiment.

This research indicates that the initial and critical step towards achieving change is the necessity of engaging with the stories that shape the ways we see ourselves and others. Therefore, change has got to come from the individual's ability to act in the world, but the study in a group community setting also shows that individuals need to be in a dialogue with others, and it is this moving back and forth between the two axes which promotes self and collective growth, and hopefully from this, genuine change transpires.

My methodological approach mindfully places theory at the centre of my teaching practice. Due to this approach, I decided to engage with my own creative life writing practice (away from the group setting in the salon), initially to have a greater understanding of the participants' experience with the creative process, but the experience of fictionalising my own memories revealed the importance of engaging with my own self-reflexive process. Natalie Goldberg always tells her creative writing students to open up their minds 'to the possibility that 1 + 1 can equal 48' (Goldberg, 1986, p. 82). I also needed to see my research beyond the limits of my own embedded discourses and explore the wider possibilities of 1 + 1. As I engaged with the complexities and ambiguities of my own identity I felt that I brought a more authentic self to my teaching practice.

Marilyn Chandler describes the fictionalising of memories as a *healing art*, a 'deeply regenerative human activity … an impulse to communicate linked with survival itself' (Chandler, 1990, p. 3). The group work in the salon enabled the participants to use their creative life writing to work towards a more fluid relationship with life-held narratives which had become embedded and unhelpful. The holding environment of the workshop and the writing itself enabled the writers to let go of their grounding in familiar identities and explore less familiar material of the self, which served to be expansive and empowering.

> You're never really a whole person if you remain silent, because there's always that one little piece inside of you that wants to be spoken out, and if you keep ignoring it, it gets madder and madder and hotter and hotter, and if you don't speak it out one day it will just up and punch you in the mouth from the inside.
>
> (Lorde, 1984, p. 42)

References

Adiche, CN 2009, 'The danger of a single story', [online] TED.com. Available at: http://www.ted.com/talks/chimamanda_adichie_the_danger_of_a_single_story [Accessed 24 November 2009].

Bolton, G (2004), Introduction: *Writing Cures, in: Writing Cures: An Introductory Handbook of Writing in Counselling and Therapy: An Introductory Handbook of Writing Counselling and Psychotherapy*: eds G Bolton, S Howlett, C Lago, J Wright, Brunner-Routledge, East Sussex.

Bruner, J 2003, *Making Stories: Law, Literature, Life*, Harvard University Press, Massachusetts.

Chandler M 1990, *A Healing Art: Regeneration Through Autobiography*, Garland Publishers, London.

Christensen, L 2009, *Teaching for Joy and Justice: Re-Imagining The Language Arts Classroom*, A Rethinking Schools Publication, Milwaukee.

Conway, JK 1995, 'Points of departure', in: *Inventing the Truth: The Art and Craft of Memoir*, ed. W. Zinseer, Houghton Mifflin Company, New York.

Davis, CB 1994, *Black Women, Writing and Identity: Migrations of the Subject*, Routledge, London.

Dubois, WEB 1903, *The Souls of Black Folks*, 1997 edition, Bedford Books, Boston.

Elbow, P 2000, *Everyone Can Write: Essays Toward a Hopeful Theory of Writing and Teaching Writing*, Oxford University Press, Oxford.

Fanon, F 2009, 'Frantz Fanon: The Fact of Blackness', in: L. Back and J. Solomus, *Theories of Race and Racism, The Reader*, (2009 edition), Routledge, London.

Gendlin, E 1996, *Focusing-Oriented Psychotherapy: A Manual of the Experiential Method*, Guildford Press, New York.

Gilroy P 2005, *Postcolonial Melancholia*, Columbia University Press, New York.

Gilroy, P 2009, 'The dialectics of diaspora identification', in: *Theories of Race and Racism. The Reader*, 2nd edition, eds L Back and J Solomous, Routledge, London.

Goldberg, N 1986, *Writing Down the Bones: Freeing the Writer Within*, Shambhala, Massachusetts.

Grewal, S, Kay, J, Landor. L, Lewis, G. & Parmar, P 1988, *Charting the Journey: Writing by Black and Third World Women*, Sheba Feminist Publishers, London.

Hall, S 1987, 'Minimal Selves', in: *ICA (Institute of Contemporary Arts), Documents 6, Identity the Real*, ICA, London.

Hall, S 1989, 'Ethnicity: Identity and difference', [Lecture to Hampshire College, Amherst] Spring 1989, Massachusetts.

Hall, S 1990, *Cultural Identity and Diaspora: Identity: Community, Culture, Difference*, Lawrence & Wishart, London.

Hall, S 2000, What is Britain? *The Guardian* [online]. Available at: http://www.theguardian.com/uk/2000/oct/15/britishidentity.comment1 [Accessed 2 October 2013]

Hooks, b 1991, *Yearning: Race, Gender, and Cultural Politics*, Turnaround, UK.

Hooks, b 1999, *Remembered Raptures: The Writer at Work*, Holt and Company, New York.

Hoving, I 2001, *In Praise of Travellers*, Stanford University Press, California.

Hunt, C 1998 'Writing with the voice of a child: Fictional autobiography and personal development', in: *The Self on the Page*: eds C Hunt, F Sampson, Jessica Kingsley, London.

Hunt, C 2000, *Therapeutic Dimensions of Autobiography in Creative Writing*, Jessica Kingsley, London.

Hunt, C 2001, 'Assessing Personal Writing', *Auto/Biography*, vol. 9, nos. 1-2, pp. 89-94.

Hunt, C, 2004, 'Reading Ourselves: imagining the reader in the writing process' in: *Writing Cures: An Introductory Handbook of Writing in Counselling and Therapy: An Introductory Handbook of Writing Counselling and Psychotherapy*: eds G Bolton, S Howlett, C Lago, J Wright, Brunner-Routledge, East Sussex.

Hunt, C 2013, *Transformative Learning through Creative Life Writing*, Routledge, London.

Hunt, C & Sampson, F 1998, *The Self on the Page: Theory And Practice of Creative Writing for Personal Development*, Jessica Kingsley, London.

Hunt, C & Sampson, F 2006, *Writing: Self and Reflexivity*, Palgrave, London.

Hurston, ZN 1928, 'How it feels to be colored me', in: *I Love Myself When I Am Laughing And Then Again When I am Looking Mean and Impressive: A Zora Neale Hurston Reader*, 1979 edition, ed. A. Walker, The Feminist Press, New York.

Jiménez Muñoz, GM 1995, 'Joining our differences: The problems of lesbian subjectivity among women of color', in: *Moving Beyond Boundaries*, Volume 2: *Black Women's Diasporas*, ed. B. Davis, Pluto Press, London.

Lamott, A 1995, *Bird By Bird: Some Instructions on Writing and Life*, Anchor Books, New York.

Leiper, R & Maltby, M 2004, *The Psychodynamic Approach to Therapeutic Change*, Sage, London.

Lorde, A 1984, *Sister Outsider: Essays and Speeches from Audre Lorde*, 2007 edition, Crossing Press, Berkley.

Morrison, T 1995, 'The site of memory', in: *Inventing the Truth: The Art and Craft of Memoir*, ed. W. Zinseer, Houghton Mifflin Company, New York.

Neisser, U 1994, 'Self-Narratives: True or False' in: *The Remembering Self: Construction and Accuracy in the Self Narrative*: eds U Neisser, R. Fivush, Cambridge University Press, Cambridge.

Patel, F & Lynch, H 2013, 'Glocalization as an alternative to internationalization in higher education: Embedding positive glocal learning perspectives', *International Journal of Teaching and Learning in Higher Education*, vol. 25. no 2, pp. 223–230

Soja, E 1996, *Thirdspace: Journeys to Los Angeles and Other Real- And Imagined Places*, 2nd edition, Blackwell, Oxford.

Stanley, L 1992, *The Auto/biographical I: The Theory and Practice of Feminist Auto/Biograph*, Manchester University Press, UK.

Thompson, K 2006, 'What people need to write', in: *Writing Works: A Resource Handbook for Therapeutic Writing Workshops and Activities*, eds G Bolton, V Field & K Thompson, Jessica Kingsley Publishers, London.

Walker, R 1995, *To Be Real: Telling the Truth and Changing the Face of Feminism*, Anchor Books, New York.

Wetherall, M 2012, *Affect and Emotion: A New Social Science Understanding*, Sage, London.

Winnicott, D 1965, *The Maturational Process and the Facilitating Environment: Studies in the Theory of Emotional Development*, The Hogarth Press, London.

Winnicott, D 1971, *Playing and Reality*, Routledge, London.

10 Social Sculpture Through Dreams and Conversations
Creating Spaces for Participatory and Situation-Specific Art-Based Methods

Lott Alfreds and Charlotte Åberg

In 2012, we, Lott Alfreds and Charlotte Åberg, co-founded the artistic collective ArtAgent, based in Stockholm, Sweden, focusing on participatory and situation-specific art. Through art practices in the public realm, we aim to develop an increased awareness of the potential and capacity of art to impact society and we have created artistic projects at various locations such as neighbourhoods, schools, social institutions, workplaces, public squares and art institutions, both in Sweden and internationally. The works include different international contexts such as social sculpture (Beuys & Harlan 2004), participatory art (Milevska 2006), and situation-specific and new genre public art (Lacy 1994). In addition to these concepts, we have used a stream of questions and experiments undertaken by thinkers and art practitioners that have influenced the condition of local communities in a global change. Referring to Arjun Appadurai's (2000) belief, we now live in globally imagined worlds and not simply in locally imagined communities. We also live in a world in which deterritorialisation, the breaking down of existing territorial connections, affects us on a daily basis as well as a parallel vision where we are moving towards a more comprehensive and internationally inclusive approach. In this shift, we see the enhanced possibility of sharing thoughts, feelings and imagination through art.

We wish to contribute to this section on methodological reshaping and spatial transgression in glocalised social work by introducing strategies that we have been using in our artistic practice with marginalised communities in Albania, Macedonia, Croatia and Sweden. In particular, we wish to describe the interplay between practice and theory in our projects, to discuss theory by way of practice, and in so doing highlight how artistic practice embodies and modifies theory. This will be demonstrated by bringing to attention different situations and conditions for art projects in Sweden and in the Western Balkans. We will begin by introducing a theoretical framework to our methodology, building on Joseph Beuys ideas of social sculpture (Beuys & Harlan 2004; Sacks 2016) and Grant Kester's notions of the potentiality of conversations in art practices (Kester 2005). We then present examples of our interpretation of what a 'social sculpture' can be the basis of our artistic and social practice. We have heterogeneous artistic backgrounds as visual artists working with sculpture, graphic art, textile design, video and photography.

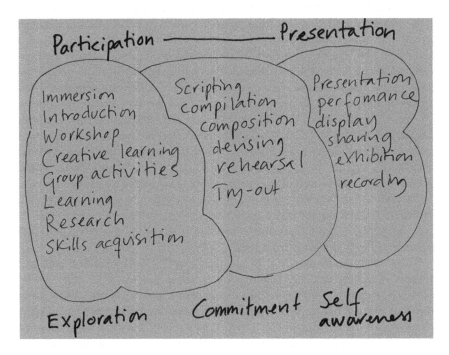

Figure 10.1 Participation model. Graphics.
Photo: Lott Alfreds 2014.

The figure attempts to describe in a simple form the journey that both the artists and participants can take. The timescale can vary from days to months and the creative inputs and outcomes are hugely variable. What we have tried to make clear is that process and product are entangled and must be understood as a whole. While a final presentation or event must be artistically credible, it is also informed by the process that created it (Arts Council England, 2010).

Social Sculpture and Conversation in Art Practices

Creativity isn't the monopoly of artists. This is the crucial fact I've come to realize, and this broader concept of creativity is my concept of art. When I say everybody is an artist, I mean everybody can determine the content of life in his particular sphere, whether in painting, music, engineering, caring for the sick, the economy or whatever

(Haks 1995, p. 53).

'Social sculpture' is a term promoted by the German conceptual artist and politician Joseph Beuys (1921–1986) in a series of open lectures in the late 1970s. In an interview with Frans Hak, illustrated in the citation above, Beuys expresses the main idea of the concept. Thus, 'social sculpture' is used to describe an expanded concept of art that embodies the artist's understanding of art's potential to transform society. As an art form grounded in the social, it includes a human activity that strives to form and shape society. Beuys believed that society as a whole could be regarded as a work of art in which each person contributes creatively by stating the well-known phrase – 'everyone is an artist' (Beuys & Harlan 2004, p. 2). This statement, however, is not an end – Beuys meant that every conscious act made by an individual is part of a larger construction of society, which is the larger work of art. The artist as a social 'sculptor', that is, a subject that actively creates and shapes structures in society, is engaged in a process of social transformation by using language, thoughts, actions, objects and aesthetic situations. Therefore, *everyone* is an artist insofar as each individual's activities are part of what constitutes a larger whole. This marks a shift from people as *spectators* of art (whereby art is one of the many activities in society) to people as *participants* in a larger work of art, whereby society is the resulting artwork. As such, everyone is equally accountable for what society is and stands for, and there are no outsiders to the work of art itself.

Beuys' concepts are infused with a utopian belief fuelled by political hope and spiritual values and are very inspiring for an entire generation of artists whose aspirations extend beyond the exclusivity of the so-called 'art world'. With this in mind and aware of our backgrounds as trained artists, we wondered what it means to incorporate these social and collective values outside the usual art contexts of art schools, museums and galleries. How could we use artistic methods as a way of reaching out into society at large and consider life as a social sculpture that everyone helps to shape? ArtAgent became interested in understanding both the conditions of participation, that is, how to involve people in collective artistic actions, and artistic materials, that is, the tools and means of participation. For instance, if it is true that speech is a sculptural material, as Beuys stated, then what can happen during group discussions with members of a particular community that may activate speech in the form of an artwork? In this case, the discussion itself *is* the artwork created by a series of conversations, dialogues and speech acts, which together are the materials that *shape* the artwork.

We are equally informed by Grant Kester's ideas about conversation where he identifies a number of contemporary artists and art collectives that have defined their practice precisely around the facilitation of dialogue among diverse communities (Kester 2005). By breaking with traditions of object- and picture-making solely for display on museum and gallery walls, many artists, like us, have adopted a performative and process-based approach (Kester 2005). They are what British artist Peter Dunn has called context providers rather than content providers, whereby the orchestration of creative dialogues extends beyond the institutional walls and acquires a political and social resonance in society at large (Lovejoy *et al.* 2011). This involves creating contexts where exchanges can take place which have the potential to 'catalyse surprisingly powerful transformations in the consciousness of their participants' (Kester 2005, p. 76). Some of the questions raised that we have been interested in are about understanding how collective or communal identities can be formed. Today we are confronted with a lot of uncertainties and are thrown into many complex situations in the formation of a glocal community. A contemporary global interest does not refer to local points of view in a shift to a large-scale economical and societal global order. On the other hand, there is an ongoing countermovement at the grass-roots level as, for example, emancipatory politics by smaller groups and NGO organisations with a focus on people's education and participation for the promotion of their interests. Appadurai (2000, p. 18) writes:

> A new architecture for producing and sharing knowledge about globalization could provide the foundations of a pedagogy that closes this gap and helps to democratize the flow of dialogue between academics, public intellectuals, and policymakers in different societies. The principles of this pedagogy will require significant innovations. This vision of global collaborative teaching and learning about globalization may not resolve the great antinomies of power that characterise this world, but it might help to even the playing field.

The practice of social sculpture and participatory art works very well with the grass-roots globalisation 'from below' because it's trying to empower different people to participate and live together in a more pluralistic society. Therefore, instead of centring our activities in how spectators respond to a particular work of art, we are concerned with collaborative, and potentially emancipatory, forms of dialogue and conversation as a starting point for an artistic experience.

Facilitating Collaborations

We first came together as independent artists working on collective projects in 2005 and 2006 with two projects in Botkyrka municipality, Stockholm. The main idea was to let artists and artworks interact with groups of staff members from different workplaces. Our first project was carried out during six months at the Botkyrka Municipal House, twenty kilometres south of Stockholm, together with a group of consultants from Botkyrka (Konstfrämjandet 2011). Botkyrka municipality is unique since it is the most multicultural municipality in Sweden, with a high percentage of immigrants living there. Politically, it is quite progressive and its slogan 'Far from Ordinary' reflects its openness and innovation towards embracing multiculturality as an asset for the region. The municipal house in Botkyrka has over one hundred employees and reflects the diversity of its population. We worked with a group of approximately ten administrators who volunteered to the project, mostly women.

We used role play, installations and mobile films as artistic expressions that inspired the group in working towards a common working process and a collaboration between artists and civil servants inside their working premises. This means that our site of intervention was not primarily a location meant for displaying art, but a site where art enters the visual and cognitive realm of the workplace by way of these conversations. When groups were defined, we started out with a few questions regarding what the employees would like to see improved at their working place. In parallel, we held smaller sessions and workshops for painting with watercolours, and creating objects in clay as forms for expressing and interpreting thoughts. This initial conversation aimed to ask the participants about their needs and to investigate whether we – artists and employees – could build something together that became 'art'. Our role as artists was challenged, as we became facilitators of an artistic process whose goal was to become an agent for change within the workplace. The participants reacted to our interventions and the sessions in many different ways.

Certain key inspirational elements were found in the work produced in the workshop sessions that created a strong connection between the participants and ourselves. In the discussions about the clay objects, for example, we agreed that poetry was a subversive force as well as a tool of resistance. We wanted to use poetry in a wider sense, not through written words but through the making of art objects. In this very action we focus on the listening processes, and what we don't often think about is that listening is a form of learning as well as the pictures that form between us. When working in a territory of oppression, you cannot avoid being radicalised by people's expression (Donovan 2012). Play was also mentioned as an important ingredient where chance is a welcome guest. In the interactions between people, there must be room for chance, because in the arts we can't follow a pre-written agenda and hope that an equal dialogue will occur in the workshops. Chance and the new possibilities that come with it are just around the corner when the conversation is free and vivid.

The above-mentioned workshops propose what Arjun Appadurai (2000, p. 5) calls 'relations of disjuncture', proposing a new process and new possibilities against the traditional ways of moral discipline while reconsidering local problems. ArtAgent and its partners operate on the belief that contemporary art is a means to intersubjective knowledge and presentation. Creative discourses benefit from self-reflexivity. The workshops are feasible as all parties act within an understanding that new process geographies and places of imagination for the socially marginalised are possible (see also Bekteshi 2014, pp. 14–16).

The Upside-Down Day

In 2005, we worked together with a group of ten consultants, responsible for consultative support to managers and employees in areas such as labour law, safety and health, rehabilitation, equality and diversity in the Botkyrka municipality. We asked the consultants if there was anything at their workplace that they wanted to improve, and paid attention to their needs. They were disappointed with the social environment at the workplace at Botkyrka Municipal House. The consultants were sitting in their own corner of the building, they never interacted with other coworkers and their supervisors were never seen in the huge building complex.

We made a day called 'the upside-down day' at the municipal house. The environment was shaped into a new form where people could meet in unexpected ways. For instance, the politicians at the municipal house were invited to have a meeting without agenda in a 'cushion room' together with children from a nearby kindergarten.

Together with employees at the Botkyrka Municipal House, we created situations where the normal routines in their working place were questioned. In group discussions, we, the artists, came up with 'worst-case scenarios', which were used as a dramaturgical source of inspiration for further conversations and activities.

The female employees in the group played around with ideas reflecting critically on the municipality's slogan, which could be seen in all official printed matter and communication material: 'Botkyrka Municipality: Open, Brave, and far from Ordinary'. One woman reacted strongly against these values and at the 'the upside-down day' she didn't bother to change from her pyjamas before going to work: 'I still laugh at what we did that day, we dressed ourselves in strange outfits and just stopped obeying. I was acting as a closed person, instead of being open and available as usual'.

Working with Dreams

In several projects, we have been working with dreams as a way to form a social sculpture. In 2006 we created 'The Dream Garden' with employees at an elderly care centre that had requested an artistic intervention to transform the smoking lounge into a winter garden where they could have a new meeting room. At this time we felt it was important to bring something out of the situation that was close to our own artistic practice. We made a contract with the group whereby they would 'donate' their stories of nightly dreams, which later could be turned into a movie script. There was a vision of 'flooding' the workplace with moving pictures, and dreams being whispered behind and between plants.

We held meetings with nurses of all ages, most of them with a background from other countries such as Ecuador, Ethiopia, Turkey and Finland. One of the participants told us a dream in which she had seen roads and the environment in Sweden before she even had any thoughts of migration. In the dream, she passed by small roads and big highways in an endless route in the unknown country that later would become her residence. A young woman had recurrent dreams where she met a tiger, and the spectacular thing was that her twin brother also had the same dreams at the same times. In the end, she decided to stop and face the tiger, her fear, and in the same moment she did so, it disappeared. All sorts of dreams came up; they were based on everyday events, families, cultural adaptations and all the range of emotions that people carry inside. There was a strong presence in those moments when we exchanged dreams with each other.

Another example of working with dreams is from our network collaboration in Albania. Within this framework, in 2007–2008, the director of Ali Demi Women's Prison in Tirana, Albania invited us. The invitation entailed conducting workshops with staff working in this prison, with support from the Swedish Institute in collaboration with Refraction Association, an Albanian human rights organisation working with issues concerning inmates and their families. Prison director Marinela Sota wanted to see if a working method based on the concept of social sculpture and dreams could be used when working with staff suffering from work-related stress syndrome.

In Albania, they have a tradition of sharing dreams with each other, which we had no idea about when we came there; it was a pure fluke. Some of them also believed in prophetic dreams and the dreams were also related to the landscape, which plays an important role in Albanian folklore. Mountains surround the city of Tirana and these often appear in dreams. One woman stated that you can get rid of nightmares if you get up early in the morning, get up to the top of the mountain and whisper the dream quietly to the mountain.

With the project 'Social Sculpture, Dreams and Gender Issues' at the women's prison, we continued to focus on dreams and their pictorial language as a uniting force. We had learnt from previous projects that it was very useful to have a tactile angle in the process as well. Boxes were made in which the content of the dream was expressed in a non-narrative way by using delicate materials such as Japanese rice paper. These were exhibited in a cultural centre in Tirana and the staff's families were invited to participate.

After the conversations and exhibition at the women's prison in Albania we wished to document the experience to be able to share it with a wider audience among artists, but also with the social sector and for knowledge building. We made a publication about the experience, which also became a way of expressing our subjective experience, both in terms of writing as well as in pictures (Alfreds & Åberg 2010). We also created an exhibition together with the book release, consisting of

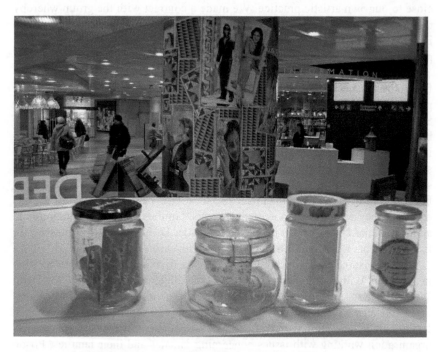

Figure 10.2 The Dream Laboratory. An exhibition by Lott Alfreds and Charlotte Åberg at the House of Culture, Stockholm.

Photo: Lott Alfreds 2010.

films and dream collections that were shown in several art institutions in Stockholm such as Candyland Gallery, Studio 44, the House of Culture and Botkyrka Art Hall.

'The Use of Art Where it's Hard to Talk'

Clothes have in all times been a sign of class, gender and group belonging. They are a part of one's identity and show the persona of the individual. Old clothing remains as a part of a memory and might tell a story of the past. By working with clothes we hope to receive different stories and memories connected with the objects. The workshop is an example of how we can use art in order to make people talk more freely (Clothes Workshop on Vimeo 2016).

In 2011, the Albanian human rights organisation Refraction Association invited us, together with two other artists, Helena Byström and Pontus Lindvall, to take part in the Western Balkan project 'The Use of Art Where it's Hard to Talk' (2016). The working method was again a collaborative approach, with practical artistic works mixed with conversations. In the 'Clothes workshop', participants were asked to bring three clothing items and to tell stories about them. In the context of post-war, the experience of wars and trauma surfaced as central. Stories and memories came up in relation to the armed conflict in Kosovo (1998–1999) by the forces of the Federal Republic of Yugoslavia (by this time, consisting of the republics of Montenegro and Serbia) and the Kosovo Liberation Army, the North Atlantic Treaty Organisation and the Albanian army.

In this project, we trained local artists and organisations in conducting these workshops, which resulted in further collaborations in the region. These local artists went on to produce their own projects together with vulnerable groups in different locations in the Balkan countries.

Visualise the Invisible

The organisation ArtAgent, as such, was founded in 2012, after these successful experiences on the occasion of the Creative Europe Programme of the European Union grant used to independently manage and create new projects. By then, we had already established a network of collaborators between small NGOs from Croatia, Macedonia, Sweden and Albania. Countries such as Albania, Croatia and Macedonia have low funding for cultural organizations and artists and the access to culture for all citizens is still limited. Projects in each country have worked on creating new ways for bringing art into direct contact with groups that normally do not have much contact with it. In the project 'Visualize the Invisible' (2013–2014), organisations in Sweden and the Balkans implemented participatory art projects in Sweden, Croatia, Albania and Macedonia (Alfreds & Åberg 2014). The artists used different art forms such as video, installations, performance and dance in cooperation with people in residential areas, Roma communities and those in social institutions such as prisons, schools and care institutions, and reached a wider discussion about art's impact on societal change. All participants were part of a mutual artistic creative process, both the artists and the people

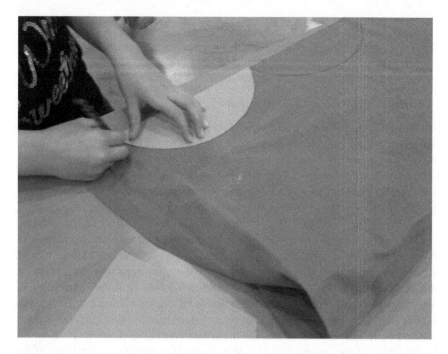

Figure 10.3 Sewing Workshops. Subtopia, Alby, Sweden. From the project 'Visualize the Invisible', a cooperation project between art organisations in Sweden, Albania, Macedonia and Croatia, 2013–2014.

Photo: Charlotte Åberg 2013.

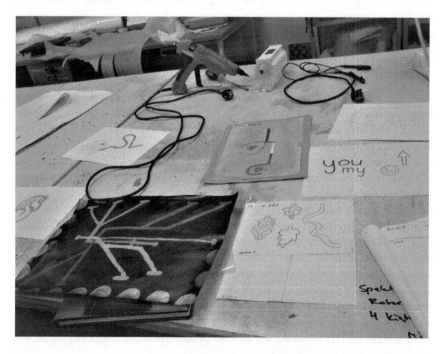

Figure 10.4 The Neon Workshop. Västerås, Sweden. 'Visualize the Invisible', 2013–2014.

Photo: Lott Alfreds 2014.

they were interacting with. An important aspect of the project was to widen the art market in the specific area and make it visible in a European context. The artists shared their experiences with each other through workshops in the Balkans and, finally, in an international exhibition and book release in Sweden. The outline was to examine art's role in society, to give artistic tools, concept and theories and to build interdisciplinary and international networks. There were many advantages in bringing artists to institutions, communities and working places. In this project, art acted as a different role model; the relationship to the artist was more equal than to that of someone in authority. The artists inspired and gave confidence to the participants with new approaches and provided extra 'tools in the toolbox'.

Concluding Reflections

Art can be shared in a broader sense, through the practice of the German artist Joseph Beuys' concept 'social sculpture' (Beuys & Harlan 2004) or in other ways, where the 'immaterial material', as thoughts and conversation, are sculptural material and be used to bridge gaps within society as well as transfer knowledge production through cultural barriers. The investigation is pursued by contrasting the way in which we are seeing art as non-movable objects or as information leaving space for context-responsiveness. In a global context, the 'immaterial materials' such as thoughts, feelings and imagination can be part of a social force and form new collective patterns against the state or market-driven interests. In this way, we can be united by a desire to create new forms of understanding through creative dialogue that crosses boundaries of ethnicity, gender, religion and culture. In an interview with Moira Roth (1990, no page), Susanne Lacy express this potential in the following way:

> For example, the notion that art was communication, a link, a crossover mechanism, caused us to want to deal with people of different races, people of different ages. Collaboration also came out of the sensibility that if art was a communication, the process of making art and the communication that occurred between the artists was an important and integral part of the work itself.

One strength that we possess as artists is that we continuously work with the unknown – something that is often unspoken or that cannot be easily described with words and therefore needs other means in order to be expressed. To let this imaginary world take part in the often dull and repetitive actions at a workplace, we create a possibility of exchange based on thoughts.

References

Alfreds, L & Åberg, C 2010, *Sossial Skulptur – A Collection of Dreams from Ali Demi Prison*, Harakulla Press, Stockholm.
Alfreds, L & Åberg, C (eds.) 2014, *Visualize the Invisible*, ArtAgent Press, Stockholm.

Appadurai, A 2000, 'Grassroots globalization and the research imagination', *Public Culture*, [online] vol. 12, no. 1, pp. 1–19. Available at: http://muse.jhu.edu/article/26176 [Accessed 12 May 2016].

Arts Council England 2010, 'Adults participatory arts. Thinking it through. A review commissioned from 509 Arts', [online] *Arts Council England*, p. 20. Available at: http://www.artscouncil.org.uk/sites/default/files/download-file/adult_participatory_arts.pdf [Accessed 23 August 2016].

Bekteshi, A 2014, 'Participatory art as a tool for dialogue and change', in *Visualize the Invisible*, ed. Alfreds L & Åberg C, ArtAgent Press, Stockholm, pp. 14–16.

Beuys, J & Harlan, V 2004, *What is Art? Conversations with Joseph Beuys*, Clairview Books, West Sussex.

Clothes Workshop, 2012 (video file), Available at: https://vimeo.com/87954758 [Accessed 11 January 2016].

Donovan, T 2012, '5 Questions for Contemporary Practice with Suzanne Lacy', [online] ART 21.org. Available at: http://elgg.leeds.ac.uk/libajn/weblog/ [Accessed 9 May 2016].

Haks, F 1995, 'Interview with Joseph Beuys' in *Joseph Beuys: Diverging Critiques*, ed. Thistlewood D, Liverpool: Tate Gallery Liverpool and Liverpool University Press, Liverpool, p. 53.

Kester, GH 2005, 'Conversation pieces: The role of dialogue in socially engaged art' in *Theory in Contemporary Art Since 1985*, eds. Kucor Z & Leung S, Blackwell, University of California Press, Berkeley and Los Angeles, California, pp. 76–88.

Konstfrämjandet 2011, *SKISS – Art, Workplace, Research*, Publikum, Stockholm

Lacy, S (ed.) 1994, *Mapping the Terrain: New Genre Public Art*, Bay Press, Seattle.

Lovejoy, M, Paul, C & Vesna, V 2011, *Context Providers. Conditions of Meaning in Media Arts*, The University of Chicago Press, Chicago.

Milevska, S 2006, 'Participatory art – A paradigm shift from objects to subjects', *Theory Now*, [online] issue 2, no pages. Available at: http://www.springerin.at/dyn/heft_text.php?textid=1761&lang=en [Accessed 12 May 2016].

Roth, M 1990, 'Oral history interview with Suzanne Lacy, 1990 March 16-September 27', Archives of American Art, Smithsonian Institution (Tape 1, side A [30-minute tape sides]) Available at: http://www.aaa.si.edu/collections/interviews/oral-history-interview-suzanne-lacy-12940 [Accessed 12 May 2016].

Sacks, S 2016, 'Social sculpture research unit.' *The Territory*, [online]. Available at: http://www.social-sculpture.org/category/territory [Accessed 11 January 2016].

The Use of Art Where it's Hard to Talk. Available at: http://uawht.blogspot.se. [Accessed 12 May 2016].

Part III

Responses from Social Work as a Glocalised Profession

11 Community Work as a Socio-Spatial Response to the Challenge of Glocal Segregation and Vulnerability

Päivi Turunen

Across the world, globalism, urbanization, migration, new technologies, and neoliberalized markets, as discussed in this book, have brought about glocal changes, constantly transforming both socioeconomic and socio-spatial conditions for human life and action. Regardless of the geographical, societal, and historical differences between nations and regions, globalization and urbanization in the Global North and South are becoming increasingly similar, discussed even as Cocacolonization and McDonaldization (Soja 2013). At the same time, cities are becoming more heterogeneous and differentiated, even creating juxtapositions of extreme wealth and extreme poverty that are found locally in almost every one of the more than 500 megacity regions of the world (ibid., p. 693). Contemporary neoliberal capitalism strives for innovation, economic growth, and high classic design of attractive and smart cities. On the other side, it will also lead to greater geographical and cultural sorting of people and places, even by skill, talent, and ability (Florida & Melander 2015). Additionally, the neoliberal transformation of welfare states in Western countries has, since the 1980s, involved a decreased public responsibility for welfare policies and services alongside an increased reliance on the market and the informal sector (Khan & Dominelli 2000; Meagher & Szebehely 2013; Larsson et al. 2012), including the decreasing public funding of community work in Britain as well as in Sweden and other countries (Mayo 2016; Popple 2015; Turunen 2004).

A great deal of the contemporary scientific discussions on socio-spatiality are focused on the worldwide urbanization, even called the planetary urbanization (ct. Brenner & Schmid 2015; Soja, 2013). But the issue of socio-spatiality concerns even smaller settlements such as cities, towns, suburbs, villages, remote areas, or small islands (Madanipour 2014; Listerborn 2013; Turunen 2002), as well as diverse spaces and places in which social workers are working and acting (Hutchinson 2009; Matthies et al. 2001; Spatscheck 2012). Even in the Nordic context, cities and towns are increasingly divided into wealthy and poor areas where migration, residential segregation, and inequality intersect and increase, despite the good intentions of comprehensive welfare policies (Björkdahl & Strömbom 2015; Andersson et al. 2016; Righard et al. 2015). In the most segregated and marginalized residential areas in Sweden, a large number of people lack labor, the demanded skill and competence for the labor market, and access to income-based social security (ct. Andersson et al. 2016; Edling 2015). The most excluded are referred to basic welfare benefits or social security, which are becoming less and less generous. Therefore, an increasing number of the population is exposed to greater structural and personal vulnerability for social exclusion, discrimination, and stigmatization. In fact, the segregated residential areas even in Sweden have existed in the shadow of the market and not benefited from the welfare state's priorities for decades. This macro exposé raises many questions, also about the role of community work in a transformed world that is highly differentiated and socially divided.

The chapter aims to present a conceptual framing of socio-spatiality and how it has been discussed in urban design, human geography, and social work with a specific focus on community-orientated practices. The inquiry is focused on the question of which kinds of socio-spatial perspectives and responses to segregation and vulnerability have been discussed, emerged, and developed? The specific aim is to reactualize and revitalize the discussion of community work as a socio-spatial response to segregation and vulnerability within glocal social work, including Nordic community work. The research method used in this chapter is the deliberation of diverse arguments about socio-spatiality and community work, based on a selection of literature, scientific articles, and practical examples from a Nordic perspective, which I am influenced by. The chief aim is to highlight, extend, and deepen our understanding of both the socio-spatial discourses and practices.

The Framing of Socio-Spatiality

Both the Global Agenda for Social Work and Social Development (ISW 2014) and the International Association for Community Development (IACD 2007) have shed light on widening social and economic inequality across the world and the need for both global and local platforms for discussion and development of responses to common future challenges, with claims to promote change, social justice, and sustainability. However, these two networks have not explicitly discussed issues of socio-spatiality, even if they have paid attention to the need for sustainable development in economic, social, and ecological respects. The focus has been laid on enhancing social development and well-being, while the spatial dimensions have not explicitly been highlighted or problematized.

In the globalization processes, traditional distinctions between the physical and the social constituent parts of human settlements have blurred, covering economic, ecological, cultural, political, aesthetic, or gender aspects of living environments (Madanipour 2014; Matthies et al. 2001; Listerborn 2013). This blurring has resulted in the increased need for inter-, multi- and transdisciplinary and -sectoral cooperation between professionals and scholars in architecture, design, planning, engineering, human geography, and social policy as well as in the social sector, which I will stress. According to Madanipour, the critical socio-spatial approach in urban design explores both the material and social relationships of human settlements. It does not replace one with the other, but brings these two together. It also requires us to think of the human environment (e.g., a city or a town) as a whole.

Urban design is not only concerned with aesthetics and practicalities of design-ing urban spaces, but also with the pursuit of social inclusiveness, participatory democracy, cultural meanings, and ecological sustainability. Madanipour does not mention social workers or community workers in the cooperation outlined by him. Therefore, I will reactualize the socio-spatial aims and roles of community work from the end of the nineteenth century when the pioneering social workers, particularly within the settlement movement, started to discuss social issues and problems in relation to the urban environment and the inhuman living conditions in residential areas inhabited by the working class poor and immigrants of the day (cf. Cox et al. 1987; van Heugten & Gibbs 2015; Matthies et al. 2001; Popple 2015; Seltzer & Haldar 2015; Turunen 2004).

Theorizing Socio-Spatiality

In human geography, there are both old and new theories about socio-spatiality that are interconnected and derive from Lefebvre to scholars of today such as Soja (1996, 2010); Massey et al. (1999); or Amin (2002). All of them raise human geographical concerns and evoke a consciousness of spatiality in conjunction with social and historical aspects of human life by claiming that the spatial dimen-sion is something more than a physical-material environment. It was Lefebvre who politicized the discussion of the production of space during the 1960s by recognizing that space and society are mutually constituted, i.e., that social and spatial relations are dialectically inter-reactive and interdependent (Gromark 1982; Haas 2012; Lefebvre 1982). His books, *The Right to The City* (Le Droit à la Ville), originally published in 1968, and *The Production of Space* (La Production de l'Espace), in 1974, still make important contributions as sources for today's postmodern and post-structural human geographical discussions on spatiality. Lefebvre's theory is philosophical, abstract, and complex. In more simplified words, he lifted the focus from physical spaces to social spaces by describing how spaces have become colonized by capitalism and governed by the state through science, planning, and other practices. On the other hand, he also claimed that spaces can be decolonized through political action in everyday life, where the forces of change are able to be mobilized. Lefebvre presented a spatialized version of Marxism by widening the scope of Marxist theory from production systems to social reproduction, in particular, the spatial construction of everyday life and its practices, stressing that capitalism does not only affect labor at working places but also the diverse spaces where people live and produce their everyday life, from home to public spaces. For Lefebvre, space was not only a material or a scientific object but also a political and strategic space for diverse types of social practices, for both governing practices from above and for struggling practices from below (Agnew 2011; Haas 2012; Lefebvre 1982). This idea of social space for action, mutual interplay, mobilization, and top-down and bottom-up strategies has been discussed in community work since the end of the nineteenth century, even if not directly articulated in Lefebvre's spatial words (cf. Addams 1910/1981; Cox et al. 1987; Hutchinson 2009; Mayo 2016; Popple 2015).

Spatiality refers to a variety of spaces, from the universe to the psychological space of the mind, from the conscious to the unconscious, and from Marx to Freud and Foucault. The spectrum is huge, requiring an extended and dynamic understanding of socio-spatiality according to which both spatial and social relations have "stretched out" from their traditional meanings (Amin 2002; Massey et al. 1999; Soja 1996, 2010). We live and act in spaces such as homes, neighborhoods, streets, working places, cities, regions, countries, etc., and transgress them daily, tending to take spaces and places for granted without theoretical reflection. Listerborn (2013), who has studied suburban women and the glocalisation of their everyday lives in underprivileged areas in Sweden, uses the concept of "glocal life" in order to capture the dialectic relationship between global influences and local everyday life. When people migrate, cross borders, live with people from different countries, keep long-distance contact with countries of origin, or have families and friends all over the world, they shape glocal lives. People interact both locally and globally in diverse social spaces and places, create the meanings of these relationships, and construct life expressions to make sense of their own world. There are both real and imaginary spaces (Soja 1996).

Amin (2002) points out that globalization marks a new ontology of place/space relations. The spatiality of the social needs has to be theorized and problematized in new ways, because there is no consensus on it. Amin's criticism is directed toward the geometrical, more or less positivistic scale theories in geography. She agrees with human geographers (e.g., Doreen Massey, David Harvey, and Nigel Thrift) that space, place, and time have come to be seen in relational terms, in more non-territorial ways, as "co-constituted, folded together, produced through practices, situated, multiple and mobile" (ibid., p. 389). Globalization, diaspora, and transnationalism have intensified in the late-modern context through an increased "time-space compression," originally discussed by Harvey and redeveloped by Massey (Listerborn 2013, p. 291). Time-space compression refers to the speed of the postmodern global and local changes in the economy, technology, communication, and social life, where place and space and time are interconnected. Massey has defined place as a set of physical boundaries, with space as the social construction of what happens in that place and time as being both linear and relative (Stevens & Hasset 2012, p. 508). Feminists reassert the concept of place, not by revalorizing place as the site of domesticity but as a meeting place for a progressive political agenda to challenge oppression (Agnew 2011, p. 325).

Agnew (2011) presents four theoretical directions of human geography: the neo-Marxist (e.g., Henri Lefebvre), the humanist or agency-based (e.g., Yi-Fu Tuan), the feminist (e.g., Doreen Massey), and the performative direction (e.g., Nigel Thrift). Agnew finds out both problems and potential in each of the four directions, but concludes that it is the construction of places through social practices which they share. These theoretical orientations offer a potential route toward overcoming the space-place conundrum, and much of the revived interest in place has to do with its process-orientation. Agnew himself conceives place as a location or a site in space (e.g., a city, a town, a village), a series of locals and settings where everyday life activities take place (e.g., workplace, home, association), and a sense of place (a unique community, landscape, or moral order). He also assumes that some sense of place (with a locality, nation-state, or world) is a necessary prerequisite for social solidarity and collective action (ibid., p. 23). These three dimensions are astonishingly similar to the three dimensions of the concept of community as it has been conceived within community work from the end of the 1960s (ct. Goetschius 1969, pp. 215–219; Turunen 2004, p. 45, 2009 pp. 49–50): as a geographical territory (e.g., a city, a suburb, a village, an island, etc.), as a social unit for social interaction (e.g., an association, a working place, an organization, etc.), and as a sense of symbolic togetherness (e.g., ethnicity, class, gender, religious, lifestyle, etc.). These different conceptions of community highlight a central problem that "at the core of defining community lies a paradox that the term is as much an aspiration as it is a reality" (Stepney & Popple 2008, p. 7). In summary, there are a number of connections between human geography and community work concerning the notion of place. What human geographers stress is that places are not static or closed, but relational and open for change. In community work, a place requires human agency for social action and change. Additionally, the communities of today also include virtual communities and the discussion of so-called third places, spaces, and thirdspaces.

Third Place, Third Space, or Thirdspace?

These three concepts are interconnected, even if they are not equivalent. They shed light on emerging processes between opposing forces in social spaces creating something new. A starting point for Soja (1996) is the spatial triad of space of Lefebvre, who conceived the social space as perceived (spatial practice), conceived (representations of space), and lived (spaces of representation). Soja's "trialectics" of spatiality are influenced by hook's explorations of the margins as a space of radical openness, feminist interpretations of the interplay of race, class, and gender, the postcolonial critique of colonialized spaces and the new cultural politics of difference and identity. This also links to Foucault's heterotopologies and trialectics of space, knowledge, and power. In short, it is in the thirdspace in which everything comes together, subjectivity and objectivity, the abstract and the concrete, the real and the imagined, the knowable and the unimaginable, the repetitive and the differential, structure and agency, mind and body, consciousness and the unconscious, the disciplined and the transdisciplinary, everyday life and unending history. The concept of thirdspace combines a three-sided interplay of spatiality-historicity-sociality. This combination has implications for bringing about a profound change in the different ways of thinking about space. It is also thought to lead to major revisions in how we study history and society. "The challenge being raised in Thirdspace is therefore transdisciplinary in scope. It cuts across perspectives and modes of thought, and is not confined solely to geographers, architects, urbanists and others for whom spatial thinking is a primary preoccupation" (Soja 1996, p. 3). Thirdspace is, according to Soja, a purposively tentative and flexible term: "It is to encourage you to think differently about the meanings and significance of space and those related concepts that compose and comprise the inherent *spatiality of human life*: place, location, locality, landscape, environment, home, city, region, territory, and geography" (ibid. p. 1). The concept of thirdspace also includes "thirding-as othering," meaning a creative process of restructuring that draws selectively and strategically from the two opposing categories to open new alternatives.

Soja (2010) has developed further his human geographical thinking for encompassing the theory of spatial justice—how it is created, maintained, and brought about. According to him, justice has also a geography, including the equitable distribution of resources, services, and access to them as part of a commitment to basic human rights. Spatial justice has its emphasis on the struggle over geography, combining both social and power elements, respectively. The most contemporary example of this type of struggle is the migration crisis in Europe, in particular, the contemporary situation of Syrian refugees and its consequences in global politics and glocal lives. This struggle has also impacted on community workers who have started discussing and comparing both theoretical and practical aspects of migration and its challenges in diverse glocal spaces where thirding of othering is going on. The international conference of the International Federation of Settlements and Neighborhood Centers in Berlin 2016 gives some examples of these processes where both people and practices are on the move.[1]

Besides the concept of thirdspace, even concepts of third place and third space figure within the socio-spatial discourses. The concept of third place by Oldenburg (1989, 1999) is pragmatic in its performance, referring to public places, between the first place (home) and the second place (work), for the informal gathering of people. The third places can be post offices, pubs, cafés, and parks but also diverse community centers, providing public places on neutral ground for gathering and interacting. According to Oldenburg, third places have come to replace the lost communities of the past, providing important spaces for civil society, democracy, participation, and even for establishing feelings of a sense of place. Third places, according to Oldenburg, promote community vitality, local democracy, and even social equity. They are importantly open for all. Jeffres et al. (2009, p. 334) note that urban centers cannot any longer ignore the search for community. Therefore, the concept of a third place (even discussed as a third space) is today vital in a number of contexts from businesses to urban planning and community work.

Within the International Association for Community Development (IACD 2007, pp. 14–16), the third space is discussed as a tension between exogenous and endogenous forces, for example, concerning participation, a crucial dimension of community development, in this case, focused on environmental issues. Participation can be initiated endogenously (starting from the internal resources within a community, i.e., community-initiated) or exogenously (starting from resources located outside of a community, i.e., externally initiated, usually by a state body, a funded organization, or a corporate entity). To my mind, community workers have, since the settlement work, created third places and spaces in the tensions of opposing forces. This may be seen as "thirding as othering," most often between local people and the state/public sector in both place-bound and non-place bound communities, but also between the public and the private sector, as will be discussed further in the chapter.

Socio-Spatiality in Social Work

Within social work, "socio-spatial" issues have primarily been discussed as a social environment and later as an eco-social environment, as in eco-social work (Matthies & Närhi 2001); a local living environment, as in community-based social work (Närhi 2002); a sustainable environment, as in eco-social practice (Peeters 2012); a spatial sensitivity, as in social space-orientated social work (Spatscheck 2012); a dynamic and nonlinear assessment in social care (Stevens & Hasset 2012); and a broad multidimensional community perspective, as in community work (e.g., Cox et al. 1987; Hutchinson 2009; Popple 2015). Eco-social work is a transnational combination of casework, community work, ecological social work, and eco-criticism. Within case work, the "socio-spatial" aspect of human life has primarily been discussed as "person-in-environment," by focusing on individual's unique situation in her/his environment. Within community work, the socio-spatial aspects have chiefly been discussed in relation to "urban environment," with emphasis on the living conditions and level of social services in the built and physical environment, especially in segregated and disadvantaged suburbs. For example, Jane Addams and her female colleagues, who grounded the Settlement Hull House in Chicago in 1889, conducted the first urban studies (Hull-house Maps and Papers) before the University of Chicago was established (Addams 1910/1981; Deegan 1990; Turunen 2004, pp. 48–54). The first settlement, Toynbee Hall, was established in East London in 1884 in an area where 44 percent of the population still live in poverty.[2] Both of these settlements were so-called university settlements, forming a kind of university-community partnership (a kind of third space, as I see). Settlement workers were engaged in both research and social change in people's everyday lives.

Jane Addams was also internationally engaged in the peace movement as well as in the citizen and women's rights movements. The settlement movement took a number of sociopolitical initiatives and activities including services and reforms from tackling poverty to community arts and planning, by starting day care, youth clubs, adult education, and art galleries and by improving local infrastructure. They even initiated the first schools of social work. The settlement movement spread to Europe, the United States, Russia, and Japan, and even to the Nordic countries. Settlements still exist today, as socioculturally orientated neighborhood centers (see further Deegan 1990; Kreutziger et al. 2001; Turunen 2004, pp. 48–54).[3] In this way, community work can be seen as a form of settlement work first established more than a hundred years ago as a mode of glocal socio-spatial response to segregation and vulnerability.

What Matthies et al. (2001) did, in their discussion of eco-social work, was to make a transnational shift from the "social question" to the "eco-social question" by synthetizing the German tradition of the social space thought and community work, the Finnish tradition of social policy and social planning, and the

British tradition of community work with an emphasis on social action. This transgressing eco-social perspective was developed within a European research project, "Making New Local Policies against Social Exclusion in European Cities," financed by the Targeted Socio-Economic Research Programme (TSER) program within the European Union. The project was conducted in socially excluded residential areas of three European cities (Jyväskylä in Finland, Leicester in Britain, and Magdeburg in Germany) by means of three types of action research modes (Matthies et al. 2000; 2001). Närhi (2002) has studied further how the local living environment is related to social exclusion and how social workers discuss it within community-based social work. According to Närhi, social workers do reflect on the environmental issues in their work but they do not analyze them theoretically. She discusses human geographical theories and designs a multidimensional model for reflection on sustainable living environments by highlighting an interdependency of diverse factors and forces connected to community structure, population, living conditions, housing policies, city planning, economic transformation, and local social policy. According to Närhi, there is a need for constructive social work in which all stakeholders are jointly involved in bringing about change in residential areas (ibid., p. 265). In Belgium, Peeters (2012) has developed his variant of eco-social work for sustainable development within social work, influenced by eco-social work thought developed by Matthies & Närhi (2001) and Närhi (2002). For Peeters, sustainable development is both an ethical and political concern, implying both global changes and a change-orientated social work practice, including global redistribution of resources as well as the emancipation and empowerment of both people and communities. Social work must, according to him, develop a structural analysis, advocacy, networking, and alliances with wider social movements, i.e., eco-social practice for eco-social justice.

Social-spatiality is most explicitly discussed in human geographical terms by Spatscheck (2012) in the article "Socio-spatial approaches to social work" stressing the need for a multilevel understanding of social spaces beyond the individualistic, clinical, and case-orientated concepts of social work. In his mode of social space work, Spatscheck transgresses the social work tradition from Jane Addams by combining it with the German social space and ecological thought in youth work, community work, and social development. Social spaces are regarded as dynamic fabrics of social and material practices that are (re)produced constantly on different levels of (inter)action. The space analysis can be done by means of both quantitative and qualitative analysis, and the social space work brings three areas of public activities together: individual perspectives on citizens and residents, administrative perspectives on social services, and town planners and architectural perspectives on planning and infrastructure. Finally, Stevens & Hassett (2012) examine risk assessment in social care, which they criticize and replace by concentrating on the complexity of theory in social geography that, according to them, looks at the interconnectedness of people and places through triangulation with space, place, and time. The focus is lifted from individual pathology to the complex human environment by stressing the need to depart from traditional cause/effect and linear models of analysis to nonlinear models that seek to understand complexity, interconnectedness, and change as a complex process. The authors encourage practitioners to focus on processes and not on procedures or outcomes alone.

In my own study, "A life-political aspect on community work," the research focus was based on processes of community development and planning (Turunen, 2002). I studied a local project called the Vågspelet (the Bold Venture) on a tiny island (Vrångö) in Gothenburg's Archipelago during the 1990s. The symbolic name of this project in Swedish implied a double connotation, a geographic reference to waves around the island and a challenge of risk-taking. The project was initiated by a group of women and aimed to rescue and enhance future life chances for all generations of the island by means of the rebuilding of a deteriorated school into a multiservice center for both public and community services. The processes included both power struggles and economic "ProbRisking" of the whole project. Despite encountering a number of risks and problems, local women succeeded in reconstructing the house and services. From a gender perspective, women developed their role as policy makers instead of policy takers in socio-spatially orientated community development and planning. The house was given the name Vrångö-Bygdegård (Vrångö Neighborhood Centre) and became a kind of third place and space for the everyday life of the entire island.[4]

Community Work as a Socio-Spatial Response

Community work has a long history in the colonial type of community development and North-American type of community organization as well as in diverse social movements from labor and women rights movements to contemporary social movements (Stepney & Popple 2008; Popple 2015; Mayo 2016). It can be conducted by both professionals and nonprofessionals, i.e., not only by social workers. A central tenet of community work has been its commitment to tackling poverty and empowering disadvantaged local communities to promote social change and social justice. Within the context of professional social work, community work has comprehended and developed structural analyses of living conditions as well as the improvement of these through both planned and direct actions with those involved (Cox et al. 1987; Matthies et al. 2001; Turunen 2004, 2009). Methods have included identifying problem areas, analyzing causes, formulating plans, developing strategies, mobilizing material and immaterial resources, and involving local people and encouraging the interrelationship between them to facilitate their aims, efforts, and dreams. There are both top-down, bottom-up, and mixed approaches, depending on the context (Hutchinson 2009; Popple 2015; Sjöberg et al. 2015).

Community work is viewed by Stepney & Popple (2008, p. 132) as a broad, inclusive term "used to describe a wide range of activity and interventions that take place in a variety of settings and usually in neighborhoods." Further, it is used by Popple (2015, pp. 93–96) to denote a generic term for a range of diverse models encompassing community care, community organization, community development, community education, community action, community economic development, feminist community work, ethnic minority and anti-racist community work, environmentalism, and the green movement critique within professional social work or beyond it. Popple goes on to describe community work as a collective form of practice that aims to help people to articulate the dilemmas they face in their everyday lives and to work together for a more just, sustainable, and equal society in a critical, participatory, and democratic manner. Community work, in his view, is primarily seen as a support for the civic society.

Community work within the Nordic context has been influenced by international traditions of community development and community organization, but also by the Dutch and Nordic tradition of community planning. In chief, it has been conducted within the welfare state, and since the 1990s, to a greater degree within civic society. Since the 1980s, Nordic community work has been in reflexive transition toward increasing differentiation (Hutchinson 2009; Turunen 2004; 2009, 2013). Nordic community work was introduced within the professional social work arena during the 1960s and the first projects were conducted around 1970. Since then, it has had two main aims, to analyze societal problems and, from this analysis, to start mobilizing both immaterial and material resources for social development and change in urban and rural contexts. The Nordic directions have varied from locality development and social planning to social action: "[...] helping and stimulating oppressed, victimized and unorganized people to come together so that they can take better care of their interests or together change a problem in their reality and conditions of life" (Ronnby 1994, pp. 209). Locality development has comprehended village and neighborhood development, social planning has been focused on service extension and participation in community/ city planning, and social action on radical bottom-up mobilization.

Nordic community work has primarily made a complementary contribution within welfare state policies for preventing social problems and improving living conditions in disadvantaged environments (Hutchinson 2009; Swedner, 1983). During the neoliberal restructuring of welfare services since the 1980s, the first practice casualty of the modernization and reform was to cut off community work and preventive social work from the mainstream. Since then, partly new types of community-orientated approaches have reappeared in other sectors such as public health, tenant and housing, crime prevention, voluntary organization, social economy, etc., and in diverse terms such as local public health work, locality development, local crime prevention, voluntary work, social economy, and even as soci(et)al entrepreneurship (Turunen 2004, 2009, 2013).

Paradoxically, in Sweden, which has a radical social law (The Social Service Act)[5] from 1982, revised in 2001, community work has almost ceased in social work education and practice as in Great Britain (cf. Turunen 2004, 2009; Stepney & Popple 2008; Popple 2015). According to the Social Service Act, the public social services shall, on a basis of democracy and solidarity, promote people's economic and social security, equality of living conditions, and active participation in the life of the community. There is a mandate to be familiar with living conditions, improve them, prevent social problems, and even participate in community planning for promoting good environments in the municipality

(Hutchinson 2009; Turunen ibid.). Regardless of the law and its mandate, the "socio-spatial" tasks have not been the first priority of social work in 35 years. One reason for this is that the law is a framework law that gives municipalities strong liberties and discretion to decide their own priorities for social services and directions of social work.

Despite the neoliberal context and associated reforms since the 1980s, there are some examples of community work to illustrate such as the Fritidsforum (the Leisure Forum), the umbrella organization for youth and neighborhood centers, developing community work since 1912 when the first settlement (Birkagården) was founded in Stockholm, the capital of Sweden.[6] The CESAM (Foundation Community Development and Social Mobilisation) in Örebro (in the middle of Sweden) has enhanced community development and community work transnationally in Europe since 1984, and lately toward social innovation.[7] The municipality of Mölndal, close to Gothenburg (the second largest city on the east coast), conducts community work in four residential areas for wellbeing, participation, and security.[8]

Since the end of the 1980s, a new type of social and societal entrepreneurship has emerged between the public, the private, and the civic sector, encompassing diverse types of enterprises with social aims such as cooperatives, community and social enterprises, corporative social responsibility (CSR), fair trade, etc. in diverse parts of the country (Gawell et al. 2009, pp. 13–15; Turunen 2013). New entrepreneurial experiments have also been promoted by the Coompanion, an organization for cooperative enterprising,[9] and the Forum for Social Innovation for commercial and community-orientated social enterprising at international, national, and local levels.[10] One concrete example of these new types of enterprises is the Yalla Trappan (the Yalla Stairs), a cooperative social enterprise of immigrant women in Rosengård, a segregated residential area in Malmö.[11] A similar type of enterprise is the cooperative food store and neighborhood services in Skattungby, in a pre-rural area of the County of Dalarna, northwest of Stockholm.[12] There are also local examples such as neighborhood associations (Stadsdelsföreningar) engaged in neighborhood work and local development in segregated suburbs, e.g., in Skäggetorp in Linköping, in the southwest of Sweden from Stockholm.[13] Recently, a more radical form of community work, such as the urban justice movement for struggling against racism, segregation, gender and ethnic and religious discrimination, has emerged in segregated suburbs in the southern part of Sweden, in Gothenburg, Malmö, and Stockholm (Schierup et al. 2014).[14] This type of radical community work reminds us of social action within community work from the 1970s, but is more diasporic than social action in the 1970s in Sweden (ct. Ronnby 1994; Swedner 1983; Stepney & Popple 2008).

I myself was engaged in community work at the Information Skarpnäck 1984–1988 (Turunen, 1988), in a new residential area, Skarpnäcksfältet (Skarpnäck Field), in south Stockholm. This community work was conducted in keeping with the Social Service Act from 1982 for preventive social work and active participation in community planning. Skarpnäcksfältet was designed for 10,000 inhabitants and intended to be something better than the residential areas built during the

Million Home Programme (1965–1974), when one million new dwellings were constructed over ten years in Sweden.[15] Today, a great number of these residential areas across the country are deeply socio-spatially segregated and stigmatized, representing a social and environmental scar on the urban landscape (ct. Andersson et al. 2016; Edling 2015). The specificity of the socio-spatial design of Skarpnäcksfältet emphasized a move from the mass production style of the Million Home Program to a variation of buildings, apartments, population, social services, and a community center in the middle of the area, creating a kind of "third place and space" in a postmodern suburb. The design combined both city and neighborhood planning.[16] Community workers at the Information Skarpnäck, established by the Department of Social Services and the Department of Leisure and Culture, followed up on the construction processes and investigated emerging needs and problems for change. Both the social planner within social services and community workers participated in collaborative committees at the municipal level as well as in committees established for social services and other activities at the local level. Both vertical and horizontal networks and community groups were established. A neighborhood committee (Stadsdelsgrupp) was initiated by community workers at the local level, and this committee and the local residents became the main agency for identifying and articulating the everyday needs and problems of the area. The same kind of socio-spatial experiments is in progress once again today, e.g., in Vallastaden (the Valla City), a new residential area close to the university of Linköping. It is designed to "be a vibrant place full of life and activity—almost like a town within the town. An area where all kinds of different buildings, people, styles, and backgrounds will converge to create a place where people can come together – and grow together."[17] The future will show, of course, whether this residential area will provide socio-spatial access to places and spaces for all segments of the population.

Summary and Conclusion

The chapter shows that social work is challenged not only by globalism and urbanism, but also by new socio-spatial conditions, demands, and discourses. In seeking theories on socio-spatiality, human geographers have shed light on spatial aspects of human environment, particularly on the transformed relationship between space, place, and time. They have also emphasized the need for a new spatial consciousness and perspective on human life and environment beyond the social and historical perspectives that social scientists have traditionally highlighted. The spatial aspect of human life has conventionally been treated as a kind of fixed background, a materially and physically formed environment that is politically neutral. The postmodern and poststructural theorists in human geography challenge this and provide theoretical concepts, modes of empirical analysis, and even strategies for the socio-spatial conception and promotion of change and justice. They transgress given normative spatial assumptions and open new critical perspectives on the understanding of glocal life and unjust geographies. Among other things, Soja (2010) has developed a theory of spatial justice by stressing that justice also has a geography. The contemporary glocal capitalism tends to favor and legitimize the wealthiest residential spaces across the world—the gated communities of Beverley Hills, not residential areas like the Bronx. On the other side, the increasing polarization between rich and poor pushes regions and cities to literally tear themselves apart and risk a worrying descent into battlefields of violent social, racial, and cultural conflict (ct. Abrahamsson 2015). Some of these battles have recently happened, as I see, in Syria, Paris, and Brussels as well as the social unrest in places like Ferguson, Missouri in the United States. It is the most segregated residential areas in Europe that have become the socio-spatial spaces for Islamic radicalization and recruiting of ISIS soldiers, a fact we can't shut our eyes to. The European Union, too, is deeply concerned about socio-spatial issues in housing and the risks associated with increasing inequality (Boverket 2016).[18]

In this chapter, socio-spatial theories, thought, and practices have been recounted to reconceptualize social work in the form of eco-social work, social-space work, and socio-spatial community work. In the future, social workers must challenge their own given perspectives and assumptions on viewing socio-spatial phenomena. The dominant perspectives that shape our vision of the future must be widened and radicalized in a glocalized world. Community workers have, since the settlement movement at the end of the nineteenth century, tried to develop social-spatial perspectives on and responses to segregation and vulnerability, without succeeding in making a decisive breakthrough in reshaping the mainstream of social work. Regardless of this fact, community workers must also revisit and renew their own theoretical thinking and practices in a transformed world. One way to do this is to gain inspiration from human geography. On the other hand, community workers should not become too downcast but must also be proud of their persevering efforts, since the end of the nineteenth century, at developing more critical socio-spatial approaches and promoting socio-spatial justice.

Notes

1 http://www.onthemove2016.com/en/
2 http://www.toynbeehall.org.uk/what-we-do
3 See even http://www.ifsnetwork.org/
4 See further http://www.vrango.com/, http://www.vrango.com/vrangohuset/
5 Socialtjänstlagen SFS 2001:453 http://www.riksdagen.se/sv/Dokument-Lagar/Lagar/Svenskforfattningssamling/Socialtjanstlag-2001453_sfs-2001-453/
6 http://www.fritidsforum.se/internationellt/short-presentation-of-the-swedish-settlement-movement/#.Vxzkb03Vy71
7 http://www.cesam.se/, http://www.cesam.se/samarbeten/eucdn/
8 http://www.molndal.se/medborgare/byggaboochmiljo/samhallsarbeteibostadsomraden.4.16eccd66132d06f5218800034145.html
9 For more about contemporary Swedish cooperatives, see http://coompanion.se/, http://coompanion.se/english
10 http://www.socialinnovation.se/en/
11 http://www.yallatrappan.se/
12 http://www.svt.se/nyheter/lokalt/dalarna/stor-drivkraft-i-lilla-skattungbyn
13 http://www.skaggetorp.info/
14 http://unescolucs.se/wp-content/uploads/2015/11/UnescoMOST-12-december-2015-program-och-inbjudan.pdf

15 https://en.wikipedia.org/wiki/Million_Programme
16 https://en.wikipedia.org/wiki/Skarpn%C3%A4cksf%C3%A4ltet
17 http://www.vallastaden2017.se/english/
18 See even http://jpi-urbaneurope.eu/

References

Abrahamsson, H, 2015, 'The great transformation of our time' in *Social Transformations in Scandinavian Cities: Nordic Perspectives on Urban Marginalization and Social Sustainability*, eds. E Righard, M Johansson & T Salonen, Nordic Academic Press, Lund, pp. 21–40.

Addams, J, 1910/1981, *Twenty Years at Hull-House*, Penguin Books, Signet Classic, New York.

Agnew, JA, 2011, 'Space and place' in *The Sage Handbook of Geographical Knowledge*, eds. JA Agnew & D Livingstone, Sage, London, pp. 316–330.

Amin, A, 2002, 'Spatialities of globalisation', *Environmental and Planning*, vol. 34, pp. 385–399.

Andersson, R, Bengtsson, B & Myrberg, G, (eds.) 2016, *Mångfaldens dilemman, boende-segregation och områdespolitik*, Gleerups, Malmö.

Boverket, 2016, *EU och bostadspolitiken: Rättsutveckling och samarbete inom EU av betydelse för svensk bostadspolitik*, [online] Available at: http://www.boverket. se/globalassets/publikationer/dokument/2016/eu-och-bostadspolitiken-2015.pdf [Acccessed 28 April 2016].

Brenner, N & Schmid, C, 2015, 'Towards a new epistemology of the urban', *City*, vol. 19, no. 2–5, pp. 151–182.

Björkdahl, A, & Strömbom, L, (eds) 2015, *Divided Cities: Governing Diversity*, Nordic Academic Press, Lund.

Cox, FM, Ehrlich, JL, Rothman, J & Tropman, JE, (eds) 1987, *Strategies of Community Organization*. 4th ed, FE Peacock Publishers, Inc., Itasca.

Deegan, MJ, 1990, *Jane Addams and the Men of the Chicago School, 1892–1918*, Transaction Books, New Brunswick.

Edling, J, 2015, *Förorterna som modern Svea glömde: en dokumentation av en obefintlig integrationspolitik*, [online] Flexicurity-Verdandi. Available at: http://www.flexicurity. se/skrifter/fororterna-som-moder-svea-glomde/ [Accessed 28 April 2016].

Florida, R & Mellander, C, 2015, 'Talent, cities, and competitiveness' in *Oxford Handbook of Local Competitiveness*, eds DB Audretsch, DB, AN Link & M Lindenstein Walshok, University Press, Oxford, pp. 34–53.

Gawell, M, Johannisson, B & Lundqvist, M, 2009, *Entrepreneurship in the Name of the Society: Reader's Digest of A Swedish Research Anthology*, [online]. Available at: http://www.kks.se/om/Lists/Publikationer/Attachments/151/Bok%20KKS%20eng.pdf [Accessed 28 April 2016].

Goetschius, GW, 1969, *Working with Community Groups: Using Community Development as a Method of Social Work*, Routledge & Kegan Paul, London.

Gromark, S, 1982, 'Henri Lefebvre: Vardagligheten och staden' in *Staden som rättighet*, H Lefebvre, Bokomotiv, Stockholm.

Haas, O, 2012, 'Socio-spatial theory: Space, social relations, difference', [online]. Available at: https://www.academia.edu/6133569/Sociospatial_theory_Space_Social_ Relations_Difference [Accessed 28 April 2016].

Van Heugten, K & Gibbs, A, (eds) 2015, *Social Work for Sociologists: Theory and Practice*, Palgrave Macmillan, Basingstoke.

Hutchinson, G, (ed) 2009, *Community Work in the Nordic Countries: New Trends*, Universitetsforlaget, Oslo.

IACD (International Association for Community Development), 2007, 'What in the world …? Global lessons, inspirations and experiences in community development', [online]. Available at: http://www.iacdglobal.org/publications-and-resources/iacd-publications/ what-world-global-lessons-inspirations-and-experiences-community-development [Accessed 28 April 2016].

ISW (International Social Work), 2014, 'Global agenda for social work and social development: First report – Promoting social and economic equalities', *International Social Work* 2014, vol. 57 no. S4, pp. 3–16.

Jeffres, LW, Bracken, CC, Jian, Q & Casey, MF, 2009, 'The impact of third places on community quality of life', *Applied Research in Quality Life*, vol. 4, no. 4, pp. 333–345.

Khan, P & Dominelli, L, 2000, 'The impact of globalization on social work in the UK', *European Journal of Social Work*, vol. 3, no. 2, pp. 95–108.

Kreutziger, SS, Ager, R, Lewis, JS, England S, 2001, 'A critical look at a contemporary welfare-to-work program in the light of the historic settlement ideal', *Journal of Community Practice*, vol. 9, no. 2, pp. 49–69.

Larsson, B, Letell, M & Thörn, H, (eds) 2012, *Transformations of the Swedish Welfare State*, Palgrave Macmillan, New York.

Lefebvre, H, 1982, *Staden som Rättighet*, Bokomotiv, Stockholm.

Listerborn, C, 2013, 'Suburban women and the "glocalisation" of the everyday lives: Gender and glocalities in underprivileged areas in Sweden', *Gender, Place & Culture*, vol. 20, no. 3, pp. 290–312.

Madanipour, A, 2014, *Urban Design, Space and Society*, Palgrave Macmillan, Houndmills.

Massey, M, Allen, J & Sarre, P, (eds) 1999, *Human Geography Today*, Polity Press, Cambridge.

Mayo, M, 2016, 'CDJ 50 years anniversary conference presentation: Looking backwards, looking forwards – from the present', *Community Development Journal*, vol. 51, no. 1, pp. 8–22.

Matthies, A-L, Turunen, P, Albers, S, Boeck, T, & Närhi, 2000, 'An eco-social approach to tackling social exclusion in European cities: A new comparative research project in progress', *European Journal of Social Work*, vol. 3, no. 1, pp. 43–52.

Matthies, A-L, Närhi, K & Ward, D, (eds) 2001, *The Eco-Social Approach in Social Work*. Jyväskylä University, Department of Social Sciences and Philosophy, Working Papers no. 106.

Matthies, A-L & Närhi, K, 2001, 'What is the ecological (self-)consciousness of social work Perspectives on the relationship between social work and ecology.', in *The Eco-Social Approach in Social Work*, eds. A-L Matthies, K Närhi & D Ward, Jyväskylä University, Department of Social Sciences and Philosophy, Working Papers no. 106, pp. 15–53.

Meagher, G & Szebehely, M, (eds) 2013, *Marketisation in Nordic Eldercare: A Research Report on Legislation, Oversight, Extent and Consequences*, Stockholm University, Studies in Social Work 30.

Närhi, K, 2002, 'Social workers' conceptions of how the local living environment is related to social exclusion', *European Journal of Social Work*, vol. 5, no. 3, pp. 255–267.

Oldenburg, R, 1999, *The Great Good Place: Cafés, Coffee Shops, Bookstores, Bars, Hair Salons, and Other Hangouts at the Heart of a Community*, Da Capo Press, Cambridge, MA.

Oldenburg, R, 1999, *Celebrating the Third Place: Inspiring Stories About the "Great Good Places" at the Heart of our Communities*, Marlowe, New York.

Peeters, J, 2012, 'The place of social work in sustainable development: Towards ecosocial practice', *International Journal of Social Welfare*, vol. 21, no. 3, pp. 287–298.

Popple, K, 2015, *Analysing Community Work: Theory and Practice*, 2nd ed, Open University Press, Maidenhead.

Righard, E, Johansson, M, & Salonen, T, (eds) 2015, *Social Transformation in Scandinavian Cities. Nordic Perspectives on Urban Marginalization and Social Sustainability*, Nordic Academic Press, Lund.

Ronnby, A, 1994, *Mobilizing Local Communities*, Mid Sweden University, Regional and Rural Development, Rapport 1994:17, Östersund.

Schierup, CU, Ålund, A & Kings, L, 2014, 'Reading the Stockholm riots – A moment for social justice', *Race & Class*, vol. 55, no. 3, pp. 1–21.

Swedner, H, 1983, *Human Welfare and Action Research in Urban Settings; Essays on the Implementation of Social Change*, Delegation for Social Research, Swedish Council for Building Research, Stockholm.

Soja, EW, 1996, *Thirdspace: Journeys to Los Angeles and Other Real-and-Imaged Places*, Blackwell Publishing, Malden.

Soja, EW, 2010, *Seeking Spatial Justice*, University of Minnesota Press, Minneapolis, MN.

Soja, EW, 2013, 'Regional urbanization and third wave cities', *City*, vol. 17, no. 5, pp. 688–694.

Spatscheck, C, 2012, 'Socio-spatial approaches to social work', *Social Work and Society. International Online Journal*, [online] vol. 10, no. 1. Available at: http://www.socwork.net/sws/article/view/314/659 [Accessed 1 December 2015]

Stepney, P & Popple, K, 2008, *Social Work and the Community: A Critical Context for Practice*, Palgrave Macmillan, Basingstoke.

Stevens, I & Hassett, P, 2012, 'Nonlinear perspectives of risk in social care: Using complexity theory and social geography to move the focus from individual pathology to the complex human environment', *European Social Work*, vol. 15, no. 4, pp. 503–513.

Seltzer, M & Haldar, M, 2015, 'The other Chicago school – A sociological tradition expropriated and erased', *Nordic Social Work Research*, vol. 5, no. 1, pp. 25–41.

Sjöberg, S, Rambaree, K & Jojo, B, 2015, 'Collective empowerment: A comparative study of community work in Mumbai and Stockholm', *International Social Welfare*, vol. 24, no. 4, pp. 364–375.

Turunen, P, 1988, *Jippo eller medborgarinflytande? En studie av samhällsarbete i ett nybyggt bostadsområde – Skarpnäck i Stockholm*, D-uppsats, Socialhögskolan-Socialt arbete, University of Stockholm.

Turunen, P, 2002, 'A Life-political Aspect on Community Work' in *Does Social Work Pay?* eds A Carlsson & EC Franzén, FoU-Södertörns skriftserie nr 20/01, Tullinge.

Turunen, P, 2004, *Samhällsarbete i Norden: diskurser och praktiker i omvandling*, [online] Acta Wexionensia no. 47/2004, Växjö University Press, Växjö. Available at http://lnu.diva-portal.org/smash/get/diva2:206461/FULLTEXT01 [Accessed 28 April 2016].

Turunen, P, 2009, 'Nordic community work in transition: A change toward diversity and reflexivity' in *Community Work in the Nordic Countries: New Trends*, ed. G Hutchinson, Universitetsforlaget, Oslo.

Turunen, P, 2013, *Deltagardemokratiska och systemiska metoder för komplexa samhällsfrågor och samhällsentreprenörskap*, [online] Working papers – Department of Sociology and Work Science 2013:1, Göteborgs universitet, Göteborg. Available at: http://www.socav.gu.se/digitalAssets/1459/1459397_turunen-deltagardemokratiska-130923.pdf [Accessed 28 April 2016].

Internet Resources

http://coompanion.se/english [27 April 2016]
http://unescolucs.se/wp-content/uploads/2015/11/UnescoMOST-12-december-2015-program-och-inbjudan.pdf [27 April 2016]

http://www.cesam.se/samarbeten/eucdn/ [27 April 2016]

http://www.ifsnetwork.org/ [27 April 2016]

http://www.fritidsforum.se/internationellt/short-presentation-of-the-swedish-settlement-movement/#.Vxzkb03Vy71 [27 April 2016]

http://www.molndal.se/medborgare/byggaboochmiljo/samhallsarbeteibostadsomraden.4.1 6eccd66132d06f5218800034145.html [27 April 2016]

http://www.onthemove2016.com/en/ [27 April 2016]

http://www.skaggetorp.info/ [27 April 2016]

http://www.svt.se/nyheter/lokalt/dalarna/stor-drivkraft-i-lilla-skattungbyn [27 April 2016]

http://www.socialinnovation.se/en/ [27 April 2016]

http://www.vallastaden2017.se/english/ [27 April 2016]

http://www.yallatrappan.se/ [27 April 2016]

https://en.wikipedia.org/wiki/Million_Programme [27 April 2016]

http://www.vrango.com/vrangohuset/[27 April 2016]

http://www.vrango.com/ [27 April 2016]

12 Protecting the Rights of Overseas Filipino Workers

Social Work Beyond National Borders

Nilan Yu and Mary Lou Alcid

Introduction

This chapter outlines work done by social workers in protecting the rights and welfare of land-based (as distinct from sea-based) overseas Filipino workers – hereinafter referred to as OFWs, an acronym that now forms part of everyday language amongst Filipinos, given the extent to which labour migration permeates Philippine life and culture. It is hoped that this account of some of the work being done to promote the rights and welfare of OFWs will contribute towards the charting of social work in what is increasingly a globalised world and the mapping out of what may be conceived as transnational social work, represented by this volume. This chapter is informed by a critical conception of the problems manifested in the lives of OFWs and their families which may be seen as arising from individual choices and inadequacies, even by the very people who experience them. Such a conception embraces the view that the life chances of poor Filipinos – many of whom are forced to take the very difficult decision of embarking on overseas contract work and countless more who can only dream of being able to do so as a way of escaping their lot in life – are, to a significant extent, shaped by the way resources and opportunities are distributed among members of society in various spheres of social existence: within the family, the community, the state and the global capitalist order. It recognises the far-reaching influence of international political economic dynamics – global capital movements, balance of trade, international lending – on the lives of people at the base of the global economic pyramid who, to some, may seem far-removed from the complex, meta-state processes in what is now a highly globalised world. Social work practice that is not informed by this conception could very well be confined to remedial interventions addressing the residual effects of these macro processes by way of problematizing the lives, decisions and living conditions of the people adversely affected. For OFWs, this may include questions such as: Was it a smart decision to seek overseas work? Did they fully consider the implications to their families and their own wellbeing? Did they consider other options? Did they make full use of the resources they had? And once having embarked on the journey, OFWs are often seen as having knowingly and wilfully subjected themselves to the laws and employment regimes of their countries of employment, abrogating some of their rights in the process and thereby justly earning the benefits as well as costs of such decision. Drawing on this critical conception of the problems, this chapter speaks of social work practice which recognises the need to transcend what are arbitrary national borders in the context of international standards on human rights and labour protection in protecting the rights and welfare of OFWs. In that sense, we can speak of transnational social work, that is, social work theory and practice that recognises and addresses relevant interconnections between local realities – the lived experiences of people – and the broad structures and processes that generate structural inequality across the globe, engendering the disadvantage and exclusion of certain populations.

More than ever in human history, we are seeing significant international shifts in the world's population as a result of migration (Castles & Miller 2009). A big part of these population shifts involves the overseas employment of skilled workers, placing millions in social environments where they have yet to acquire the status of citizens or, by design embedded in migration law, are systematically barred from obtaining citizenship status in their host countries. This renders many of them vulnerable to labour, criminal and sexual exploitation (Global Migration Group 2013). For many such foreign workers, a key objective is to preserve their employment – often purchased at great social and financial costs to themselves and their families (Harper & Martin 2013). Consequently, some are compelled to preserve their employment at whatever cost, even if it means allowing themselves to be subjected to unfair practices of and abusive treatment by employers. It is difficult enough for such workers to seek relief from unfair treatment and abuse in countries where legal systems are stacked against what may be seen as easily replaceable and therefore dispensable (Mahdavi 2011) foreign contract workers in favour of local employers. But even if workers were successful in mounting a legal case against abusive employers, they still face the real risk of not having their employment contracts renewed and, perhaps, even forfeiting future employment prospects in that country. After all, employers are not bound by law to renew the employment contracts of non-citizens and resentful employers can strike them with trumped-up charges in retaliation. And so, such workers end up losing even in those rare instances when they do succeed in seeking legal redress. Many workers may be inclined to suffer inequities in their workplaces rather than risk jeopardising what may well be everything that they are worth and owe. Those who feel aggrieved enough to seek legal redress often do not have the resources and institutional support to do so. We are then faced with the question of how the rights of such workers as embodied in the Universal Declaration of Human Rights can be protected in these circumstances.

The chapter begins with an outline of a critical conception of social work, the one that informs the analysis of the challenges and practice presented here. This is followed by a discussion of labour migration as a global issue requiring a global response. The chapter then focuses on Filipino labour migration, with an account of the background of and challenges faced by OFWs. The heart of the chapter is an account of some of the work being done in promoting the rights of OFWs and the social workers who have played a key role in these initiatives. The chapter ends with a note on how such work can be seen as representing a form of transnational social work practice and a discussion of the implications of such conceptualisation for social work practice, education and research.

Critical Social Work in a Globalised World

There are various and – in some cases – conflicting conceptions of social work. The one-hundred-year debate in social work is underpinned by competing conceptions of social problems and, with this, competing conceptions practice. One end of the spectrum, where mainstream social work leans toward, is founded on a highly individualist understanding of social problems accompanied by practice emphasising individual reform, while a highly structural understanding of social problems underpins the social reform-oriented practice at the other end (Mullaly 2007). This chapter is informed by a structural understanding of social problems and a critical conception of social work referred to variously as critical social work, radical social work, political social work and structural social work (Mullaly 2007). Critical social work recognises that many of the issues manifested as personal problems in people's lives arise out of social inequality and disadvantage. In other words, many of the challenges social work professionals encounter in their work that, in mainstream forms of practice, are regarded and then treated as personal and intrapersonal problems are rooted in the way society is structured, particularly in terms of how certain members of society – distinguished along various social lines including class, gender, sexuality, race and ethnicity, and ability – are privileged over others to the point of making living and survival difficult for disadvantaged members of society. The focus of social work, from a critical perspective, is the challenging of social inequality, disadvantage and oppression (Mullaly 2007). This is implied in definitions of social work that speak of the promotion of social change, human rights, social justice, empowerment and the liberation of people as central tenets (see, for example, International Federation of Social Workers 2014).

Where they are recognised in literature, different forms of structural disadvantage along the lines of class, gender, race and ethnicity, sexual orientation and ability are often understood in particular national contexts even when they are acknowledged as pervading issues (see, for example, Wall's [2014] analysis of gender inequality in Australia and Chang & England's [2011] account of gender inequality in East Asia). These issues are, quite understandably, often analysed within the confines of specific political economic orders, given how particular forms of disadvantage and discrimination are of specific concern to a localised audience and lend themselves to analyses within localised contexts such as families, communities, organisations and institutions embedded in nation-states. But even when issues potentially involving transnational social dynamics such as class inequality and racism are discussed, they are – more often than not – framed in terms of the inequality between privileged groups and disadvantaged populations within particular political economic contexts (see, for example, Croll's [2013] and Saperstein & Penner's [2012] discussions of racial inequality in the US). And yet we know of the intersectionality of disadvantage and oppression (Bose 2012). We know of the significant economic differences between countries that result in unequal life chances and drive population flows across national boundaries. In the economies that host them, many migrant workers and their families – often distinguishable by social markers such as skin colour and language – then go on to experience disadvantage linked to their place of origin and racial identity (see, for example, Oikelome & Healy's [2013] analysis of differences in outcomes for doctors in the United Kingdom linked to migration and gender). What is being argued here is that certain forms of structural disadvantage transcend national boundaries and therefore must be understood from a transnational, if not international, perspective. And if social work is about the challenging of social inequality, disadvantage and oppression, then it must be conceptualised in such a way as to encompass inequality, disadvantage and oppression on such a scale.

Initially, we framed this account using the term 'global social work'. The meaning we attached to this term is not relevant here. What is relevant is how the use of the term raised the question: Can we then, in contrast, speak of a non-global social work? We can speak of social work practice limited to the local (family, community or even nation-state) context. However, the critical conception of social work outlined here leaves little room for a highly localised conception of lived realities of people in this globalised world. A critical conception of many of the problems manifested in the lives of people in developing countries like the Philippines requires an understanding of the global structures and processes that engender these. To suggest the notion of a 'global social work' would be to tacitly accept the notion of a 'non-global social work'. But a critical perspective would put into question a conception of social work that does not necessitate an understanding of the links between the lived realities of people and the global forces that shape their lives. In other words, to suggest a conception of social work that requires and involves no understanding of relevant global geopolitical dynamics that bear upon the lives of the people we work with would be antithetical to a critical conception of social work. It was for this reason that we opted not to make any reference to 'global social work' here but, instead, chose to speak of transnational social work. By transnational social work, we simply mean practice that transcends national boundaries which may or may not be informed by a critical perspective. This chapter advances a conception of transnational social work informed by a critical perspective.

Theoretical and philosophical groundwork around the internationalisation of social work provides us with the foundations for theory building in this direction. A good starting point is the common ground embodied by internationally accepted definitions of social work such as the one adopted by the International Federation of Social Workers (2014) and the International Association of Schools of Social Work. But we have yet to transcend the heavily national-bounded conceptualisations of social work, with national legal frameworks figuring prominently in definitions of professional practice in many countries. A big step forward came with the development of literature on international social work (see, for example, Hokenstad *et al.* 1992; Midgley 2001). Midgley (2001) noted different uses of the term, including (1) practice in international agency settings, (2) practice with immigrants and refugees, (3) exchanges between social work professionals from different countries and (4) a conceptualisation of social work that accords it a role in the global setting. The third and fourth uses provide us with the conceptual handle for what is referred to here as transnational social work.

Labour Migration as a Global Issue

There are 231.5 million international migrants in the world – 3 per cent of the global population (International Labour Office 2014). There has been an exponential increase in the world's migrant stock over the decades and, while growth slowed with the impact of the global financial crisis, migration is expected to continue to rise in the foreseeable future. Differences in economic growth and standards of living between countries are the main drivers of international migration (Ryder 2014). The substantial inequality that we find between individuals in particular political economic contexts mirrors and is magnified by the stark inequality between nations (Joyce 2010; Ortiz & Cummins 2011; van Zanden *et al.*, 2014). Despite global efforts to foster economic development in the least developed countries, global inequality today is as vast as it was some 200 years ago (van Zanden *et al.*, 2014). Global inequality is represented in various ways such as by conceptual divides between the North and South, developed and developing economies and Western and non-Western countries.

Beyond simply recognising the existence of inequality between countries, there are those who call attention to how this forms an integral component of the current global political economic order (see, for example, Sison & De Lima 1998). Countries like the United States have profited and are profiting massively from their economic relations with developing countries, even in cases where supposedly beneficent foreign aid is concerned (see, for example, Hiatt's [2007] and Perkins' [2004] accounts). Economic inequality between nations is an integral element of the existing global economic order in the way it rationalises the distribution of human and natural resources between nations. Economic imbalance between countries fuels out-migration from weaker economies to more economically robust countries which, in turn, results in what is described by some as a brain drain (Camacho 2010). This process exacerbates global inequality in the way it creams off some of the best human resources from weaker economies, with advanced industrialised societies benefitting from the in-migration of skilled workers even as multinational corporations capitalise on low wages in their operations in less-developed economies. But migration dynamics is much more complex than the North-South, developed-developing binary. While developed countries currently host more than half of all migrants, migration to these countries has slowed in recent years, even as South-South migration has accelerated (Ryder 2014).

The experience of disadvantage populations from less developed economies does not end when they acquire employment elsewhere. Even in countries where strong anti-discrimination and labour protection laws are in place, such populations of migrant workers can face daunting challenges. In the United States, female immigrant workers are often pictured as 'brood mares' and immigrant workers, in general, are routinely portrayed as a burden on the economy and as probable 'welfare cheats' (Chang 2000: 7). The language we use in reference to migrants reflects the global imbalance described above. Westerners who live and work in other countries – whether it be in another Western country or in a non-Western country – are frequently referred to using a special term almost exclusively reserved for them: expats. Non-Westerners who live and work in Western countries are routinely referred to using such terms as 'migrants', 'labour migrants' and 'economic migrants' (McDowell 2009: 19; Parutis 2014: 36), and are often yoked with a heavy burden of proof of their economic utility to their host countries. Layered on top of the racial and citizenship divide is the differentiated migration experience on account of gender. While women roughly account for about half of the migrant population, there is a clear pattern of gendered labour migration in terms of the field of employment and, by default, country of destination (International Organization for Migration 2009; Sijapati 2015).

A global economic order that allows for the systemic privileging of citizens from certain countries over others, to the extent of compromising the life chances of disadvantaged populations, represents the very kind of structural inequality and oppression that is seen as a challenge for critical social work. And in the way that a critical perspective would point out that structural disadvantage embedded in policies, practices and culture of organisations, institutions and societies requires action beyond the individual level, a critical understanding of some of the issues faced by migrant workers and the countries where they come from necessitates a response that goes beyond the national level. Structural inequality at the global scale requires a transnational if not a global response. If the challenging of inequality and oppression is seen as central to social work and some forms of inequality and oppression occur at the international level, then social work practice would have to be conceptualised at a global scale, providing space for professional intervention beyond and across national boundaries and politico-legal frameworks. Social work should not simply be thought of as a professional activity confined within the boundaries of the nation-state such that the legitimacy of professional action stops the moment national borders are crossed. If social work is to be true to claims of protecting human rights and promoting social justice in what is now a globalised world, it is, by necessity, a global profession. At the very least, social work practice – that is, practice that challenges structural inequality and oppression – should transcend national boundaries. The work involved in protecting the rights and welfare of OFWs presented here can be viewed as a sketch of what such form of practice can be.

Filipino Labour Migration and the Challenges Faced by OFWs

Filipino labour migration is set in the context of the Philippines' place in the global economy. Centuries of Spanish and American colonial rules established a highly unequal society inextricably embedded in the global capitalist order

(Yu 2006). While direct colonial rule was ostensibly ended with the grant of Philippine independence in 1946, the political and economic ties that bound Philippine society to the United States has been firmly kept in place (Thornton 2008) and have since extended to America's allies – Australia for one (Laforteza 2007).

Extreme social inequality and a highly individualist welfare state system denies tens of millions quality education and decent employment opportunities (Yu 2006). Even those who manage to complete tertiary education are left with very limited job prospects in a gaunt economy marked by an oversupply of skilled and semi-skilled workforce and low labour costs. These conditions impel many, including professionals, to seek out employment overseas, even at the risk of their safety and lives (Vilog & Ballesteros, 2015). For those who manage to do well in overseas employment, the economic pay-off can significantly improve the family's standard of living, with the impact going beyond the family. Personal remittances to the Philippines from migrants around the world exceeded US$ 28 billion in 2014 (World Bank 2015). Such is the significance of labour migration to the Philippine economy that the state has taken a proactive role in its governance with the aim of facilitating the employment of Filipino workers abroad (Battistella, 2012). This *de facto* labour export policy has been carried forward by successive governments over the last several decades, legitimised by discourse portraying OFWs as the country's 'new heroes', even in the face of concerns over its heavy social costs to OFWs and their families (Encinas-Franco 2013: 97).

There were over 10 million OFWs as of December 2013 (Commission on Filipinos Overseas 2013). Most (96 per cent) were overseas contract workers (Philippine Statistics Authority 2015), with the majority (57 per cent) working in Western Asia – primarily Saudi Arabia (almost 25 per cent of all OFWs), United Arab Emirates, Qatar, and Kuwait (Philippine Statistics Authority 2015). They formed part of the 83 per cent of overseas contract workers working in Asia, with only a minority employed elsewhere – Europe (6.7 per cent), North and South America (6.1 per cent), and Australia (1.7 per cent). The distribution is roughly equal between the genders (Philippine Statistics Authority 2015) although there are gendered differences in the kind of employment engaged in and, as a consequence, the countries of destination. For example, the bulk of overseas contract workers in Hong Kong are domestic helpers – more than 170,000 come from the Philippines – and virtually all of them are females (Mandap 2015; Mission for Migrant Workers 2015; Wong *et al*. 2008). One in every three (33 per cent) OFWs is employed as a labourer or unskilled worker (Philippine Statistics Authority 2015).

Migrant workers can face serious exploitation and abuse including trafficking and forced labour, labour exploitation, non-labour (including sexual) exploitation and brutal conditions in employment that can result in serious injury and death (Global Migration Group 2013; Migrant Forum in Asia 2014). Undocumented or so-called 'irregular' migrants are routinely detained as punishment and as a means of deterrence (Migrant Forum in Asia 2013a). Issues that affect OFWs working as domestic workers include extensive work hours (more than 16-hour work days are not unheard of), physical or sexual assault by employers, non-payment of wages, excessive employment agency fees, premature termination of contracts and the confiscation of their passports and contracts (Mission for Migrant Workers 2015). The market-driven character of labour migration renders Filipino migrant workers vulnerable to abuse and exploitation (Tigno 2014).

Social Work Practice in Promoting OFW Rights

Having been among the first labour-sending countries, the Philippines pioneered the development of programs and services to respond to international labour migration issues and concerns such as illegal recruitment, trafficking in girls and women, excessive placement fees by labour recruitment agencies, contract substitution, oppressive working and living conditions of workers in destination countries and discriminatory policy frameworks. Churches – most notably the Roman Catholic Church and the National Council of Churches in the Philippines (NCCP) – provided the auspices for responses to the problems and issues of OFWs. Professional social workers have also played key roles in these initiatives.

The NCCP helped set up non-governmental organisations (NGOs) such as the Batis Center for Women Inc. (Batis) that was set up in 1988 to address the abuse of female Filipino entertainers in Japan. From its very beginnings, Batis was transnational in character. It was a joint initiative between the NCCP and the Asian Women's Shelter of the Japan Women's Christian Temperance Union. Its first executive director, Violeta Marasigan, was a social worker. So is its current executive director, Rose Otero. Another NGO that the NCCP helped set up the following year (1989) was the Kanlungan Centre Foundation Inc. (Kanlungan). Kanlungan was established to provide direct services such as legal assistance, case management, education on migrants' rights and feminist counselling to potential, onsite and returned OFWs, particularly women. A social worker, Mary Lou Alcid, served as the founding chair of its board of trustees and executive director for more than eight years. The NGO hired social workers as case managers, researchers, policy advocates and community organisers. A Filipino social worker, Agnes Matienzo, has been the coordinator of the Migrant Domestic Workers West Asia Program of the Migrant Forum in Asia (MFA) since 2008. Founded in 1994 and based in the Philippines, the MFA is the first regional network of NGOs, associations, trade unions of migrant workers and advocates established to work for the promotion of the rights and welfare of Asian migrant workers.

Various auspices were also established abroad, with social workers at the forefront. For example, the Mission for Migrant Workers Ltd. (MFMW) in Hong Kong, previously called the Mission for Filipino Migrant Workers, was founded in 1981 to provide pastoral care and social services to Filipino domestic workers. The NCCP was a founding member while the Anglican Church of England provided it with office space. Since its founding, a Filipino social worker, Cynthia Abdon-Tellez, has been the MFMW's executive director. From a sole focus on Filipino migrants, the MFMW has since evolved to include other Asian migrant workers. It prides itself on being the longest existing independent service provider for migrants in Hong Kong and Asia (Mission for Migrant Workers 2013).

Maria Angela Villalba, a social worker who started her professional practice as a community worker in rural areas in the Philippines, founded the Asian Migrants Centre in Hong Kong in the early 1990s with seed money from her former church-based agency.

Because social problems usually manifest at the personal level, case management is a key aspect of the response of social workers. Case management of international labour migration cases by Philippine-based organisations may involve supporting prospective and actual migrant workers who have been victimised by unscrupulous recruiters and abusive employers and are seeking legal remedies to human rights violations in the form of unfair labour practices, gender-based violence and discriminatory policies, and/or access to social services such as medical assistance and temporary shelter. It may also involve working with families of OFWs who are experiencing extreme difficulties abroad, including those who have to be rescued from abusive employers, have been arrested and/or are facing criminal charges and in need of legal services, have been abandoned by labour brokers, are stranded in transit countries or are facing repatriation because of labour, immigration, medical and/or psychiatric reasons. The repatriation of the remains of dead OFWs is also a common concern of case managers. In cases of deaths under suspicious circumstances, NGOs support families in seeking and seeing through the appropriate action of the country's department of foreign affairs. And should there be counterpart citizens' groups or NGOs in the destination country, transnational linkage and coordination are established for concerted efforts to facilitate investigation, prosecution of the perpetrator(s) and repatriation of the remains.

Case management involves transnational coordination work. Churches have the advantage of having their own congregational and inter-congregational networks all over the world. They can help facilitate case management. However, case managers need to follow official protocol and work through government channels such as the Department of Foreign Affairs Office of the Undersecretary for Migrant Affairs (OUMWA). The OUMWA, in turn, informs the Philippine embassy or consulate about the case so it can make the necessary representation with its counterparts in the country of destination. The non-governmental networks in the destination country concerned can follow up on the progress of the case and, if necessary, put some pressure on the duty bearers – in many cases, the government of the host country – to facilitate access to needed services, legal redress and repatriation. With current advances in information technology, it has also become possible for case managers in the Philippines to work with migrants in destination countries on specific areas of concern.

Social work practice in support of migrant workers invariably runs into questions of geopolitics. There is the broad question of why labour migration is a necessary choice for many who come from particular racial, ethnic, gender and class backgrounds. Then there are questions relating to the status and treatment of such workers in their host countries. Hong Kong does not set limits on foreign domestic workers' stays in the territory but such workers do not have the right of abode. In March 2013, the Hong Kong Court of Final Appeal ruled that foreign domestic workers were not eligible for permanent residency, essentially excluding them from a rule that allows foreigners to obtain permanent residency in the city after seven years of uninterrupted stay ('Hong Kong court denies domestic workers residency' 2013). Singapore bans foreign domestic workers from marrying Singaporeans (Varia 2007). Such workers are expected to go back to their country of origin after their contract or their employment careers, which may span decades. Such policies discriminate against a particular set of foreign workers, largely identifiable with certain racial and ethnic identities, and constitute them as non-entities with regard to citizenship rights.

To be able to influence policy and legal frameworks as well as combat xenophobia and racism in the destination countries, it is vital for migrant workers to unite and collectively voice their experiences and concerns. NGOs working with migrant workers facilitate this process by providing support services such as education and training to migrant workers' associations and alliances, thereby enabling them to engage duty bearers in the sending and destination countries and among the public at large. Such efforts have allowed migrant workers to organise themselves and forge partnerships within and across nationalities. In Hong Kong, the Asian Migrants Centre facilitated the establishment of the Asian Domestic Workers Union (ADWU) in the 1990s. Over time, other international networks of foreign domestic workers emerged such as the Asian Migrants Coordinating Body, an alliance composed of associations of Sri Lankan, Nepali, Indonesian, Filipino and Thai domestic workers in Hong Kong.

Apart from sectoral organising at the national and international level, it is equally important to form coalitions of migrant workers' organisations, NGOs and individual advocates that can push forth the agenda for the protection of the rights and welfare of migrants. The MFA, for example, serves a vehicle for engagement with intergovernmental bodies at the regional level and with international bodies towards the adoption of agreements, standards and instruments (such as a standard employment contract for foreign domestic workers) that are consistent with human rights standards. The MFA has actively taken part in successful global campaigns including the call for countries to ratify the United Nations Convention on the Protection of the Rights of All Migrant Workers and Members of Their Families, and the adoption and ratification of the International Labor Organization Convention No. 189, Domestic Workers Convention of 2011 which came into force on September 5, 2013. Through the strengthening of people-to-people understanding and transnational cooperation in advocacy and networking, the MFA seeks to achieve its vision of 'an alternative world system based on respect for human rights and dignity, social justice, and gender equity, particularly for migrant workers' (Migrant Forum in Asia 2013b). These initiatives complement broader efforts such as those represented by the work of the International Labour Organization in promoting decent work across borders and a rights-based protection of international labour migrants (International Labour Office 2010; Public Services International 2015). They also resonate with a rights-based approach to practice, as a critical conception of social work would argue.

Social Work Beyond National Borders

Migrant workers are the embodiment of the people we speak of when we define social work as a profession and discipline that promotes social change and development, empowerment and liberation in line with principles of social justice and human rights. Many of them bear the burden of layer upon layer of disadvantage along the lines of race, class, gender and other social lines. Thus, promoting the rights and welfare of migrant workers represents a challenge for social work practice. With the globalisation of labour and employment comes the need for a transnational social work response.

Securing the rights and welfare of migrant workers necessitates a broad approach that addresses conditions in sending and receiving countries. The task requires the fostering of development and decent work in developing countries as well as the promotion of safe, non-exploitative labour policies and work conditions in the countries that host migrant workers (Global Migration Group 2013). A strategic response – the first policy response as far as the International Labour Organization is concerned (Ryder 2014: 6) – is the promotion of decent work opportunities for all across the globe. In countries of origin, there is a need to eliminate the conditions that generate the kind and level of global labour migration that puts socially and economically disadvantaged citizens in precarious overseas employment conditions. In and of itself, this represents a challenge for social work practice that requires a critical understanding of national realities set in the context of global geopolitics and relations. The task of promoting local environments that do not push citizens into international labour migration, even at the risk of their health and safety, requires a critical understanding of the global balance of power and resources such that local efforts that support local employment and workers are accompanied by international efforts to promote fair relations between countries in international politics, finance and trade. In situations where labour migration is necessary and viable, the aim is for fair migration for all (Ryder 2014). This is being done in the Philippines through a multi-level and multi-strategy approach in the governance of labour migration through national policies and the pursuit of bilateral and multilateral agreements (Alcid 2006; Battistella, 2012).

Assistance and protection are needed where we find migrant workers subjected to oppressive and exploitative practices. This will involve identifying exploited migrants, protecting them from further harm – including the non-criminalisation of exploited migrants – and assisting exploited and abused labour migrants in preventing further abuse and exploitation and obtaining justice for the wrongs they have suffered (Global Migration Group 2013). This requires social work practice that transcends national borders. This realisation has tremendous implications on how we conceptualise social work, how we practice social work and, by extension, how we teach social work as well as the scope of social work research. It requires a rethinking of what hitherto were geopolitically bounded conceptions of social work that discursively circumscribed the application of its theoretical and philosophical base to particular national contexts. There is a need to reconceptualise social work as a professional discipline whose legitimacy and sanction are confined within the limits of particular political economies. It provides an argument for the fostering of stronger links between social workers in other countries, towards the promotion of decent work and a decent life for all. It impresses upon us the need to view the conditions of foreign workers in one's own country as an integral concern and to view foreign workers as being no different from our own. It reminds us that our philosophical mandate calls for the protection of the rights and welfare of workers, regardless of where they are and where they are from, which would require a paradigm that transcends the socially constructed geopolitical boundaries that currently inform our thinking and practice. In applying this insight to social work education and research, we are reminded of the need for a strong human rights and social justice orientation. For some, this may go without saying but it is only when we start talking about people from and in other countries that such a claim is truly tested. A strong human rights perspective would argue that all workers deserve to have their rights and welfare protected, wherever they may be. This requires a corresponding conceptualisation of social work that goes beyond the confines of the imaginary lines that have been drawn across the globe. It is hoped that the notes outlined above, relating to a critical conception of social work in the context of a globalised world, contribute towards the construction of social work theory and practice transcending national boundaries that, in the absence of a better term, can be referred to as transnational social work.

References

Alcid, M. L. L. (2006). NGO-labor union collaboration in the promotion of the rights and interests of landbased overseas Filipino workers. *Asia and Pacific Migration Journal*, 15(3), 335–357.

Battistella, G. (2012). Multi-level policy approach in the governance of labour migration: Considerations from the Philippine experience. *Asian Journal of Social Science*, 40, 419–446.

Bose, C. E. (2012). Intersectionality and global gender inequality. *Gender & Society*, 26(1), 67–72.

Camacho, J. V., Jr. (2010). International migration, brain drain and the Philippine economy's rocky road to development. In P. Kee & H. Yoshimatsu (eds), *Global Movements in the Asia Pacific* (pp. 201–224). New Jersey: World Scientific.

Castles, S., & Miller, M. (2009). *The Age of Migration: International Population Movements in the Modern World* (4th edition). Basingstoke: Palgrave Macmillan.

Chang, C.-F., & England, P. (2011). Gender inequality in earnings in industrialized East Asia. *Social Science Research*, 40, 1–14.

Chang, G. (2000). *Disposable Domestics: Immigrant Women Workers in the Global Economy*. Boston: South End Press.

Commission on Filipinos Overseas (2013). *Stock Estimate of Filipinos Overseas as of December* 2013. Mandaluyong: Commission on Filipinos Overseas.

Encinas-Franco, J. (2013). The language of labor export in political discourse: 'Modern-day heroism' and constructions of overseas Filipino workers (OFWs). *Philippine Political Science Journal*, 34(1), 97–112.

Global Migration Group (2013). *Exploitation and Abuse of International Migrants, Particularly Those in an Irregular Situation: A Human Rights Approach*. Vienna: United Nations Office on Drugs and Crime.

Harper, S. E., & Martin, A. M. (2013). Transnational migratory labor and Filipino fathers: How families are affected when men work abroad. *Journal of Family Issues*, 34(2), 272–292.

Hiatt, S. (ed.) (2007). *A Game as Old as Empire*. San Francisco: Berrett-Koehler Publishers.

Hokenstad, M. C., Khinduka, S. K., & Midgley, J. (Eds.). (1992). *Profiles in international social work*. Washington, DC: National Association of Social Workers.

'Hong Kong court denies domestic workers residency' (2013, March 25) [online]. Available at: http://www.bbc.com/news/world-asia-china-21920811 [Accessed dd mmm yyyy]

International Federation of Social Workers (2014, August 6). *Global definition of social work* [online]. Available at: http://ifsw.org/policies/definition-of-social-work/ [Accessed 05 Jun 2015].

International Labour Office (2010). *International Labour Migration: A Rights-Based Approach*. Geneva: International Labour Office.

International Labour Office (2014). *World of Work Report 2014: Developing with Jobs* (2nd ed.). Geneva: International Labour Office.

International Organization for Migration (2009). *Gender and Labour Migration in Asia*. Geneva: International Organization for Migration.

Joyce, J.P. (2010). *Globalization and inequality among nations. In S. Asefa (ed), Globalization and international development: Critical issues for the 21st Century* (pp. 57-72). Kalamazoo, MI: W.E. Upjohn Institute.

Laforteza, E. (2007). White geopolitics of neo-colonial benevolence: The Australia-Philippine 'partnership'. *Australian Critical Race and Whiteness Studies Association*, 3(1), 1–17.

Mahdavi, P. (2011). 'But We Can Always Get More!' Deportability, the State and gendered migration in the United Arab Emirates. *Asian and Pacific Migration Journal*, 20(3–4), 413–431.

Mandap, D. C. (2015, April 17). Number of Filipino domestic workers in HK at all-time high [online]. Available at: http://www.rappler.com/move-ph/balikbayan/90186-filipino-domestic-workers-hk [Accessed 19 January 2017]

McDowell, L. (2009). Old and new European economic migrants: Whiteness and managed migration policies. *Journal of Ethnic and Migration Studies*, 35(1), 19–36. doi:10.1080/13691830802488988.

Midgley, J. (2001). Issues in international social work: Resolving critical debates in the profession. *Journal of Social Work*, 1(1), 21–35.

Migrant Forum in Asia (2013a). Detention of undocumented migrants in Asia. *Policy Brief No. 4*. Quezon City: Migrant Forum in Asia.

Migrant Forum in Asia (2013b). The organization [online]. Available at: http://www.mfa-sia.org/about-mfa/the-organization [Accessed 19 January 2017]

Migrant Forum in Asia (2014) The role of missions in protecting and promoting the rights of migrant workers. *Policy Brief No. 8*. Quezon City: Migrant Forum in Asia.

Mission for Migrant Workers (2013). *What is the mission* [online]. Retrieved from http://www.migrants.net/what-is-the-mission/ [Accessed 19 January 2017]

Mission for Migrant Workers (2015). Casework Report 2014. Hong Kong: Mission for Migrant Workers.

Mullaly, B. (2007). *The New Structural Social Work: Ideology, Theory, Practice* (3rd ed.). South Melbourne: Oxford University Press.

Oikelome, F., & Healy, G. (2013). Gender, migration and place of qualification of doctors in the UK: Perceptions of inequality, morale and career aspiration. *Journal of Ethnic and Migration Studies*, 39(4), 557–577. doi:10.1080/1369183X.2013.745233.

Ortiz, I., & Cummins, M. (2011). *Global Inequality: Beyond the Bottom Billion*. New York: United Nations Children's Fund.

Parutis, V. (2014). 'Economic migrants' or 'middling transnationals'? East European migrants' experiences of work in the UK. *International Migration*, 52(1), 36–55. doi:10.1111/j.1468-2435.2010.00677.x.

Perkins, J. (2004). *Confessions of an Economic Hit Man*. San Francisco: Berrett-Koehler Publishers.

Philippine Statistics Authority (2015, May 27). 2014 Survey on Overseas Filipinos [online]. Available at: https://psa.gov.ph/content/2014-survey-overseas-filipinos%C2%B9 [Accessed 15 Nov 2015].

Public Services International (2015). Working in Finland: Pre-Departure Information for Filipino and Indian Migrant Health Workers Bound for Finland. Ferney-Voltaire Cedex: Public Services International.

Ryder, G. (2014). *Fair Migration: Setting an ILO Agenda*. Geneva: International Labour Migration.

Saperstein, A., & Penner, A. M. (2012). Racial fluidity and inequality in the United States. *American Journal of Sociology*, 118(3), 676–727.

Sijapati, B. (2015). Women's labour migration from Asia and the Pacific: Opportunities and challenges. *Issue in brief*. Geneva: International Organization for Migration.

Sison, J. M., & De Lima, J. (1998). *Philippine Economy and Politics*. Philippines: Aklat ng Bayan Publishing House.

Thornton, S. H. (2008). People Power and neocolonial globalism in the Philippines. *Asia Journal of Global Studies*, 2(2), 20–34.

Tigno, J. V. (2014). At the Mercy of the market?: State-enabled, market-oriented labor migration and women migrants from the Philippines. *Philippine Political Science Journal*, 35(1), 19–36. doi:10.1080/01154451.2014.914999.

van Zanden, J. L., Baten, J., d'Ercole, M. M., Rijpma, A., Smith, C., & Timmer, M. (eds). (2014). *How Was Life? Global Well-Being Since 1820*. Paris: OECD Publishing.

Varia, N. (2007). *Globalization Comes Home: Protecting Migrant Domestic Workers' Rights*. New York: Human Rights Watch.

Vilog, R. B. T., & Ballesteros, M. D. M. (2015). Overseas Filipino workers in conflict zones: Narratives of Filipino nurses in Libya. *Bandung Journal of the Global South*, 1(4), 1–21. doi:10.1186/s40728-015-0018-6.

Wall, L. (2014) Gender equality and violence against women: What's the connection? *Australian Centre for the Study of Sexual Assault Research Summary* (pp. 1–14). Melbourne VIC: Australian Institute of Family Studies.

Wong, S.-L., Moore, M., & Chin, J. K. (2008). Hong Kong: Demographic change and international labor mobility. Paper presented at the PECC-ABAC Conference on Demographic Change and International Labor Mobility in the Asia Pacific Region, Seoul.

World Bank (2015). Personal remittances, received (current US$) [online]. Available at: http://data.worldbank.org/indicator/BX.TRF.PWKR.CD.DT [Accessed 19 January 2017].

Yu, N. (2006). Ideological roots of Philippine social welfare. *International Social Work*, 49(5), 559–570.

13 Migration: National Welfare Institutions

Doulas as Border Workers in Obstetric Care in Sweden

Sabine Gruber

It's a difficult situation: I'm there and I hear what the doctor says. He says, 'Can you explain that we'll do it this way; that it's what's best for her and her baby'. And I tell her and she refuses. And he understood me, but he didn't understand her. And she understood me, but not him, and won't listen to me. […] He looked at her, she looked at me and I looked at her [sighs and laughs].

The opening quotation describes how a culture interpreter doula translates and conveys information between a woman in labour and an obstetrician. A central aspect of her narrative is that the woman and the physician speak different languages, so they have difficulties understanding each other. Her statement also tells us that she is expected to act on behalf of both the patient and the physician, and the final sigh and laughter testify that it can be a really challenging task to navigate between different desires and expectations.

In this chapter, I explore the complexity that is associated with the doula mission. Doulas are cultural interpreters that provide support and information to migrant women during their pregnancy and childbirth.[1] The task of the doulas is to translate and manage language and cultural obstacles between women in labour and the Swedish obstetric care. In this text, I intend to analyze this work in the context of the Swedish welfare state. By drawing on critical border studies research (e.g. Johnson *et al.* 2011; Paasi 2009), I will approach the culture interpreter doula's work as border work between a national welfare institution and migrant women. Thus, rather than scrutinizing the explicit translation work done by the doulas, I intend to explore how an arrangement like the doula-project tends to maintain and reproduce national boundaries even far away from territorial borders. Through analysing interviews that address culture interpreter doulas' work (specifically with regards to how they explain, translate and bridge different languages and cultural backgrounds), I attempt to shed light on how national borders are negotiated, opposed or taken for granted. My overall ambition is to highlight how projects aimed to provide equal welfare to all citizens, regardless of ethnic and linguistic background, simultaneously produce processes of inclusion and exclusion.

This chapter is an empirical contribution that relies on interviews with culture interpreter doulas, midwives, physicians and managers of the relevant doula project as well as communication officers and participant observations at a training session for culture interpreter doulas.[2] The interviews dealt with policy and daily routines at the respective institutions, with a special focus on contexts where ethnicity, cultural background and language were considered important. However, the illustrations I use in this chapter are limited to the doulas' specific duties as described and understood by the informants. Although the study primarily relates to the healthcare sector, it also contributes to the field of social work in a globalizing world. Through its focus on welfare responses to international migration, in the intersection of national welfare institutions, local practices and migrants, the analysis will connect to several key issues in this book concerning contemporary challenges for social work in a globalized world. In the next section, I describe the welfare-state context for the doula project, with emphasis on the migration policy development in Sweden from the 1970s onwards. I will also discuss Sweden's welfare responses to international migration, and how these policies affect migrants' conditions in the Swedish welfare state.

National Welfare Institutions and International Migration

For many decades, the Swedish welfare system has served as a symbol for an inclusive and non-discriminatory social democratic welfare system striving to uphold universal rights for its citizens (Esping-Andersen 1990). In keeping with this, the immigration policy introduced in Sweden during the 1970s aimed to ensure migrants' social citizenship and the same welfare rights as the native population. These policies have been viewed as one of Europe's most progressive and egalitarian approaches to migration (Borevi 2012; Schierup *et al.* 2006). From an international and historical perspective, there is no question that the Swedish welfare system has been highly successful in large part as the result of a wealth redistribution policy that has successfully combated poverty and bridged major income disparities. However, critical researchers have challenged and re-evaluated this uniformly positive view, pointing out that the Swedish welfare system has been much less successful in counteracting racism and ethnic discrimination (e.g. de los Reyes *et al.* 2003; Keskinen *et al.* 2009; Pred 1998; Pringle 2009). Their research has made essential contributions to show how the welfare system's organization, practice, and ideas have produced a host of different categories of women, men and families based on conceptions of ethnicity/race, gender and sexuality. Moreover, these studies reveal that homogenized conceptions about categories such as migrant women, migrant men and migrant families have been fused with specific culturalized problems and needs that have legitimized various welfare institution's discriminatory and racialized initiatives (Carbin 2010; Gruber 2011; Ålund & Schierup 1991). The inherent paradox that has been uncovered within the Swedish welfare system, in which formal rights go hand in hand with ethnic discrimination, characterizes not only the healthcare sector but also practically all welfare areas (e.g. de los Reyes 2006; Groglopo & Ahlberg 2006; Hertzberg 2003; Sawyer & Kamali 2006; Öhlander 2004). This contradiction has been defined as a 'subordinated inclusion' (Mulinari & Neergaard 2004). In other words, migrants' and racialized groups' civil rights have been appended to a hierarchized relationship to the ethnic majority, resulting in these groups being assigned a sub-ordinate position in both the welfare state and labour market (ibid.).

Categorizations such as migrant women, migrant men and migrant families capture a welfare-state nationalism (e.g. Keskinen *et al*. 2009; Mulinari 2010) that has been described as typical of Sweden (and of other Nordic countries). This nationalism is characterized by the welfare system and its institutions' inti-mate interweaving with conceptions of the nation and who belongs within it and who does not (ibid.). In Sweden, welfare state nationalism is in part upheld by a strong notion of gender equality. For example, Sweden is often portrayed as one of the world's most gender-equal countries (de los Reyes *et al*. 2003; Eduards 2007). As a consequence, gender equality emerges as something men and women identified as the nation's majority population obviously comprises, while migrant women, migrant men and migrant families are identified with gender oppression and patriarchal cultures (Carbin 2010; Gruber 2011, 2015). Gender equality is likewise a key feature of the new assimilation-based integration policy that in the 1990s replaced the pluralistic, multicultural ideology of the 1970s. Hence, demands on migrants to adapt to values defined as 'Swedish' or 'western' have increased (Bredström 2008; Brubaker 2001; Hansen & Hager 2012; Schierup & Ålund 2011). In line with this shift, issues related to Swedish gender equality are now addressed in practically every introductory programme and course designed for migrants (Carbin 2010; Larsson 2015).

The Swedish Welfare State's Response to International Migration

Although the former Swedish multicultural policy strived to achieve inclusion, cultural freedom and partnership, the policy has been criticized for culturaliz-ing migrants, an approach that reduces migrants' problems and needs to their cultural background, ethnicity or religion (Ålund & Schierup 1991). In practice, this 'culturalist' understanding generated a new field of knowledge in the 1970s and 1980s. This new field, 'immigrant knowledge' (Sandberg 2010), encouraged social workers, healthcare workers, teachers and other welfare workers to learn about and address cultural differences as well as migrants' needs and problems. For instance, cultural competence has figured as a key concept in social work (e.g. Ahmadi & Lönnback 2005; Aune 1983; Hessle 1984; Soydan 1984). The term 'immigrant knowledge' also clearly illustrates who is designated as being problematic in the meeting between welfare institution and citizen. Thus, cultural competence has been established as both a strategy and a solution in welfare insti-tutions' meetings with migrants in order to make the client understandable to the institution (Eliassi 2015; Gruber 2015; Kamali 2002).

Culture interpreter doulas, bridge-builders, health communication officers and integration pedagogues are examples of occupations that have recently emerged in Swedish welfare institutions (e.g. Abrahamsson & Agevall 2009; Modin 2016). The starting point and common denominator for all these new welfare jobs is a need formulated in terms of cultural and linguistic competence. Irrespective of the welfare area or institution, these professions are mostly paraprofessionals. They are expected to bridge, explain, translate or interpret differences linked to cultural background and language, and so are expected to facilitate meetings and deal with communication problems between various welfare institutions and citizens with migrant backgrounds (ibid.). These kinds of front-line workers are playing increasingly key roles in delivering welfare services to migrants, in Sweden as well as in other Western countries (Bauder & Jayaraman 2014). However, their importance is not reflected in terms of status and career opportunities. Studies suggest, for example, that migrants are locked into these jobs with few chances to advance (Abrahamsson & Agevall 2010; Bauder & Jayaraman 2014, Gruber 2015). Moreover, the employees are often hired on contract positions with low-paid part-time work, organized in projects as sort of short-term solutions to long-term needs (Abrahamsson & Agevall 2010). After ten years of activity, the doula project analysed here is still financed one year at a time, and hence is not a permanent feature of regular obstetric care.

National Borders as Social Practices

Criticism towards ideas that assert notions that globalization creates a borderless world has contributed to the development of a broader theoretical understanding of borders, emphasizing the importance of understanding borders not only as territorial bounded, but also as the sum of a large number of social, cultural and political processes (Johnson *et al.* 2011; Paasi 2009; Parker 2009). Researchers in the field of critical border studies argue that borders are limited neither to the state's sovereignty nor to national geographic demarcations but are phenomena that are also produced and maintained far beyond a nation's static and fixed borders. This concept of borders is understood in terms of social practices infused with power and ordering, whereby demarcations among different groups emerge and are maintained. Consequently, borders are spread all over the society, not merely confined to territorial national borders, security or national flags, but multiplied and reduced in their location and function and thus both thinned out and doubled (Paasi 2009). This approach also enables complex analyses of the links between territoriality, border drawing practices and the roles of borders as barriers and mediators of contacts at the level of local institutions and social practices (Paasi 2009). In line with these thoughts, I conceptualize the meeting between migrant women and the Swedish obstetric care system as a border practice. That is, I conceptualize the doulas' translating, interpreting and bridging as border work. A central concern deals with how the doulas navigate in the border area between national maternity care and obstetric care and migrant women with respect to processes of inclusion and exclusion. Before the analysis, I will briefly describe the doula project.

Striving for Equal Maternity Care for All Women

Historically, maternity healthcare was already a crucial institution of the Swedish welfare system when it was established in the 1940s. In a way, maternity healthcare also stands out in the context of the Swedish official gender equality ideology, as it is by tradition women-centred (Jansson 2008). Both maternity care and obstetric care are financed through taxes. These services are provided free of charge and are primarily organized as part of the public sector. However, under the current restructuring of the welfare state, private maternity care alternatives have become more widely available and this care is provided to pregnant women for a fee. However, generally speaking, maternity care, whether public or private, is organized in line with national recommendations as a basic national programme (Socialstyrelsen 1996). Some regional authorities have also developed special programmes for 'at-risk pregnancies' (SFOG 2008). These programmes target groups of women such as migrant women, young mothers and single mothers from vulnerable groups (Darj & Lindmark 2002; Fabian *et al.* 2004).

The doula project highlighted in this chapter was started by two midwives in a private maternity reception. They were upset by the fact that migrant women, due to language difficulties and discrimination, were not offered the same quality of maternity and obstetric care as native Swedish women. This experience of ine-quality in maternal healthcare and obstetric care has been strongly confirmed by national as well as international research, showing that migrant pregnant women experience more maternal difficulties than native-born women (Esscher 2014; Essén *et al.* 2000; Robertsson *et al.* 2005; see also Katbamna 2000). For example, in Sweden, women from Somalia and Ethiopia run a higher risk of losing their baby during pregnancy or childbirth than native Swedish women. Additionally, Swedish obstetric care often does not use interpreters, a condition that adds to the vulnerability of these women (Bredström & Gruber 2015; Esscher 2014). Thus, with an ambition to offer migrant women more equal maternity and obstetric care, the two midwives applied for and received money from the regional Public Health Committee (Folkhälsokommittén) to start and lead a project organized as a quality improvement project with culture interpreter doulas giving support and information to migrant women during their pregnancy and childbirth. The goal of equality is clearly stated and permeates various texts about the project: 'to develop new methods to strengthen the foreign-born women's health in accord-ance with public health goals', 'to create social conditions for good health on equal terms for the entire population', and 'to provide foreign-born women [with] equal access to safe care, as [for] native Swedish women'.[3] Nevertheless, the ini-tiative for more equitable maternal and obstetric care is taken by a private actor and not by public health. It is also striking that immigrant women's serious com-plications during pregnancy and childbirth are addressed with culture interpreter doulas and not efforts, changes or method development within the institutions and their organization. The doula project is accordingly a collaboration between the Public Health Committee and the region's public maternity and obstetric care providers, although the private maternity clinic is responsible for the project, for organizing the doulas' assignments and for paying their salaries. The doulas are employed by the hour, and the amount of service they can provide is determined by the amount of funding the project receives from the Public Health Committee. Consequently, the availability of culture interpreter doulas is not need-driven but governed by available financial resources. According to the project managers, the title 'culture interpreter doula' reveals an important difference with respect to 'ordinary Swedish doulas'. Doulas categorized as ordinary Swedish doulas are hired to provide (Swedish) women (or couples) with emotional and practical support during delivery. But culture interpreter doulas, in addition to providing emotional and practical support, are also expected to bridge different languages and supposed cultural differences between healthcare providers and migrant women. In other words, they are expected to provide support during delivery to the woman giving birth as well as to the midwife and physician. Moreover, ordinary Swedish doulas are hired by the pregnant woman (or couple), as these doulas are privately organized and work for a fee. Culture interpreter doulas, however, are contracted by the maternity care clinic, are paid by public funds and are free for pregnant women. This doula service is also free of charge for the obstetric clinic, which is of importance at a time when obstetric care in Sweden is heavily understaffed (e.g. Björk 2013). In the analysis that follows, I begin by examining who the doulas are and how their work tasks are described in the interviews.

Migrant Background and Well-Integrated Into Swedish Society

As Diana Mulinari (2010) has pointed out, that there is a clear division of labour between white, native Swedish women and migrant women within the Swedish public sector. Native Swedish women tend to work in professional jobs (such as midwives, nurses, social workers and teachers) whereas migrant women typically work in the lower ranks of the public sector (such as cleaners and assistant nurses) (see also Gruber 2013, 2015). This division is also confirmed in our empirical material; the midwives are native Swedes and the doulas involved in the project have a racialized migrant background. While some of the doulas have lived in Sweden since childhood, the majority of them migrated to Sweden as adults. The project included approximately 20 doulas with different cultural and national backgrounds, and they spoke a wide range of languages (Arabic, Farsi, Serbo-Croatian, Sorani, Turkish, Urdu and Somali). Many of the doulas also worked as interpreters and had been recruited to the project via the interpreting agency. Several of them had academic qualifications and degrees from their home countries but were unable to secure work in Sweden that matched their education. Hence, they had trained to become assistant nurses or childminders to secure employment. Others had run the mill on various courses, projects and trainee employments organized by the Swedish Public Employment Service before they began to work as doulas.

Almost all the doulas had personal experience with Swedish maternity and obstetric care as they themselves had given birth to children in Sweden.[4] This experience was viewed as important by both the doula project's managers and the policymakers we interviewed. These informants emphasized the importance of the doulas being integrated into Swedish society. The managers' statements about being integrated underline that the doulas are expected to be familiar with the societal structure in Sweden as well as with Swedish norms and values with respect to maternity care and obstetric care. A typical manifestation of this view is the fact that the doulas were expected to encourage the father-to-be to attend the delivery. Consequently, the father's presence was made an issue in itself, a point that I will return to later in the chapter.

An element in the training programme for culture interpreter doulas intended to compare obstetric care in Sweden with the obstetric care in the doulas' native countries, highlighting the differences between Sweden and the doulas' native countries. Those who had no personal experience of giving birth in their country of origin were encouraged to interview a relative with such experience so they could educate themselves about childbirth traditions in their 'home country'. This approach of contrasting obstetric practices in different countries is also reflected in the doulas' comments. For example, they often talked about obstetric care in their native country in a problematic way – such as being authoritarian, harsh and painful – whereas Swedish obstetric care is described as developed, modern and emphasising women's participation. The comments below, made by two doulas, show how differences are not only generalized, but also are polarized and localized to different national contexts – 'here in Sweden' and 'there in another country'.

> And at a maternity ward in Iraq there's more than one woman, there are several. That is, two, three, four, like in Gambia, [...] and they [...]. But here, in Sweden, the women can make demands. Here they listen to the woman and aren't as harsh.
>
> Swedish women are goal-oriented; they know everything that's going on around them. But our women [...] in their case it's the doctor who makes all the decisions. There, the woman isn't proactive. Some women don't even know that you need to undergo check-ups when you're pregnant and some don't do so. It's so very different there.

Obstetric care, of course, can differ in many respects. Of interest here is that the differences are framed in terms of national differences and that obstetric care in Sweden is portrayed as being more developed than in the other country, almost without reflection. In the interviews, it was stressed that the doula's assignment was to be active and that they have to communicate with both the birth-giving woman and the maternity ward staff. Furthermore, based on linguistic and cultural competences, the culture interpreter doula's assignment was described as involving a good deal more than the ordinary Swedish doula's assignment, since they were required to provide support both to the woman in labour (and the couple) and to the maternity care and obstetric staff. Accordingly, the cultural interpreter doula is positioned as a representative for a cultural and linguistic community, which limits her assignments to a specific ethnic group. This is also confirmed by the fact that the doulas we talked with were neither members of Sweden's national doula association nor saw any reason to join it.[5]

Communication in Swedish seems to be the norm in maternity and obstetric care, even when the maternity care institution uses an interpreter (Bredström &

Gruber 2015) and this was not problematized at all in any of the interviews we conducted. Managing difficulties or misunderstandings in the communication between the woman giving birth and the midwife or physician due to language barriers is, instead, the specific task of the cultural interpreter doula. As result of their role, the doulas were often referred to as 'the most important person in the room'. In the next section, I will deepen the analysis of the double mission in the doula practice and the tensions this may produce.

'We Always Act as a Provider of Civic Information, Mother and Sister'

> The staff receive help from the doula to make themselves understood to the expectant mother. It may be a matter of performing a C-section, for example, [...] if they say she needs a C-section and she is a Somali woman – Somali women most often don't want a C-section – and she says 'Absolutely no C-section', and flat-out refuses. In this instance, it's the doula who can be the one to properly explain why it is necessary – that it is important for the baby to survive, and so on. And, yes, that's the way it is: the doula is the one who can explain why the hospital staff decide one thing or the other.

The comment above, made by one of the project managers, illustrates the responsibility that doulas may bear and how this responsibility is all about helping both the woman in labour and the obstetric staff. The doulas' accounts of the work they perform are generally similar to this reasoning and provide insight into the border work they perform when they mediate, bridge or balance the communication and information during childbirth. One doula described it in this way:

> Also, I think we understand Swedish well, too. We have a good knowledge of the Swedish language. We don't know everything, of course, but we know enough that it becomes easier to try to use humility and to take the midwife's side. At the same time, we're good at Arabic and know how to angle things so we also appear to be on her [the woman in labour's] side. Like, you can transform the conflict into more, into something funny, and I'm very good at doing that.

This quotation shows how the doula strikes a balance between complying with the midwife's instructions and the woman's needs. But more than that, it emphasizes the doula's central role; she can be the only one who has a grasp of the communication in the delivery room. The twofold assignment and its framing in national terms are further expounded in the following two quotations:

> Yes, it's also the case that our women need guidance because they don't know, they don't have the ability, or rather haven't been taught that they should make their own decisions, that in this room [...] we teach them that this

is your room; you can lie on the floor, you can scream, you can do whatever you want in your own way. You can make a plan; you can be in pain. Simply put, you can express yourself in any way you like.

I tell them [the women] that that's the way we do things. Swedish midwives sew up the wound if they need to make an incision.

The reasoning linked to 'our women', 'we' and 'Swedish midwives' demonstrates how the doula has to make herself a representative of different national 'we's' and how she navigates between them. The first quotation captures how an independent and active approach is connected with a Swedish way of giving birth, whereas a submissive approach is connected with norms and values in the woman's home-land, as in the following quote from one of the doulas:

Instead of them sitting there and waiting for the midwife to do something. They [the women] say 'Thank you, thank you', but it's the midwife's job; they're supposed to help her [...] and some kiss the midwife's hand because she went and fetched an aspirin.

Here, subordinating oneself to the midwife or displaying excessive gratitude is framed as a non-Swedish behaviour. This excessive gratitude is seen as an expression that the woman is stuck in her cultural background and traditions. Thus, the doulas want to support women to set requirements, as women do in Sweden, and to not just be grateful for everything. However, the ambition to introduce the women to 'the Swedish way' is not only an approach to teaching them that women in Sweden can make demands but is also an attempt to emphasize women's rights in the Swedish healthcare system. It conveys a desire to protect the women from being poorly treated by the maternity care and obstetric care staff and thereby to counteract discrimination:

They [midwives and physicians] have more power over our women, especially when they don't understand the language; they [migrant women] might not know the rules. And when it comes to Swedish women, they [midwives and physicians] know that they can be reported [if they don't respect the woman's wishes]. But they [migrant women] don't know that they can report them and they're not going to complain. We help them because they don't know these things.

Experiences where women were treated better by maternity care and obstetric care staff when they were accompanied by a doula are described throughout the interview material. These examples illustrate that the women receive more detailed information from the midwives when a doula is present. The statements also make clear that the doulas act as a kind of representative, not only for the individual woman but for the entire ethnic or linguistic community. That is, when a woman in labour is treated poorly, the doulas perceive this as a disrespect to the entire ethnic and linguistic community, and thus also to her.

According to the interview material, midwives rarely ask about issues linked to cultural aspects or the women's experiences. Instead, it is the doulas who call attention to, discuss and manage cultural aspects and the expectant mothers' experiences (see also Gruber 2015).

'Here in Sweden, the Father Attends the Birth'

The doulas provide support not only during the delivery but also to the expecting woman before the delivery. Migrant women, for example, are not always offered parental training due to their lack of Swedish language skills (Bredström & Gruber 2015; Fabian *et al.* 2004). Instead, the doulas educate them about pain relief, breathing exercises and different birthing positions. At the time of the interviews, each doula had participated and assisted between 20 and 45 women during childbirth. They often talked about how they, by now, were well known by the obstetric staff and that the midwives appreciated the help they provided in the delivery room and exhibited great confidence in the doula's ability.

Doula:	Many people trust us nowadays, so when we're there, the midwife is not there so much. She just says 'Call me if you need anything'. And when she comes, she asks 'How did it go? Everything OK'? And so I tell her 'She's had a little bleeding and has been to the toilet and emptied her bladder'. 'Great', she says and leaves and doesn't intervene so much.
Interviewer:	Does she talk more with you than with the mother?
Doula:	Yes, she talks with the woman. But because often when she comes in, I might already have put the woman to bed, you know; tucked her in nice and warm and she's breathing nice and calmly and it's dark in the room, she doesn't talk so much with her. Then she talks to me, whispering.

The interviews reveal that the midwife communicates with the doula rather than with the woman. This may be due to the existing language difficulties, but as the above dialogue demonstrates, it also seems to be a result of the fact that the midwives seem to hand over some of their work tasks to the doula. The doula's auxiliary function in relation to the obstetric staff is apparent not least of all when arranging the father's presence in the delivery room. As the two quotations below illustrate, it falls to the doula to convince the father to attend and participate in the delivery. That is, the doulas have to convince the father-to-be to undertake the responsibility that is the norm for men in Sweden – to participate in the delivery of their child:

> We understand this Arabic culture. In some cultures, the man is not allowed to be present in the delivery room and perhaps the [Swedish] midwife tells him 'You have to be here'. But perhaps she does so through us, so that we can broach the subject tactfully with the father, try to persuade him in a good way.

You know, in his language. We can explain how important it is to be with the mother, perhaps just to hold her hand because there's a big difference between our culture and Swedish culture. And then we end up in the situation where we try using both Swedish and Arabic cultures.

I have also succeeded in convincing men who would never enter a delivery room to do so even though they know that in our countries, or where they come from, under no circumstances do men enter a room where a woman is giving birth. But I've succeeded in convincing them to come in now and then and to hold her hand and just show her their love and support.

Some doulas told with pride how they had managed to convince 'Arabic men' to attend the birth of their child. Some doulas, however, expressed frustration that some staff were unable to understand how deeply rooted the traditions are that a delivery room is 'a female room' where men should not go. The doula acting as a mediator between the woman (and couple) and the obstetric care staff is prominent in the case with current fathers. That is, at the same time as they act as the Swedish obstetric cares' extended arm by conveying expectations that the fathers should be actively involved in the delivery, they also act in a sensitive way regarding the gender-based traditions that the single woman and man are comfortable with and used to. As the quotations suggest, it is the doula who takes responsibility for this practice, while the midwives are more or less absent during the doula's talk about men's presence and participation in the delivery room.

Front-Line Workers in the National Welfare Institution

They have become much more than just doulas. They also function as resources; they can call the Social Insurance Agency, schools, and preschools. They have become informal disseminators of knowledge. These women are well integrated into Swedish society and they possess this cultural competence, so they are recruited to many different projects. This strong position they hold and this network of contacts they have allows them to spread this information. Attend various events and speak with the women in their own language.

The above quotation is taken from an interview with a communications officer in the relevant county council region and provides a telling picture of how the culture interpreter doulas are viewed as a resource and guide migrant women's communication and contacts with various welfare institutions. Consequently, their assignment is not seen as limited to maternity care and obstetric care; it is much broader. Furthermore, the communications officer's statement suggests a heavy workload for the doulas, duties often undertaken on a voluntary basis. The doulas are expected to be available when various institutions request their assistance or when the women ask for help communicating with different public agencies and welfare services, such as social services, healthcare centres or their children's school. In these situations, the doula's work takes on an almost activist character, ensuring that the women have access to various welfare services. Hence, the access to welfare is ensured by the doulas, not the institutions themselves:

> The woman had not even a single garment for her new-born baby. She could not speak the language, she was there all alone, and she had two kids since before. I started this that we collected clothes, not only for the baby but also for the older children.

However, more than providing material help and support in contact with welfare institutions, the doulas are mobilized as a kind of gate-opener to various ethnic linguistic networks, when welfare institutions initiate actions targeting racialized migrant groups. For example, in one project that was aimed to improve migrant women to do cell samples, the doulas were also asked to serve as informers about the cell samples project.

The doulas are undoubtedly often positioned as a kind of expert in facilitating the meeting between the maternity care and obstetric care and migrant women. But this expert position seems to be a rather weak, informal and uncertain institutional position in the border zone between the national obstetric care and the national 'others'. However, as an agitated head of obstetrics argues in the next quotation, a program such as this doula project may also create conflicts for the institution:

> We have always said no, no, no: parental training [as opposed to education provided by the doulas] is our thing. Parental training should be provided by professionals. Untrained people should not explain to others how childbirth works because they [the doulas] are not midwives. They have no medical training. But the problem is that they don't really understand that. They think, like, but we can do the job a lot better and it's better that they come to us [the doulas] than that they don't come at all. And yes, you could make that case. But at the same time, if you [...] if, so to speak, the doulas were to take over the entire antenatal education bit, and actually get the women to attend, which we don't always manage to do, then you could say that, yes, there is a small benefit. But imagine if they tell them the wrong thing. Is it reasonable to assume that people without training can hold parental trainings that are correct and sensible? Why should we accept lower quality instructors, just because they have another ethnic background? So it turns into a case of warped equality. Suddenly we will accept, like, any old rubbish, just because they have black skin. I have a problem with that. Or rather, we have a problem with that.

With the assistance from doulas, the maternity care midwives reach women who the institutions have obvious difficulties in establishing contact with. This physician's concern is with the quality of the maternity care; she is not convinced that the quality offered to migrant women is of the same quality offered to native Swedes. The physician's reasoning portrays the inherent conflict in the doula project. An initiative like the doula project, which is not integrated with ordinary maternity and obstetric care but is instead organized as an external appendage to these institutions, will remain an exception to the institution's ordinary activities. As a result, the institution will produce both differing standards of care for citizens and unequal terms among different groups of employees within the welfare system.

Responses to International Migration in a National Welfare Context: Concluding Remarks

The culture interpreter doula project, as with similar projects such as bridge builders and integration pedagogues (e.g. Abrahamsson & Agevall 2009; Modin 2016), is considered to be successful in reaching and offering welfare services for migrants. The objective of these types of activities is to enable equal access to various welfare services, which no doubt is a lofty ambition. However, the critical border perspective on the doula project identifies a number of problematic aspects, which ultimately may counteract the project's laudable goals. Seen from this perspective, the analysis reveals that maternity care and obstetric care, concerning the doula project, are constructed as Swedish monolingual institutions. Consequently, the institutions are not expected to change in order to produce a more culturally sensitive and appropriate welfare service or adapt to migrants' needs and circumstances. The solution advocated is rather to employ doulas with various ethnic and linguistic backgrounds who work in the institution's front line, that is, in direct contact with migrant women. This front-line work means not only that the women's needs and problems are largely handled by the doulas but also that these front-line workers operate on the border of the national welfare institution. As is emphasized by the analysis, the doulas are balancing on the border of the national welfare institution, acting as a kind of border worker. They negotiate, challenge and counteract various norms, values and traditions, sometimes from a position as an insider in the Swedish institution and other times from a position as an outsider. So even if the doula's efforts are talked about as extremely important for women giving birth and obstetric care staff, they move between an insider and outsider position in relation to the maternity care and obstetric care. However, organisationally, the doula practice remains an activity located outside these institutions, in a sort of border zone between the institutions and the women. As such, more than bridging borders, the doula project also seems to maintain borders, which ultimately perpetuates a boundary between the nation's citizens and the nation's other.

Notes

1 I have translated the Swedish concept *kulturtolks doula* as 'culture interpreter doula'. The term 'doula' is derived from an ancient Greek word that, roughly translated, means a woman who gives care. In the modern age, a doula is a woman with experience of childbearing who is trained to provide ongoing support and information to a pregnant woman and her partner before, during and after childbirth (Lundgren 2010). A doula is not required to have medical training, however. They are paraprofessionals, trained individuals who are not professionals.

2 The empirical material is part of a research project I conducted together with my colleague Anna Bredström entitled 'Ethnicity and gender in primary healthcare: Understanding, practice and consequences' (2008–0513), funded by the Swedish Research Council for Health, Working Life and Welfare (FORTE). The empirical material was collected at maternity healthcare institutions, healthcare centres and youth clinics.

3 To ensure the anonymity of the informants, I give no references to the texts where these quotations are taken from.

4 Several of the doulas also had experience of giving birth in their country of origin and some of them had given birth in a number of countries, depending on where they had resided during their adult life.

5 In Sweden, the national association for doulas is called Organisation för Doulor & Förlossningspedagoger i Sverige (ODIS). The association provides information about and contact with doulas and also organizes doula training.

References

Abrahamsson, A & Agevall, L 2010 'Immigrants caught in the crossfire of projectification of the Swedish public sector: Short-term solutions to long-term problems', *Diversity in Health and Care*, vol. 7, no. 3, pp. 201–209.

Ahmadi, N & Lönnback, EB (eds) 2005 *Tvärkulturellt socialt arbete. Av socialarbetare för socialarbetare, Forsknings och utvecklingsenheten*, Stockholm: Stockholm stad.

Ålund, A & Schierup, CU 1991 *Paradoxes of Multiculturalism: Essays on Swedish Society*, Aldershot: Avebury.

Aune, A 1983 *Invandrarkunskap i högskolan. Sammanfattning av en diskussionerna vid SIV:s högskolekonferens 1979–1982*, Norrköping: Statens Invandrarverk.

Bauder, H & Jayaraman, S 2014 'Immigrant workers in the immigrant service sector: Segmentation and career mobility in Canada and Germany', *Transnational Social Review*, vol. 4, no. 2–12, pp. 176–192.

Björk, N 2013 'Det finns ingen plats för födelse', *Dagens Nyheter*, 12 September.

Borevi, K 2012 'Sweden: The flagship of multiculturalism' in *Immigration, Policy and the Scandinavian Welfare State 1945–2010*, eds G Brochman & A Hagelund, Hampshire: Palgrave Macmillan, pp. 25–96.

Bredström, A 2008 *Safe Sex, Unsafe Identities: Intersections of "Race", Gender and Sexuality in Swedish HIV/AIDS Policy*. PhD thesis, Linköping University.

Bredström, A & Gruber, S 2015 'Language, culture and maternity care: "Troubling" interpretation in an institutional context', *Nordic Journal of Migration Research*, vol. 5, no. 2, pp. 58–66.

Brubaker, R 2001 'The return of assimilation? Changing perspectives on immigration, and its sequels in France, Germany, and the United States', *Ethnic and Racial Studies*, vol. 24, no. 4, pp. 531–548.

Carbin, M 2010 *Mellan tystnad och tal. Flickor och hedersvåld i svensk offentlig politik*, Stockholm Studies in Politics. PhD thesis, Stockholm University.

Darj, E & Lindmark, G 2002 'Mödrahälsovården utnyttjas inte av alla', *Läkartidningen*, vol. 99, no. 1–2, pp. 41–44.

de los Reyes, P (ed) 2006 *Om välfärdens gränser och det villkorade medborgarskapet*, SOU 2006:37. Stockholm.

de los Reyes, P Molina, I & Mulinari, D (eds) 2003 *Maktens (o)lika förklädnader: Kön, klass & etnicitet i det postkoloniala Sverige: En festskrift till Wuokko Knocke*, Atlas: Stockholm.

Eduards, M 2007 *Kroppspolitik: Om moder Svea och andra kvinnor*, Atlas: Stockholm.

Eliassi, B 2015 'Constructing cultural otherness within the Swedish welfare state: The case of social workers in Sweden', *Qualitative Social Work*, vol. 14, no. 4, pp. 554–571.

Esping-Andersen, G 1990 *The Three Worlds of Welfare Capitalism*, Polity Press: Cambridge.

Esscher, A 2014 *Maternal Mortality in Sweden: Classification, Country of Birth, and Quality of Care*, PhD thesis, Uppsala University.

Essén, B Hansson, BS Östergren, PO Lindqvist, PG & Gudmundsson, S 2000 'Increased perinatal mortality among sub-Saharan immigrants in a city-population in Sweden', *Acta Obstretica of Gynecologica Scandinavia*, vol. 79, no. 9, pp. 737–743.

Fabian, HM Rådestad, IJ & Waldenström, U 2004 'Characteristics of Swedish women who do not attend childbirth and parenthood education classes during pregnancy', *Midwifery*, vol. 20, no. 3, pp. 126–135.

Groglopo, A & Ahlberg, BM (eds) 2006 *Hälsa, vård och strukturell diskriminering*, SOU 2006:76. Stockholm.

Gruber, S 2011 'In the name of action against "honour-related" violence: National notions, gender, and boundaries in the Swedish school's ambitions to combat violence and oppression', *Nordic Journal of Migration Research*, vol. 1, no. 3, pp. 126–136.

Gruber, S 2015 'Cultural competence in institutional care for youths: experts with ambivalent positions', *Nordic Social Welfare Research*. Available from: http://www.tandfonline.com/action/showAxaArticles?journalCode=rnsw20. [Accessed 9 November 2015].

Hansen, P & Hager, SB 2012 *The Politics of European Citizenship: Deepening Contradictions in Social Rights and Migrations Policy*, Oxford: Berghahn.

Hertzberg, F 2003 *Gräsrotsbyråkrati och normative svenskhet: Hur arbetsförmedlare förstår en etniskt segregerad arbetsmarknad*, Arbetslivsinstitutet: Stockholm.

Hessle, S 1984 'Omhändertagande av invandrarbarn' in *Socialt arbete och invandrare*, ed H Soydan Liber: Malmö, pp. 64–80.

Jansson, K 2008 *Maktfyllda möten i medicinska rum. Debatt, kunskap och praktiki svens förlossningsvård 1960–1985*, PhD thesis Södertörn University, Sekel Bokförlag: Lund.

Johnson, C Jones, R Paasi, A Amoore, L Mountz, A Salter, M & Rumford, C 2011 'Interventions on rethinking "the border" in border studies', *Political Geography*, vol. 30, no. 2, pp. 61–69.

Kamali, M 2002 *Kulturkompetens i socialt arbete. Om socialarbetarens och klientens kulturella bakgrund*, Carlssons: Stockholm.

Katbamna, S 2000 *'Race' and Childbirth*, Open University Press: Buckingham.

Keskinen, S Tuori, S Irni, S & Mulinari, D (eds) 2009 *Complying with Colonialism. Gender, Race and Ethnicity in the Nordic Region*, Ashgate: Farnham.

Larsson, JK 2015 *Integrationen och arbetets marknad. Hur jämställdhet, arbete och annat 'svenskt' görs av arbetsförmedlare och privata aktörer*, PhD thesis, Atlas Akademi: Stockholm.

Lundgren, I 2010 'Swedish women's experiences of doula support during childbirth', *Midwifery*, vol. 26, no. 2, pp. 173–180.

Modin, M 2016 'Integrationspedagog – skapandet av en efterfrågad utbildning', *Socialmedicinsk tidskrift*, 2016, no. 1, pp. 76–81.

Mulinari, D 2010 'Postcolonial encounters: Migrant women and Swedish midwives' in *Changing Relations of Welfare. Family, Gender and Migration in Britain and Scandinavia*, eds J Fink & Å Lundkvist, Ashgate: Farnham, pp. 155–177.

Mulinari, D & Neergaard, A 2004 *Den nya svenska arbetarklassen: Rasifierade arbetares kamp inom facket*, Boréa: Umeå.

Öhlander, M 2004 'Problematic patienthood. "Immigrants" in Swedish health care', *Ethnologia Scandinavica*, vol. 34, pp. 89–107.

Parker, N & Vaughan-Williams, N 2009 'Postscript: Ongoing research. Lines in the Sand? Towards an agenda for critical border studies', *Geopolitics*, vol. 14, no. 3, pp. 582–587.

Paasi, A 2009 'Bounded spaces in a "borderless world": Border studies, power and the anatomy of territory', *Journal of Power*, vol. 2, no. 2, pp. 213–234.

Pred, A 1998 *Even in Sweden: Racisms, Racialized Spaces and the Popular Geographical Imagination*, University of California Press: Berkeley, Los Angeles.

Pringle, K 2009 'Swedish welfare responses to ethnicity: The case of children and their families', *European Journal of Social Work*, vol. 13, no. 1, pp. 19–34.

Robertsson, E Malmström, M & Johansson, SE 2005 'Do foreign-born women in Sweden have an increased risk of non-normal childbirth?', *Acta Obstretica et Gynecologica Scandinavia*, vol. 84, no. 9, pp. 825–932.

Sandberg, G 2010 *Etnicitet, ungdom och socialt arbete – En analys av kulturbegreppet i et komplext och kluvet forskningsfält*, Linné University: Växjö.

Sawyer, L & Kamali, M (eds) 2006 *Utbildningens dilemma. Demokratiska ideal och andrafierande praxis*, SOU 2006:40: Stockholm.

Schierup, CU & Ålund, A 2011 'From paradoxes of multiculturalism to paradoxes of liberalism. Sweden and the European neo-liberal hegemony', *The Journal for Critical Education Policy Studies*, vol. 9, no. 2, pp. 125–142.

Schierup, CU Hansen, P & Castles, S 2006 *Migration, Citizenship and the European Welfare State. A European Dilemma*, Oxford University Press: Oxford.

SFOG [Swedish Society of Obstetrics and Gynecologi] 2008 *Mödrahälsovård, Sexuell och Reproduktiv Hälsa*, (ARG) Rapportserie nr.59, Stockholm.

Socialstyrelsen [Swedish National Board of Health and Welfare] 1996 *Hälsovård före, under och efter graviditet*, SoS-rapport 1996:7 Socialstyrelsen: Stockholm.

Soydan, H (ed) 1984 *Socialt Arbete och Invandrare*, Malmö: Liber.

14 Undoing Privilege in Social Work

Implications for Critical Practices in the Local and Global Context

Bob Pease

Introduction

Social work has been significantly constrained by the restrictions of national social policy contexts. It is the premise of the chapter that social work cannot be studied without taking into consideration the global forces shaping the profession and the problems that social workers address. This means that a critical approach to social work must interrogate the global production of inequalities, as the problems social workers engage with are not solvable within national borders. Wimmer and Schiller (2002) use the language of "methodological nationalism" to designate the practice of framing inequalities within the context of the nation-state. That is, it is assumed that nation-states provide the conceptual basis for studying both local and international problems. Within this view, all social phenomena are conceptualized within the boundaries of the nation-state. Just as this has been a limitation of the social sciences more broadly, it is also the case that much discussion of social work has been conducted within methodological nationalism, although it is not named as such.

When we move beyond methodological nationalism, how do we designate an approach to social work? The terms international, global, and transnational have all been proposed and all have different meanings. I prefer the term transnational because it seems to me to be more critically reflective of the positioning of Western social work within the international context. By transnational, I mean an approach to social work that transcends national borders (Wallimann 2014) and addresses cross-national relations. I argue that critical transnational social work must develop a set of principles to guide progressive theory and practice in the global context. In this chapter, I outline six key principles to inform critical practice at the local and transnational levels.

Acknowledge Structural Inequalities Between Countries

The Global Agenda for Social Work and Social Development (2012) espouses the global definition of social work developed by the International Federation of Social Workers (IFSW). While social workers proclaim international ideals and inter-country cooperation through their involvement in international professional associations such as the IFSW and the International Association of Schools of Social (IASSW), as well as at international conferences, they often fail to acknowledge the impact of global neoliberal ideas on their international collaborations and inequalities at the national and local levels (Midgley 2015).

The premise underpinning the development of global standards for social work is that there is a universal conception of social work that applies to all countries. However, to what extent do global standards reproduce Western dominance and a Western discourse of social work? Jönsson (2014) makes the point that the privileges associated with the West are understood as resulting from the internal political and cultural developments within the West itself rather than as a consequence of global imperialism. This framing of Western privilege has influenced social work theories and practices which often do not acknowledge the global forces shaping social inequalities and the profession.

Too much of international social work focuses on the cultural and technological differences between countries at the expense of understanding structural inequalities in wealth and power (Briskman et al. 2013). It is not possible to have a mutual exchange between countries if we do not acknowledge and address the structural inequalities in power between nations and consequently between different geopolitical forms of social work (Haug 2015). Just as it is important to understand social work transnationally, it is also crucial to locate social work within geopolitical spaces where the profession in specific contexts is shaped by power relations within geographically defined spaces. Social work has been slow to adopt sociospatial approaches to the social work. In particular, I argue that critical geography (Bauder and Engel-Di Mauro 2008) has considerable usefulness for critical social work practice at the local and transnational levels.

It is thus important to remember that international dialogues between countries are not only cross-cultural encounters but also dialogues across unequal relations of power and privilege. The construction of cultural competence for work with others across cultures, for example, can lead those in the West to ignore their own geopolitical and cultural positioning (Nadan 2014).

Challenge West-Centrism in the Social Sciences

There is a longstanding critique of Western social work educators being employed as consultants to assist in the development of social work curricula in the global South (Moosa-Mitha 2014). Such consultants not only often ignore the power differences between countries, but are also often not cognizant of their own Western privilege in international exchanges. Since Midgley's (1981) important critique of professional imperialism in the 1980s, social workers are now more aware of the problems associated with the transfer of Western knowledge to social work in the global South. Notwithstanding the growing perception among social workers around the world about the dangers of professional imperialism (Gray and Fook 2007), however, the universal applicability of social work values of justice, empowerment, and human rights, etc., continue to be fostered globally.

Haug (2015), in a major review of social work texts, found numerous examples of epistemological and cultural imperialism embedded in the documents promoting international social work. She notes, for example, the use of Western scientific knowledge in the International Code of Ethics for global social work and also that it was predominantly European men who were most involved in the framing of the global social work documents. Thus it is white Western knowledge systems that have informed the definition of international social work, which is framed as part of the discourse of international development, without any consideration of the critique of development discourses (Haug 2015).

There is a deeply internalized belief among many social work educators in the West that Western knowledge and theories are superior and such beliefs support the legitimacy of exporting Western theories to the non-West (Razack 2009). It is a fundamental requirement for Western social workers who are interested in fostering transnational social work to interrogate their own Western privilege to resist the reproduction of Western professional imperialism in social work. As Western knowledge is not objective or universal but rather shaped by a particular geopolitical space, international dialogues initiated from the West to the non-West need to approach cross-cultural exchanges with humility (Akena 2012). Midgley (2007) uses the language of cosmopolitanism as a framework for understanding social work outside of the nation-state. Such a perspective encourages cooperation and exchanges between nation-states to promote social justice and human wellbeing and invites interrogation of nationalist prejudices within the West. Cosmopolitanism is contrasted with unipolarism, which claims that imperialism has brought significant benefits to the non-West. The belief that Western models of social work have universal applicability rests upon an implicit assumption that these models are superior to any approaches that are developed in the non-West.

The adoption of Western models of social work in the non-West is, in part, a product of the globalization of social work knowledge (Jönsson 2014). To undo privilege in global social work, we must move beyond West-centrism. Social work must come to terms with its historical legacy of colonialism and acknowledge the dominance of Western epistemologies in social work knowledge, research, and practice. Given the longstanding nature of these critiques of professional imperialism in social work, it is odd that there are few links made in contemporary discussions about global and international social work to the literature on colonialism and imperialism (Schiller 2006). One strategy is to explicitly name social work in the West as Western social work to more clearly mark its geopolitical location. If we are to challenge West-centrism in social work, we will need to undermine its claim to universal relevance and understand it as a partial rather than universal foundation for the profession.

What complicates the intensification of West-centric knowledge is that it not only comes from within the West but is also fostered by leaders in the global South who believe that the goals of development and modernity in the West are what is needed in the global South (Jönsson 2014). Sewpaul (2010) also notes, for example, that countries in the South are complicit in emulating Western social work. She argues that there is a paradox here in that, while they critique the dominance of Western social work discourses, some of them also embrace theories, models, and concepts that come from the West. Thus, we witness a valorization of Western knowledge in some countries of the global South (Sewpaul 2014).

There is also a danger in contrasting Western social work with non-Western or indigenous social work in that it can suggest that both Western social work and non-Western social work are monolithic frames (Sewpaul 2007). There are many diverse forms of social work within the West. This is increasingly recognized within the non-West, as Yan and Tsui (2015) noted in their study of social work literature in the United States. They found that Western social work knowledge was quite diverse and that many Western social work concepts were contested within those national borders. They recognized that this has implications for social work theory and practice in China. If there are many different ways of constructing social work knowledge, even in the West, what Western ideas are most useful for Chinese social work? (Pease 2015).

Yan and Tsang (2008) suggest that when Chinese social workers look to Western social work knowledge, they tend to draw more upon the scientific and evidence-based practice approaches and underemphasize Western values such as human rights and social justice which inform the more progressive view of social work in the West. They are thus more likely to draw upon the more politically conservative forms of helping as opposed to critical theory-influenced political practices. Hutchings and Taylor (2007) note that clinical Western social work models such as solution-focused therapy and cognitive behavior modification are popular in social work education in Hong Kong. They suggest that these Western models may sit comfortably with the Chinese government, as they do not promote radical change. It must seem odd to Chinese social workers to read about the socialist commitments espoused by radical social workers in the West as the basis for radical and critical practice, when the espoused socialist claims of the Chinese government inhibit advocacy on behalf of oppressed clients. In this context, it is easy to see why conservative Western social work ideas which focus on evidence-based practice and counseling modes of intervention are more likely to be promoted in China (Tsang and Yan 2001).

As demonstrated earlier, there is no one expression of Western social work, as the ideological and political debates between more radical and critical forms of social work and the mainstream models and frameworks attest. It is thus important to challenge the view that Western social work is homogenous, to strengthen the anti-colonialist approaches that are developing from within the West, and to explore the implications for critical social work in the non-West.

Validate the Importance of Local and Indigenous Knowledge

Webb (2003) argues that the very notion of global social work is problematical because it implies that there is only one form of social work at the global level. Such a framing ignores the multiplicity of knowledges and practices within social work and it fails to account for the local cultural orders within which the varied forms of social work are embedded. While social work is clearly shaped by global and transnational forces and its practices transcend national borders, it is also constructed at the local level. The concept of local knowledge is based on the idea that theories of practice are best generated within the material context in which they are practiced. It is thus important to maintain links between the local and the global and to see internationalization and indigenization as not mutually exclusive but complementary (Gray and Coates 2007).

The development of local and indigenous knowledges have been one form of resistance to the hegemony of Western social work. One of the premises of professional imperialism was the view that many non-Western countries were not capable of developing their own social work knowledge and frameworks for practice (Gray 2005). While there have been very important developments in indigenous knowledge construction in social work in Australia (Bennett et al. 2013; Fejo-King 2013; Muller 2014), it is still the case that, here as elsewhere, indigenous knowledge is marginalized in the training of social workers (Tamburro 2013). At the same time, we have to be careful in promoting local indigenous traditions that we do not end up unwittingly supporting local oppressive regimes (Ioakimidis 2013). Some forms of indigenization reproduce the status quo (Young and Zubrzycki 2011) because they do not challenge the structural inequalities in the local context. Authoritarian regimes may well use local knowledge and charges of Western imperialism as defenses against examining their human rights responsibilities and to argue against social workers having legitimate roles to advocate for social change and social justice (Sewpaul 2007). Clearly, some nation-states will place greater restrictions on the potential for social workers to engage in advocacy and social action roles in relation to social justice. Thus, resistance and critical practice at the local level and within national borders are also important (Sewpaul 2005).

Be Aware of the Potential for Cooptation of International Social Work

There is a commitment by the IFSW through its global agenda to promote economic and social equality. However, while social workers are encouraged to challenge poverty and social injustice, the premises of the global agenda seem to support the current political and economic arrangements and the dominant ideologies that reproduce those arrangements (Briskman et al. 2013). Such unacknowledged contradictions contribute to the cooptation of social workers into neoliberal ways of working.

While Sewpaul was initially a reluctant architect of the global standards, she later came to argue that such standards could promote social justice if they were developed with appropriate cultural sensitivity (2005). However, in 2010, she began to question whether the global standards might be reinforcing the legitimation of Western social work (Sewpaul 2010). More recently (Sewpaul 2014), she has been more overtly critical of the whole universalizing project. Sewpaul (2014) charges the IASSW and the IFSW global standards document as reflecting new managerialist and neoliberal ideologies with their emphasis on performance appraisals, standard setting, and endorsement of notions of development and progress. While Sewpaul (2014) talks about the tension within the global standards document between the espousal of social justice and equality and the accommodation to the global patterns which produce injustice and inequality, it is more useful to see this in terms of contradictions arising from the social forces shaping the IASSW and the IFSW. The IASSW, and social work educators more generally, are part of the ideological apparatus of the state, to use Marxist language. It is understandable that they would, in part, endeavor to legitimate dominant discourses of Western social work.

Sewpaul (2014) argues that social work educators are not just victims of the economic system. They perpetuate and are complicit in the reproduction of Western hegemony and other forms of privilege. She challenges the IASSW and the IFSW to critically reflect upon the role they play in reproducing professional imperialism and neoliberalism. It remains to be seen whether they have the critical capacity to interrogate their own assumptions and world views to become aware of and challenge their complicity in the reproduction of neoliberal hegemony. Gray and Webb (2015) also charge the writers of the Global Agenda with not naming the underlying causes of the social inequalities that the document purports to be addressing. For them, it is essential to name neoliberal capitalism as the fundamental frame for understanding the social forces shaping structural inequalities around the globe. Otherwise, there is no clear strategy for challenging those inequalities. Are international social work associations prepared to openly name neoliberalism and state capitalism as the causes of inequality? Gray and Webb seem doubtful about the likelihood of this prospect. But, putting aside whether they have the moral courage to do so, they will first need to theoretically understand the global social forces shaping the world around us.

Moosa-Mitha (2014) observes that the notion of international social work is always conceived of being out "there" in the world outside of the West as opposed to being "here" *in* the West. Webb (2003) argues that the notion of international social work is a form of "ethical welfare imperialism," because in his view, there is no evidence of a convergence of culturally different forms of social work into a standardized one-size-fits-all model. If we do not critically interrogate the power of social work within the West, we are likely to reproduce power differences between countries. Privilege operates not just *within* national borders but also internationally through membership of dominant Western nations. How does social work avoid the critique of global interventions reinforcing Western theories and practices when the very concept of social work is a Western invention derived from European values of objectivism, rationalism, and humanism (Young and Zubrzycki 2011)?

Acknowledge the Complicity of State Social Work

Western social workers need to acknowledge their historical role in supporting imperialism in various contexts. This means locating social work within an understanding of postcolonial theory. Social workers cannot claim innocence in terms of their profession's association with colonization (Razack 2009). If social workers do not own their complicity with dominant ideologies and practices of imperialism, they are doomed to continue to reproduce it in their current practice. Hence, there is no politically neutral discourse of social work. The IFSW does not interrogate its own positioning within the broader context of Western hegemony and imperialism. It implicitly presents itself as an ahistorical and apolitical player who is simply fostering cross-cultural conversations premised upon a presumed equality of power. If we cannot acknowledge our complicity with the perpetuation of injustice and colonialism, how can we proclaim a space to speak in support of global justice (Haug 2015)?

Ioakimidis (2011) documents a number of historical cases where social workers proclaimed support for social justice and equality while at the same time aligning themselves with authoritarian regimes. He observes that it is at those times when social work proclaims a politically neutral role that it is most vulnerable to being complicit in oppressive practices. Systemic efforts of local and international patrons to transplant Anglo-American knowledge have been historically combined with eradicating existing grassroots welfare networks. International pioneers who preached social development contributed to the creation of a social work project that served as a tool for political oppression and imperialist politics. Ioakimidis (2013) refers to social work's historical complicity with oppressive regimes as the "dark side" of social work. He notes social work's collaboration with Nazi Germany, social work's support of apartheid in South Africa, and social work's support for the authoritarian regime in Greece as examples. In the Australian context, social workers were actively involved in "the Stolen Generation," where Aboriginal children were removed from their families as part of a policy towards assimilation (Young and Zubrzycki 2011). Ioakimidis (2013) suggests that social work's reluctance to acknowledge its "dark" past is a form of social amnesia. If we do not recognize our contradictory location within the state, we are likely to be unable to resist becoming part of neoliberalism. The key argument here is that if we do not interrogate our historical legacies with oppressive regimes, we cannot position ourselves as a social justice-based profession. Individual social work practitioners need to heed the question posed so many years ago by a critical sociologist: "Whose side are you on?" (Becker 1973).

Locate Ourselves and Situate Western Social Work in Context

The argument of this chapter is that to advance a progressive transnational social work we need to understand our own location in relation to global issues. This means that social workers in the West need to understand the impact of neoliberalism on social work and social work education. Numerous studies reveal the pervasive impact of neoliberalism on social workers' thinking and practices (Lorenz 2005; Baines 2006; Wallace and Pease 2011; Fenton 2014; Gray et al. 2015). Critical whiteness studies hold some promise for revealing social work's lack of interrogation of its own assumptions (Tascon and Ife 2008; Young and Zubrzcki 2011; Jeyasingham 2012; Zufferey 2012) because it puts the focus on the normative practices of Western white social workers rather than concentrating on racial others. Das and Anaud (2012) point out that the concept of cultural competence, in terms of knowing the "cultural other," is premised on Eurocentric ways of knowing and being that ignore understandings of colonialism and imperialism.

Young and Zubrycki (2011) have emphasized the importance of a "whiteness lens" to acknowledge both social work's historical involvement in reproducing disadvantage in indigenous communities and its ongoing role in colonial practices. They undertook a critical analysis of key social work texts to interrogate the positioning of culture and race in them. They found a lack of recognition of white privilege and what this means for the development of social work knowledge. When race and culture are mentioned, it is almost always on non-white racial identities. The racial background of white social workers is not named but rather assumed in these texts and thus reproduces the norms of the dominant culture. Taking a critical whiteness perspective provides a lens to explore their own positioning in relations of privilege and power. Nadan (2014) suggests that encouraging social work educators and practitioners to reflect upon their own whiteness and the privileges associated with it will turn the gaze back onto "us" in the West. This is critical if we are going to acknowledge white privilege and the unconscious racism that supports it. This reflexivity goes beyond critical reflection which does not explicitly interrogate privileged positioning (Pease 2006). Critical reflection does not name class, race, sexuality, gender, able-bodiedness, and geopolitical location as central categories of privilege and oppression (Pease 2010). Consequently, they are often neglected when critical reflection is used, where it is more on the exclusions and problems faced by the client than on the privileged positioning of the social worker (Mattsson 2013).

Aguila-Idanez and Buraschi (2014) use the language of "ethnocentric culturalism" as a way of naming the implicit logic underpinning Western social work models. They advocate intercultural awareness raising to expose the implicit assumptions underpinning Western social workers' blindness to their own privilege and power. It is the lack of understanding of the cultural horizon of those of us in the West that limits our capacity to understand the experiences of those in the non-West. It is because these prejudiced assumptions are often unconscious that they have some power in shaping the views of social workers in the West. Zufferey (2012) notes the usefulness of the epistemologies of ignorance literature (Sullivan and Tuana 2007) for identifying the various ways in which ignorance about privilege is reproduced. She offers a timely reminder that we cannot stand outside of the dominant discourses that construct us and that we all need the humility to acknowledge what we do not know about our own privilege and power in the West. Zufferey (2012) expresses it in terms of "not knowing that I do not know and not wanting to know." Social workers often do not know about how their unearned privilege and power arises from their membership of a privileged group. This lack of knowledge means that social workers all too often do not understand social work's historical role in professional imperialism. Social work is located in white-dominated institutions and racially unequal power relations that shape the theory and practice of the profession in fundamentally racialized ways.

Conclusion

If promoters of international social work from the West fail to acknowledge the structural inequalities between nations and their respective privileged positioning within those inequalities, they are unlikely to appreciate the local realities and local knowledge of those they are engaged with. Acknowledging and challenging the impact of dominant forces on our experiences and ideas is the first step in undoing privilege and oppression,

Good intentions are not enough to exclude social workers from the perpetuation of forms of injustice. Social workers who are committed to critical and emancipatory social work need to be open to the myriad of ways in which they may be part of the problem, even as they espouse a social justice and human rights approach to practice. They need to understand the social and political processes that produce various forms of social inequality. If they do not understand how the structures of privilege and oppression are reproduced, they will not know how best to challenge them (Blum 2008).

Social workers in the West cannot simply transcend the structures of privilege in which they are embedded. Their responsibility lies in continually interrogating the systems that privilege them. No one is innocent when it comes to complicity. We need to develop a critical awareness of how we are implicated in the perpetuation of inequality through our practices in social work.

References

Aguila-Idanez, M. and Buraschi, D. (2014) 'Educating Social Workers Without Boundaries through the Intercultural Social Intervention Model.' In *Global Social Work: Crossing Borders, Blurring Boundaries*, edited by C. Noble, H. Strauss and B. Littlechild. Sydney: Sydney University Press.

Akena, F. (2012) 'Critical Analysis of the Production of Western Knowledge and its Implications for Indigenous Knowledge and Decoloniszation.' *Journal of Black Studies*, 43 (6): 599–619.

Baines, D. (2006) 'Social Work and Neoliberalism: "If You Could Change One Thing": Social Service Workers and Restructuring.' *Social Work* 59 (1): 20–34.

Becker, H. (1973) *Outsiders: Studies in the Sociology of Deviance*, New York, Free Press.

Bennett, B., Green, S., Gilbert, S. and Besarab, D. eds. (2013) *Our Voices: Australian and Torres Strait Islander Social Work*, Melbourne: Palgrave Macmillan.

Bauder, H. and Engel-Di Mauro, S. eds. (2008) *Critical Geographies*, Kelowna, British Columbia: Praxis Press.

Blum, L. (2008) 'White Privilege: A Mild Critique.' *Theory and Research in Education*, 6 (3): 309–21.

Briskman, L., Martin, J., Kuek, S. and Jarema, A. (2013) 'Without Borders: Fostering Development Studies in Social Work.' *Policy and Practice: A Development Education Review*, 17 Autumn: 70–89.

Das, C. and Anand, J. (2012) 'Strategies for Critical Reflection in International Contexts for Social Work Students.' *International Social Work*, 57 (2): 109–120.

Fenton, J. (2014) 'Can Social Work Education Meet the Neoliberal Challenge Head On?' *Critical and Radical Social Work*, 2 (3): 321–35.

Fejo-King, C. (2013) *Let's Talk Kinship: Innovating Australian Social Work Education, Theory, Research and Practice Through Aboriginal Knowledge. Insights From Social Work Research Conducted with the Larrakia and Warumungu Peoples of the Northern Territory*, Canberra: New Millennium Printers.

Gray, M. (2005) 'Dilemmas of International Social Work: Paradoxical Processes in Indigenization, Universalism and Imperialism.' *International Social Welfare*, 14: 231–238.

Gray, M. and Fook, J. (2007) 'The Quest for a Universal Social Work: Some Issues and Implications.' *Social Work Education: The International Journal*, 23 (5): 625–644.

Gray, M. and J. Coates (2008) 'From "Indigenization" to Cultural Relevance.' In *Indigenous Social Work Around the World: Towards Culturally Relevant Education and Practice*, edited by M. Gray, J. Coates and M. Yellow Bird. Aldershot: Ashgate.

Gray, M. and Webb, S. (2015) 'No Issue, No Politics: Towards a New Left in Social Work Education.' In *Global Social Work: Crossing Borders, Blurring Boundaries*, edited by C. Noble, H. Strauss and B. Littlechild. Sydney: Sydney University Press.

Gray, M., Dean, M., Agliias, K., Howard, A. and Schubert, L. (2015) 'Perspectives on Neoliberalism for Human Service Professionals.' *Social Service Review*, 89 (2): 368–392.

Haug, E. (2015) 'Critical Reflections on the Emerging Discourse of International Social Work.' *International Social Work*, 48 (2): 126–135.

Hutchings, A. and Taylor, I. (2007) 'Defining the Profession? Exploring an International Definition of Social Work in the China Context.' *International Journal of Social Welfare*, 16: 382–390.

International Federation of Social Workers, International Association of Schools of Social Work and International Council of Social Welfare (2012) *The Global Agenda for Social Work and Social Development Commitment to Action* [online]. Available at www.iassw-aiets.org.

Ioakimidis, V. (2013) 'Beyond the Dichotomies of Cultural and Political Relativism: Arguing the Case for a Social Justice Based "Global Social Work" Definition.' *Critical and Radical Social Work*, 1 (2): 183–99.

Iokimidis, V. (2011) 'Expanding Imperialism, Exporting Expertise: International Social Work and the Greek Project 1946–74.' *International Social Work*, 54 (4): 505–519.

Jeyasingham, D. (2012) 'White Noise: A Critical Evaluation of Social Work's Engagement with Whiteness Studies.' *British Journal of Social Work*, 42: 669–686.

Jönsson, J. (2014) *Localised Globalities and Social Work: Contemporary Challenges*. Doctoral Thesis in Social Work, Faculty of Human Sciences, Mid Sweden University.

Lorenz, W. (2005) 'Social Work and the New Order: Challenging Neoliberalism's Erosion of Solidarity.' *Social Work and Society*, 3 (1): 93–101.

Mattsson, T. (2013) 'Intersectionality as a Useful Tool: Anti-oppressive Social Work and Critical Reflection.' *Affilia: Journal of Women and Social Work*, 29 (1): 8–17.

Midgley, J. (1981) *Professional Imperialism: Social Work in the Third World*. London: Heinemann

Midgley, J. (2007) 'Perspectives on Globalization, Social Justice and Welfare.' *Journal of Sociology and Welfare*, XXXIV(2): 17-36.

Midgley, J. (2015) 'Global Inequality, Power and the Unipolar World: Implications for Social Work.' *International Social Work*, 50 (5): 613–626.

Moosa-Mitha, M. (2014) 'Using Citizenship Theory to Challenge Nationalist Assumptions in the Construction of International Social Work Education.' *International Social Work*, 57 (3): 210–208.

Muller, L. (2014) *A Theory for Australian Indigenous Health and Human Service Work: Connecting Indigenous Knowledge with Practice*. Sydney: Allen & Unwin.

Nadan, Y. (2014) 'Rethinking "Cultural Competence" in International Social Work.' *International Social Work*, DOI:10.1177/0020872814539986: 1–10.

Pease, B. (2006) 'Encouraging Critical Reflections on Privilege in Social Work and the Human Services.' *Practice Reflexions*, 1 (1): 15–26.

Pease, B. (2010) *Undoing Privilege: Unearned Advantage in a Divided World*. London: Zed.

Pease, B. (2015) 'Undoing Privilege in Western Social Work: Implications for Critically-Reflective Practice in China.' *China Journal of Social Work*, 8 (2): 93–106.

Razack, N. (2009) 'Decolonizing the Pedagogy and Practice of International Social Work.' *International Social Work*, 52 (1): 9–21.

Schiller, N. (2006) 'Transnational Social Fields and Imperialism: Bringing a Theory of Power to Transnational studies.' *Anthropological Theory*, 5 (4): 439–461.

Sewpaul, V. (2005) 'Global Standards: Promise and Pitfalls for Re-inscribing Social Work into Civil Society.' *International Journal of Social Welfare*, 14: 210–217.

Sewpaul, V. (2007) 'Challenging the East-West Value Dichotomies and Essentialising Discourse on Culture and Social Work.' *International Journal of Social Welfare*, 16: 398–407.

Sewpaul, V. (2010) 'Professionalism, Postmodern Ethics and the Global Standards for Social Work Education and Training.' *Social Work Maatskaplike Werk*, 46 (3): 253–262.

Sewpaul, V. (2014) 'Social Work Education: Current Trends and Future Directions.' In *Global Social Work: Crossing Borders, Blurring Boundaries*, edited by C. Noble, H. Strauss and B. Littlechild. Sydney: Sydney University Press.

Sullivan, S. and Tuana, N. eds. (2007) *Race and Epistemologies of Ignorance*. Albany: State University of New York Press.

Tascon, S. and Ife, J. (2008) 'Human Rights and Critical Whiteness: Whose Humanity?' *The International Journal of Human Rights*, 12 (3): 307–327.

Tamburro, A. (2013) 'Including Decolonization in Social Work Education and Practice.' *Journal of Indigenous Social Development*, 2 (1): 1–16.

Tsang, A. and Yan, M. (2001) 'Chinese Corpus, Western Application: The Chinese Strategy of Engagement with Western Social Work Discourse.', *International Social Work*, 44(4): 433-454.

Wallimann, S. (2014) 'Transnational Social Work: A New Paradigm with Perspectives.' In *Global Social Work: Crossing Borders, Blurring Boundaries*, edited by C. Noble, H. Strauss and B. Littlechild. Sydney: Sydney University Press.

Wallace, J. and Pease, B. (2011) 'Neoliberalism and Australian Social Work: Accommodation or Resistance?' *Journal of Social Work*, 11 (2): 132–142.

Webb, S. (2003) 'Local Orders and Global Chaos in Social Work.' *European Journal of Social Work*, 6 (2): 191–204.

Wimmer, A. and Schiller, N. (2002) 'Methodological Nationalism and Beyond: Nation-State Building, Migration and the Social Sciences.' *Global Networks*, 2 (4): 301–334.

Yan, M. and Tsang, A. (2008) 'Revisioning Indigenization: When *Bentuhuade* and *Bentude* Social Work Intersect in China.' In *Indigenous Social Work Around the World: Towards Culturally Relevant Education and Practice*, edited by M. Gray, J. Coates and M. Yellow Bird. Farnham, Surrey: Ashgate.

Yan, M. and Tsui, M. (2015) 'The Quest for Western Social Work Knowledge.' *International Social Work*, 50 (5): 641–653.

Young. S. and Zubrzycki, J. (2011) 'Educating Australian Social Workers in the Post-Apology Era: The Potential Offered by a "Whiteness" Lens.' *Journal of Social Work*, 11 (2): 159–173.

Zufferey, C. (2012) '"Not Knowing That I Do Not Know and Not Wanting to Know": Reflections of a White Australian Social Worker.' *International Social Work*, 56 (5): 659–673.

15 Glocality and Social Work

Methodological Responsiveness to Moments of Rupture

Lia Bryant and Mona Livholts

This international edited collection actualises emergent critical questions about how social work knowledge, education and practice may develop and extend the rapidly emerging field of glocality and social work. The scholarship that informs the text is drawn from countries such as Australia, Finland, Japan, South Africa, The Philippines, Sweden and the United Kingdom from the discipline of social work. The text also includes the disciplines that inform and extend contemporary social work like art, gender studies, social and cultural geography and sociology. Throughout the text, interstices between local and globalising process are analysed in a range of contextual circumstances. Authors challenge the idea of globalising forces as monodirectional or as a view from 'above' which determine local conditions and contexts and equally challenges the local context as one that simply resists or speaks back to the global. Indeed, glocalisation in this text refers to overlaps between the local and global (e.g. Chapters 3, 4 and 8) and multidirectional multiscalar interstices (e.g. Chapters 2, 10 and 11). Each of these understandings brings to social work an in-depth consideration of spatial analyses that move between and within bodies, communities, nation-states and global institutions, processes and phenomena. Whilst there are patterns and trends showing commonality in social issues, knowledges, practices and imaginings connected to globalising processes, these are dispersed unevenly. Globalising processes are taken up in a multitude of ways across terrains of the body, communities and nations.

Understandings of the glocal as relational and immersed in political economy are evident across a number of chapters. For some of the authors in this volume, glocal conditions can give rise to grass-roots initiatives which respond to political economies and create new emancipatory spaces. Alfreds and Åberg's chapter (Chapter 10) is an example of an emancipatory space whereby art is a practice of social sculpture transforming individuals and communities. For Turunen (Chapter 11), the glocal occurs through four mutually constitutive and relational concepts or a TPSN framework, that is, place, scale, networks and polymorphic understandings of territories or bordering within a political economy. Turunen's analyses show how, over time, glocal influences shape approaches to community work. She illustrates how approaches to community development have moved from and between grass-roots to state-led initiatives and in contemporary times to models of 'innovative' entrepreneurial approaches. Turunen uses an understanding of political economy of the glocal as an axis in which to locate neoliberal policy that draws on 'developing' the individual to 'reform' communities of people. Bryant and Garnham (Chapter 2) further analyse the moralising dimensions which work within political economies – and therefore glocality – in relation to farmer distress and suicide. They argue that farmers are enmeshed within the multiple spatialities of the glocal, which include the body and subjectivity, transnational corporations, international markets, national policies and local community politics. They show how moral and political economies based on neoliberal discourses of economic success and failure locate farmers as entrepreneurs, and that this framing emotionally implicates the subject in analogous feelings of failure/shame and success/pride. Bryant and Garnham show how spatial scales and bodily encounters are mediated by glocal contexts and conditions with actions, reactions and emotions enabling moments of spatial encounters. Such encounters are imbued with power relations, which shape encounters between bodies and places. Similarly, Chapters 3 and 12 draw on glocal political economies to understand movements of migration and, in particular, exploitation and othering. In both chapters (also see Chapter 14), the glocal works within western-centric ways of being and knowing. For Yu and Alcid (Chapter 12), the glocal is framed within political economic objectives which fail to protect the rights and welfare of migrant workers – these workers become expendable to the needs of capital. For Masocha (Chapter 4), the glocal emerges as a space inherently tied to nationalism and endemic inequalities between the global north and south.

Collectively, the chapters point to the fluidity of the glocal and to spatialities in flux, which change across time. The fluidity of the glocal is particularly evident in Gordon's work (Chapter 9) on migratory experiences. She examines how movement across spaces during the life course shape, shift and reformulate identities, thereby illustrating how identities and ways of being become multiple. For Gordon, spatialities merge and become somewhat amorphous in relation to ways of being through migratory experiences where 'people oscillate and interplay between multiple spaces, crossing a myriad of frontiers, compatible with a contemporary world of constant change' (p. 144). Gordon is pointing toward a glocality that is enmeshed with self and evolves over time where spatial relations to self move beyond 'the confines of fixed racial classification and ordering; to identify diversity and difference without the need to cement it in a place' (p. 145). Livholts (Chapter 6) and Gottzen (Chapter 7) bring attention to fluidity and glocality in the ways local spaces and intimate spaces hold affective atmospheres that change across time as bodies encounter these spaces. These chapters show the *becoming* of space, that is, how space comes into being in relation to the interstices of time and space (Massey 1991, 2005).

Similarly, Anbäcken (Chapter 8) conceptualises the glocal as spatiality closely connected to time and place, arguing that natural disasters occur more readily with global climatic variability. Disasters shape the material, emotional and social ways of life for present and future generations with both landscapes and families altering and needing to be rebuilt. For Tuscon (Chapter 5), the glocal also comes into being through socio-natural disasters whereby the construction, reception and rejection of the humanitarian gaze come into play through how we come to know about troubles 'elsewhere'.

Glocality and Social Work Praxis: Facilitating Emancipatory Spaces

Understandings of glocality employed in this text problematise social spaces and, importantly, also create new spaces for social work education, research and practice. Pease's chapter (Chapter 14) scrutinises the epistemological foundations of social work and its implications for emancipatory practice. Specifically, he attends to the global standards for social work (ethics and principles). He questions whether it is possible to have global standards when there is an assumptive global premise about what social work is, emanating from western-centric theories and practices. Pease argues that the concept of global social work is problematic as it assumes a monolithic discipline and profession. In these ways, he problematises the global and its relation to localities. For social work to facilitate emancipatory spaces, Pease calls for social workers from the west to 'transcend the structures of privilege in which they are embedded… [to] continually interrogat[e] systems that privilege them' (p. 224).

The chapters by Gordon (Chapter 9) and Livholts (Chapter 6) are examples of interrogations of the politics of location whereby social workers challenge what they have learned to see. These chapters develop new approaches to enable the process of seeing differently. Gordon (Chapter 9) asks readers of her text to interrogate how we can avoid reproducing unequal global relationships through disseminated visual images. She creates new possibilities for seeing and subverting the humanitarian gaze by examining the underlying power relations encoded in images. The intertextual reading of subjects, space and culture is, for Gordon, an emancipatory space as it opens up new possibilities of engagement. She offers a series of critical questions for analysis about intended audiences, relationships between viewers and subjects and how subjects in films are constituted. Livholts (Chapter 6) similarly engages the reader in questions of the silences of privilege and, in particular, discursive silences. In Chapter 6, Livholts uses 'site writing' (Rendell 2010) as an example of writing that situates the writer. She creates spaces for possible emancipatory practice through a relational, dialogical and situated engagement with social issues, ideas, experiences and texts. Specifically, Chapter 6 illustrates how, through situated writing, subjective locations are open to exploration and insights enabling recognition of the self and others. Situated writing as writing practice, as a multiscalar social work approach, becomes an iterative bridge between thinking and doing that may lead to new knowledges, understandings and interactions which may slowly dissolve processes of 'othering'.

Iterative reflexive ways of working are central to participatory community-based approaches which, through its processes, can enable unexpected outcomes and potentially emancipatory outcomes for individuals and communities. Turunen

(Chapter 11), for example, invites us to critique community work and question whether current approaches focused on social entrepreneurship and social innovation are emancipatory. She argues that social innovation and entrepreneurial approaches are often framed in terms of government and business, especially as 'quick fix solutions to social problems, more focused on economic and technological factors than on social problem solving as a complex human activity' (p. 176). She does not reject a focus on social innovation but draws our attention to its inherent individualistic assumptions, that is, changing people and not necessarily policies and structures. Turunen draws us towards what she refers to as the 'shadows', where more radical approaches are emerging in the way social services are constituted and delivered through and with communities.

Chapter 10 reflects the work of ArtAgent and its partners in a variety of community settings. The naming of a project they worked on as 'The Dream Garden' (p. 161) captures the essence of multiple possibilities for change. Alfreds and Aberg show how the spaces of elderly care become transformed using participatory approaches that create new spaces in institutional settings. Institutional settings are a material example of the glocal–global patterning of buildings, internal colours, furniture and subsequent atmospheres which are located in, tempered and given meaning in the local. The interdisciplinary union of social work and art provides specific tools to participatory research and practice. These tools combine social work values and therapeutic facilitation alongside the arts, which enables a tapping into the body beyond the thinking self and, particularly, allows a connection to the senses. As Pink (2005, p. 9) quoting Bendix (2000, p. 41) argues, 'sensory perception and reception' requires methods that are capable of grasping 'the most profound type of knowledge [which] is not spoken of at all...'. There is extensive scholarship which explores the therapeutic benefits of the arts to social work research and practice (e.g. Bryant 2015; Hesse-Biber 2007; Huss and Cwikel 2005), and Chapter 10 brings these into our realms of knowing.

The sensory and affective aspects of the body is a recurring theme which cuts across the three parts of this edited volume. This theme draws together two inter-related spheres of enquiry. The first is the question of how new and in-between spaces emerge theoretically, methodologically and materially to shape and reshape the glocal in ways that encourage new audiences, increase participation and enable movement between academia and other sectors. The second is an exploration of how bodies move, feel, react and act in and between spaces. An understanding of how glocalisation is experienced from the lived body allows theoretical development and practice responses to the glocal that are informed by people's daily lives, emotions and practices. The following sections examine each theme and how they are explicated in the text.

In-Between Spaces: Glocality and Methodological Re-Shaping

In the introductory chapter, we (Livholts & Bryant) emphasised that social work 'as a discipline extends globalisation theories by centralizing the social'

(p. 4). Chapters in this volume show how such focus, seen through theoretical and methodological lenses of glocality, creates new and in-between spaces for writers and readers to take on challenges in research and in education, practice and activism. Of relevance for social work is that the complexity of challenges that emerge for people and communities as glocalised social issues and problems demand increased collaboration between researchers from different disciplinary fields, academia and communities, NGOs and civil society (Appadurai 2013; Hesse-Biber & Leavy 2008). Further, theories and methodologies that support anti-discriminatory and social justice perspectives are central to epistemological re-shaping beyond methodological nationalism. Leavy (2015) suggests that to be able to ask new research questions and communicate research with broader audiences, it is necessary to challenge what we see and think. By emphasising the word *shaping* when 'building research projects and representing research' (p. 2), Leavy makes links between research question, form, content and audiences (see also Gunaratnam 2007; Livholts 2012). In this book, the creating of new knowledge that develops a knowledge base for glocalised social work is intimately intertwined with thinking and shaping knowledge in new ways. Glocalisation is a conceptualisation that has been used in areas such as business, technology, sociology and education (e.g. Patel & Lynch 2013; Robertson 2013). As we have pointed out in the introduction, we regard glocalisation as an emergent theoretical framework for social work that, alongside established concepts such as global and transnational, 'enrich complex understandings of interconnections, power asymmetries and interspatial social issues' (p. 6). We consider 'glocality' to be a useful term in the final chapter to illustrate the contribution of this book. Steger (2010, p. 2) describes how the term glocality expresses 'a possible future condition that, like all social conditions, will ultimately give way to new constellations'. By identifying, conceptualising and creatively paving the way for new and in-between spaces for methodological reshaping, we see this book as a contribution to extending the social reach of glocality and social work.

Language, a term with multiple discursive, embodied and material contextualised meanings in social research, is developed as a methodological tool for re-shaping knowledge through translations and situated writing in this volume. In Chapter 6, a critical analysis of translation as language practice and the contribution of situated writing and story-telling is in focus, illustrating the complexity of power relations and possible transformation that support social justice. Inspired by Spivak's (1993) 'The politics of translation', Livholts (Chapter 6) makes use of the in-between space occurring through shifts between English and Swedish. She raises issues linked with awareness of discomfort, blocks and doubts that appears in the spaces of writing and reading. This is part of a glocalised methodology where 'translation is an active practice which places languages (words, gestures, expressions) in situations where meaning is created in complex relations of power between dominant groups, across national borders and local sites geographically' (p. 98). Gordon (Chapter 9) introduces the reader to the migratory experience and beyond and provides glimpse into the multiplicity of ways in which migratory lives are shaped through negotiation, transition and transcendence. The negotiating and re-shaping of life experience that Gordon shares with the reader by *fictionalising* stories opens up an in-between space for writers' and readers' giving them permission to fictionalise and thereby better understand the social. In Gordon's chapter, the reader is invited to visit places like the hair salon/barbershop to critically engage in re-thinking what is possible through dialogue, creative life writing and by telling an alternative story, known and unknown to the writer and the reader. Gordon's chapter is an example of how it is possible to make use of in-between spaces through the interconnectivity between (migrant) communities and research and activism that potentially brings forth the link between social work, social transformation, empowerment and social change. The active agency for social work in contemporary and future situations of disasters, particularly to tackle loss and to rebuild communities, is the focus of Anbäcken's chapter (Chapter 8). The methodological re-shaping in this chapter is autoethnography (see also Witkin 2014). It involves the situated researcher that is relationally part of the history and geopolitics of Japan, who visits and re-visits, witnesses, re-witnesses and listens to stories from a volunteer in social work. These in-between spaces of story-telling are linguistically shifting, between English and Japanese as a way of strengthening the voice of the (Japanese speaking) story-teller.

The emergence of glocality and social work also creates new and in-between spaces for 'border workers' (Chapter 13) and 'third figures' (Chapter 5). In Gruber's chapter (Chapter 13), critical border studies are used to analyse and discuss the culture interpreter doula's work as border work in the space between national welfare institutions and migrant women in a Swedish context. This kind of 'border work', which has emerged recently, is organised along unequal structures in regard to working and employment conditions and Gruber states that 'more than bridging borders, the doula project also maintain borders, which ultimately perpetuates a boundary between the nation's citizens and the nation's other' (p. 212). This chapter provides insights into how relations of power are central to language and understanding, listening, interpretation and power within and beyond territorial boundaries. In Chapter 5, Tuscon introduces readers to a 'new landscape of 'the social' (p. 71) by analysing human rights films in the intersection of social work, glocalisation theory and film studies. Images increasingly shape the social worlds in which we live, and Tuscon challenges the idea of representation as abstract discourse by stating that 'in films subjects are people, after all, and not mere objects for our needs' (p. 82). This chapter discusses 'distant viewers' and 'assumed spectators' that are often western and powerful and challenges the future of this power relation. Tuscon asks her readers to think about the 'third figure' in human rights films, often an activist characterised by complexity and agency and with a mission for social change that can be used by scholars, social workers and activists at a local level to undo unequal power relations.

Several chapters draw attention to the possibilities of analysing and acting on in-between spaces through re-conceptualisation. Gottzén (Chapter 7) makes use of atmosphere as a methodological tool to understand domestic violence and thus creates a new in-between space for acknowledging ways in which 'cities, houses, cafés and women's shelters – and the ways in which atmospheres, in a figurative sense, can refer to the tones and moods that surround such places' (p. 106). Another example is how Alfreds and Åberg, in their chapter (Chapter 10), make use of Beuys' (Beuys & Harlan 2004) social sculpture 'as an art form grounded in the social' to include 'human activity that strives to transform society' (p. 158). The new methodological space for social work is where speech, conversation, thinking and creativity become a collective process where the social is re-shaped and re-considered as social practice through the inclusion of new analytical conceptualisations. Appadurai (2013, p. 275) argues that 'the very idea of research has not been sufficiently been reflected on'. By creating new understandings of the social in social work through glocality, chapter contributions encourage re-readings and increased participation in a historical and geopolitical project that enables movement between academia and other sectors.

Reading is intimately related to the form and design of the written, and the visual in images and through words is interpreted differently by readers. As Stanley (1995) describes in her ground-breaking work on biography and auto/biography, the first encounter with a book is visual. She draws attention to the delicate task of evaluating readers as a group and how symptomatically marginalised groups are often treated as a collective of homogenised responses to readings. Also, she discusses the effect of the text as an image and ways in which it may evoke memories, thoughts, ideas and resistance. Thus, writing and reading are embodied activities that take place in between material, 'real' and imaginative spaces, and this volume invites readers to create new ways of seeing and thinking through lenses of glocality.

Emotions and Bodies in Place and Space

Probyn's (2005, p. 234) 'tripartite interrogation of the physiological-psychological-sociological' feeling body provides an integrated and complex understanding of emotions. This account removes the body and emotions from a purely discursive social construction expanding the parameters of enquiry to our embodied physiological, neurological and cognitive selves marked by social discourses and practices. Specifically, as argued by Bryant and Jaworski (2015, p. 13–14), 'Probyn is alerting us to the complexity of emotions, the existence of innate emotions, at times understood and at others incapable of acknowledgement by the human subject'. In Chapters 6–10, acknowledged and unacknowledged emotions emerge in relation to in-between and third spaces but also occur in relation to reflexive writing techniques. For example, Gordon's chapter is a good example of spaces that enable unacknowledged emotions and new narratives to emerge. Indeed, Gordon's chapter is about writing bodies where, as Holmes (2010) suggests, emotions underpin the reflexive process of thinking and writing. For Holmes (2010), it is the real and imagined dialogue with our feelings and the feelings of others that can in the present change the way of viewing the past. In this collection, we explored affective bodies suffering from violence to selves or others (Chapters 2,

4 and 7), bodies spatially enmeshed in violence and, in particular, bodies not recognised by nation-states (Chapters 3, 12 and 13). Chapter 2 focused on how farmer distress is lived as the visceral entwined with physical pain, bodies releasing tears and feelings of anger and shame, enmeshed in discursive constructions of a lack of self-worth. Indeed, Bryant and Garnham show how personal narratives of lack of self-worth in relation to farm viability and 'worthiness' to live are deeply reflective of both neo-liberal articulations of success and gendered norms around farming and 'appropriate' expressions of masculinities. Chapter 2 is an empirical example of Ahmed's (2004) understandings of emotions as discursively and, therefore, politically inscribed. Similarly, bodies inscribed by regimes of power as lacking in worth (as opposed to self-worth) are particularly evident in Chapters 4 and 12.

Masocha (Chapter 4) shows how *detaining* and/or prohibiting the entry of the bodies of asylum seekers in Australian and the United Kingdom is entrenched in ideological and political motivations to 'marginalise, constrict and exclude asylum seekers in both countries' (p. 60). Exclusion and detention become possible as national discourses create a series of emotions about who is entitled to belong to a nation and through constituting asylum seekers as a threat to culture, employment and safety (see Ahmed 2004). As Ahmed suggests, discourses of citizenship and protection of ways of life bring forth emotion, binding one group against the 'other'. Emotions are made and recreated to work in the context of bestowing a lack of worth on asylum seekers. The political production of emotions works to 'shape the "surfaces" of individual and collective bodies' (Ahmed 2004, p. 1). Masocha's chapter illustrates how framing the bodies of asylum seekers as a threat, as receptacles that induce emotions like fear, legitimates policies and practices of exclusion, detention and expulsion.

Chapter 4 focuses on a range of issues associated with gendered global violence and attention to masculine and raced bodies. The authors draw attention to scholarship based on southern sexual violence, calling to question ways in which African men have been problematised. Negative constructions of poor, black migrant men have rendered these men as dangerous. The authors argue that 'the emphasis on researching poor, migrant and black communities within and across national boundaries may service to fuel an othering of some sexualities' (p. 50). Hence, black men's bodies (violent or not) become othered and glocal subjects of fear.

Chapter 12, like Chapter 4, also provides an analysis of bodies deemed less worthy and subject to oppression as a consequence of racism. Yu and Alcid illustrate how working bodies are marked through nomenclature that privileges the west. Western bodies who migrate are often referred to as expats while non-western bodies are often called migrants, labour migrants or economic migrants. Further, the type of labour taken up by women from the Philippines in western countries for western employers is often gendered, with women taking on domestic work and other labouring or unskilled work. As Yu and Alcid show, it is the bodies of these women that are at risk of death, injury, trafficking and forced labour – these bodies become stripped of human rights. Reading in between the lines of Yu and Alcid's chapter are two narratives of emotion. The first narrative of emotion that emerges for the reader is the horror of the injustices that overseas Filipino workers experience, and the second is the emotional indifference of nation-states and capital which renders these women's bodies as tools for labour, sex and injury.

The question of bodies in trauma and emotions is evident in Chapter 8. Anbacken examines emotions associated with grief and loss as people experience the loss of homes and community and the deaths of family, friends, neighbours and community members as a consequence of a tsunami. Anabacken describes loss as embodied in sudden disasters – that is, being confronted with dead or missing bodies and feeling loss as visceral and psychologically traumatic. The author illustrates that language used in the media to describe the trauma is likened to the body, for example, an open wound, and for some, suicide is the way to end bodily suffering. Anabacken's chapter challenges social workers to consider loss and grief that incorporates the body but also material and social losses in giving care to those experiencing grief.

Collectively, the chapters draw attention to glocal social work shaped by body politics and embodied emotions that are physiological-psychological and sociological. These chapters remind us that social work at the scale of the glocal is felt at the scale of the body, and that the body is enmeshed within multidirectional global/local processes. The chapters referred to in this section provide a frame of reference for analysing research and practice to examine multiple, shifting and emerging understandings of oppression, marginalisation and hope and social justice across and within geopolitical spaces.

Concluding Remarks

This book has brought new methodological foci to understanding glocal social issues and problems using creative methodologies and theoretical understandings of spatiality to problematise social spaces where social work has had a long presence in fields like gendered violence. The collection has also brought focus to populations, for example, farmers, overseas Filipino workers, and doulas as border workers, and social issues, such as migration and natural disasters where social work as a discipline has remained largely absent. The chapters, like rooms in a house, show shifting, fluid, embodied and affective political geospatial relations. Creative approaches in social work may be likened to how air 'enters through cracked windows like some barely audible promise, and souls of banished words... [become] resurrected in...' (Grushin 2016, p. 31). In-between or third spaces, like rooms, make possible creative endeavours that are emancipatory. In this way, through writing or depicting one's dreams in photography, people come to know a little more of their fragmented and situated selves and ways to heal, develop or expand their opportunities.

Head (2016, p. 77) argues that 'moments of rupture or contexts of change and uncertainty are the conditions that can create the spaces for such possibilities to emerge' and ruptures can be thought of as 'generative moments'. If the large social questions embedded in globalising conditions, that is, disparity in wealth and respect between the global north and south, climate change, conflict and war, human impact on the health of the planet and the stripping of human rights of some, particularly asylum seekers, are ruptures, how can social workers use these ruptures to create generative moments? How can social work facilitate, advocate and contribute to glocal social change? The multiscale dimensions of social issues and therefore change require new ways of working but also require us to continually question western-centric privileging in social work. It is timely for social work to rethink its engagement in the glocal spheres working across spatialities that are multidirectional and intersecting.

References

Ahmed, S 2004, *The Cultural Politics of Emotion*, Edinburgh University Press, Edinburgh.

Appadurai, A 2013, *The Future as Cultural Fact. Essays on the Global Condition*. Verso, London and New York.

Bendix, R 2000, The Pleasures of the Ear: Towards an Ethnography of Listening, *Cultural Analysis*, vol. 1, pp. 35–52.

Beuys, J H & Harlan V 2004, *What is Art? Conversation with Joseph Beuys*. Clairview Books, West Sussex.

Bryant, L 2015, Introduction: Taking up the Call for Critical and Creative Research Methods in Social Work, in Bryant, L 2015 (ed.) *Critical and Creative Research Methodologies in Social Work*, Ashgate, Surrey, pp. 1–26.

Bryant, L & Jaworski, K 2015, Introduction: Daring to Walk on the Grass, in Bryant, L and Jaworski, K (eds) 2015 *Women Supervising and Writing Doctoral Theses, Walking on the Grass*, Lexington Books, Maryland.

Grushin, O 2016, *Forty Rooms*, G.P. Putnam's Sons, New York.

Gunaratnam, Y 2007, Where is the Love, *Journal of Social Work Practice*, vol. 21, no. 3, pp. 271–287.

Head, L 2016, *Hope and Grief in the Antrhopocene*, Routledge, Abingdon, Oxon.

Hesse-Biber, SN 2007, Feminist Research: Exploring the Interconnections of Epistemology, Methodology, and Method, in Hesse-Biber, SN (ed.) 2007, *Handbook of Feminist Research: Theory and Praxis*, Sage, Thousand Oaks, pp. 1–28.

Hesse-Biber, SN, & Leavy, P (eds) 2008, *Handbook of Emergent Methods*, Guilford Press New York.

Holmes, M 2010, The Emotionalization of Reflexivity, *Sociology*, vol. 44, no. 1, pp. 139–154.

Huss, E & Cwikel, J 2000, Researching Creations: Applying Arts-Based Research to Bedouin Women's Drawings, *International Journal of Qualitative Methods*, vol. 4, no. 4, pp. 44–62.

Leavy, P 2015, *Method Meets Art. Arts-Based Research Practice*, The Guilford Press, New York.

Livholts, M 2012, Introduction: Contemporary Untimely Post/Academic Writings – Transforming the Shape of Knowledge in Feminist Studies in Livholts, M (ed.) *Emergent Writing Methodologies in Feminist Studies*, Routledge, New York, pp. 1–25.

Patel, F & Lynch, H 2013, 'Glocalization as an alternative to internationalization in higher education: Embedding positive glocal learning perspectives', *International Journal of Teaching and Learning in Higher Education*, vol. 25, no. 2, pp. 223-230.

Pink, S 2005, *Sensory Ethnography*, Sage. London.

Probyn, E 2005, *Blush: Faces of Shame*, University of Minneapolis Press, Minneapolis.

Rendell, J 2010, *Site Writing the Architecture of Art Criticism*, Tauris and Company, London.

Robertson, R 2013, 'Situating Glocalisation: A relatively autobiographical intervention', in Drori, GS, Hollerer, MA and Walchenback, P (eds) *Global Themes and Local Variations in Organization and Management*, Routledge, New York, pp 25-36.

Steger, MB 2010, *'Globalization': The Encyclopedia of Political Thought*, 1st edn, John Wiley & Sons Ltd.

Stanley, L 1995, *The Auto/biographical I: The Theory and Practice of Feminist Auto/biography*, Manchester University Press, Manchester.

Spivak, GC 1993, The politics of translation in GC Spivak (ed.) *Outside in the Teaching Machine*, Routledge, New York, pp. 179–200.

Witkin, SL 2014, *Narrating Social Work Through Autoethnography*. Columbia University Press, New York.

Index

Milton Keynes UK
Ingram Content Group UK Ltd.
UKHW040107071024
449327UK00019B/863